Juvenile Delinquency

Juvenile Delinquency

Prevention, Assessment, and Intervention

Edited by
KIRK HEILBRUN
NAOMI E. SEVIN GOLDSTEIN
and RICHARD E. REDDING

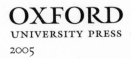

OXFORD
UNIVERSITY PRESS
2005

OXFORD
UNIVERSITY PRESS

Oxford University Press, Inc., publishes works that further
Oxford University's objective of excellence
in research, scholarship, and education.

Oxford New York
Auckland   Cape Town   Dar es Salaam   Hong Kong   Karachi
Kuala Lumpur   Madrid   Melbourne   Mexico City   Nairobi
New Delhi   Shanghai   Taipei   Toronto

With offices in
Argentina   Austria   Brazil   Chile   Czech Republic   France   Greece
Guatemala   Hungary   Italy   Japan   Poland   Portugal   Singapore
South Korea   Switzerland   Thailand   Turkey   Ukraine   Vietnam

Copyright © 2005 by Oxford University Press, Inc.

Published by Oxford University Press, Inc.
198 Madison Avenue, New York, New York 10016

www.oup.com

Oxford is a registered trademark of Oxford University Press

Library of Congress Cataloging-in-Publication Data
Juvenile delinquency : prevention, assessment, and intervention / edited by Kirk Heilbrun,
Naomi E. Sevin Goldstein, and Richard E. Redding.
p.   cm.
ISBN-13 978-0-19-516007-9
ISBN 0-19-516007-X
1. Juvenile delinquency—United States.   2. Juvenile delinquency—United States—Prevention.
3. Juvenile corrections—United States.   I. Heilbrun, Kirk.   II. Goldstein, Naomi E. Sevin.
III. Redding, Richard E.
HV9104.P454   2005
364.36'0973—dc22   2004011413

9 8 7 6 5 4 3 2 1

Printed in the United States of America
on acid-free paper

To the memory of my father-in-law, Frank Griffin.
There are old pilots, and there are bold pilots—but there are no old, bold pilots.

—K. H.

To my husband, Josh, to my sister, Marion, and to my parents, Alan and Paula.
—N. E. S. G.

To my grandmother, Effie Brown Redding.
—R. R.

Acknowledgments

There are a number of individuals who contributed to this book in various ways who deserve our thanks and gratitude. First, we were fortunate to recruit an outstanding group of contributors; collectively, they contributed chapters that are comprehensive and scholarly but practical and readable. We are very grateful to Deb Chapin, Dewey Cornell, Cindy Cottle, Dave DeMatteo, Alan Goldstein, Patty Griffin, Scott Henggeler, Barry Krisberg, Ria Lee, Fran Lexcen, Geff Marczyk, Barbara Mrozoski, Ed Mulvey, Seyi Olubadewo, Randy Otto, Lourdes Rosado, Eileen Ryan, Ashli Sheidow, David Tate, and Angela Wolf. Thanks to each of you.

Kerynne O'Malley served as our very able assistant throughout the writing and editing involved in this book. For her competence, dedication, and hard work, we are most appreciative. Both Joel Dvoskin and Tom Grisso contributed valuable ideas regarding the structure and content of the book; thanks to both of you.

Oxford University Press, particularly Joan Bossert and Maura Roessner, was terrific—competent, professional, and supportive—throughout all stages of this work. We are very appreciative of everything they brought to this project.

Patty and Anna were, as always, loving and supportive as Kirk worked on his part of this project. Naomi is grateful for Josh's patience and encouragement as she worked on this book and for Alan and Paula's willingness to serve as resources on content and format.

Contents

Contributors

DEBORAH A. CHAPIN has worked with youth in the area of alcohol and drug addiction and related mental health issues for over 15 years. In recent years, her work concerned the psychological assessment of youth involved in the juvenile justice system. She is currently working toward a doctoral degree specializing in psychological assessment of troubled youth in educational settings. She can be contacted at <debchapin50@juno.com>.

DEWEY G. CORNELL is a forensic clinical psychologist and Curry Memorial Professor of Education at the University of Virginia in Charlottesville, Virginia. His research interests include youth violence, juvenile threat assessment, and school safety. He can be contacted at <dcornell@virginia.edu> and http://youthviolence.edschool.virginia.edu.

CINDY C. COTTLE is a forensic psychology postdoctoral fellow at Dorothea Dix Hospital in Raleigh, North Carolina. Her research interests include juvenile offending, assessment of legal competencies among juvenile offenders, predictors of criminal recidivism, and malingering. She can be contacted at <cindy cottle@nc.rr.com>.

DAVID DEMATTEO is currently a research scientist at the Treatment Research Institute at the University of Pennsylvania. His research interests focus on the application of social science to the law and public policy. He can be contacted at <ddematteo@tresearch.org>.

ALAN M. GOLDSTEIN is Professor of Psychology at John Jay College of Criminal Justice–CUNY, and he is in the independent practice of criminal forensic psychology in Hartsdale, New York. Dr. Goldstein is the editor of *Forensic Psychology* (2003), a volume in the Handbook of Psychology series published by John Wiley & Sons. He can be contacted at <alanmg@optonline.net>.

PATRICIA A. GRIFFIN is a senior consultant for the National GAINS Center for Persons with Co-Occurring Disorders in the Justice System and a consultant for Philadelphia's behavioral health system on forensic issues. Her areas of expertise include policy and system issues for offenders with co-occurring mental illness and substance use disorders, diversion of persons with severe mental illness from the criminal justice system, community forensic treatment services, and linkages between institutions and the community. She can be contacted at <pgriffin@nav point.com>.

KIRK HEILBRUN is Professor and Head of the Department of Psychology at Drexel University in Philadelphia, Pennsylvania. His research and practice interests include criminal and juvenile offending, forensic mental health assessment, and violence risk assessment and risk management. He can be contacted at <kirk.heilbrun@drexel.edu>.

SCOTT W. HENGGELER is Professor of Psychiatry and Behavioral Sciences at the Medical University of South Carolina and Director of the Family Services Research Center (FSRC) in Charleston, South Carolina. The mission of the FSRC is to develop, validate, and study the dissemination of clinically effective and cost-effective mental health and substance abuse services for children presenting serious clinical problems and their families. His work on his chapter was supported by Grants DA10079, DA99008, and DA15844 from the National Institute on Drug Abuse; MH59138, MH51852, and MH60663 from the National Institute of Mental Health; AA122202 from the National Institute on Alcoholism and Alcohol Abuse and the Center for Substance Abuse Treatment; and the Annie E. Casey Foundation. He can be contacted at <henggesw@musc.edu>.

BARRY KRISBERG has been the president of the National Council on Crime and Delinquency for the past 27 years. He has been at the forefront of criminal justice reform, with an emphasis on juvenile justice. He is a proponent of community capacity building to address issues relating to youth. He can be contacted at <bkrisberg@aol.com>.

RIA LEE is a doctoral student in clinical psychology at Drexel University in Philadelphia, Pennsylvania. She completed her doctoral internship at the Federal Medical Center in Lexington, Kentucky, and is currently working on completing her dissertation. Her research interests include sexual violence, behavioral motivations, and violence risk assessment. She can be contacted at <ria.lee@drexel.edu>.

FRANCES J. LEXCEN is presently the Juvenile Forensic Psychology Fellow at the University of Washington in Tacoma, Washington. Her research interests include the mental health needs of juvenile offenders and forensic and civil competencies in adolescents. She can be contacted at <lexcefj@dshs.wa.gov>.

GEOFFREY MARCZYK is currently Assistant Professor and Director of Joint Degree Programs in Psychology and Criminal Justice in the Institute for Graduate Clinical Psychology at Widener University in Chester, Pennsylvania. His major research interests include forensic assessment and social science applications to the legal system. He can be contacted at <grmo301@mail.widener.edu>.

BARBARA MROZOSKI is a doctoral student in the Law–Psychology program at Villanova School of Law and Drexel University in Philadelphia, Pennsylvania. Her research interests include forensic assessment, risk assessment, civil commitment, and criminal recidivism. She can be contacted at <bmrozoski @comcast.net>.

EDWARD P. MULVEY is Professor of Psychiatry and Director of the Law and Psychiatry Program at Western Psychiatric Institute and Clinic at the University of Pittsburgh School of Medicine. His research is primarily focused on determining how clinicians make judgments regarding the type of risk posed by adult mental patients and juvenile offenders. His work on his chapter was done as part of the Pathways to Desistance study, funded by the Office of Juvenile Justice and Delinquency Prevention, National Institute of Justice, the John D. and Catherine T. MacArthur Foundation, the William T. Grant Foundation, the Robert Wood Johnson Foundation, the William Penn Foundation, the Pennsylvania Commission on Crime and Delinquency, and the Arizona Governor's Justice Commission. He can be contacted at <mulveyep @upmc.edu>.

OLUSEYI OLUBADEWO is a doctoral student in the Law–Psychology program at Villanova School of Law and Drexel University in Philadelphia, Pennsylvania. Her research interests include female juvenile offenders, mental health in juvenile offenders, and juvenile delinquency prevention. She can be contacted at <obo23@drexel.edu>.

RANDY K. OTTO is Associate Professor in the Department of Mental Health Law and Policy at the Florida Mental Health Institute, University of South Florida, Tampa, Florida. His research and professional writing focuses on forensic assessment. He can be contacted at <otto@fmhi.usf.edu>.

RICHARD E. REDDING is Professor of Law at Villanova University School of Law, Research Professor of Psychology at Drexel University, and Director of the J.D./Ph.D. Program in Law and Psychology at Villanova and Drexel universities. His research interests include juvenile delinquency and juvenile justice, criminal law and psychology, the use of social science in law and public policy, and biases in social science research and its use in public policy. He can be contacted at <redding@law.villanova.edu>.

LOURDES M. ROSADO is currently an attorney with the Juvenile Law Center, a nonprofit, public interest law firm in Philadelphia, Pennsylvania, that works to advance the rights and well-being of children in jeopardy. Her work centers primarily on youth involved in the juvenile justice and child welfare systems. She can be contacted at <lrosado@jlc.org>.

EILEEN P. RYAN is a forensic general and child psychiatrist and Associate Professor in the Department of Psychiatric Medicine, University of Virginia. She is also Medical Director of the Institute of Law, Psychiatry, and Public Policy at the University of Virginia. Her professional and research interests include the competency and culpability of juveniles transferred to adult court, mental illness in juvenile and criminal offenders, and female offenders. She can be contacted at <er3h@virginia.edu>.

NAOMI E. SEVIN GOLDSTEIN is co-Director of the J.D./Ph.D. Program in Law and Psychology at Villanova Law School and Drexel University and Assistant Professor of Psychology at Drexel University in Philadelphia, Pennsylvania. Her research focuses on adolescents' capacities to waive *Miranda* rights and on developing and evaluating intervention programs for female juvenile offenders. She can be contacted at <Naomi.Goldstein@drexel.edu>.

ASHLI J. SHEIDOW is Assistant Professor of Psychiatry and Behavioral Sciences at the Medical University of South Carolina. Her research interests focus on the development, prevention, and treatment of adolescent psychopathology and juvenile delinquency from an ecological perspective, with a concentration in quantitative methods. Her work on her chapter was supported by Grants DA10079, DA99008, and DA15844 from the National Institute on Drug Abuse; MH59138, MH51852, and MH60663 from the National Institute of Mental Health; AA122202 from the National Institute on Alcoholism and Alcohol Abuse and the Center for Substance Abuse Treatment; and the Annie E. Casey Foundation. She can be contacted at <sheidoaj@musc.edu>.

DAVID C. TATE is currently Assistant Clinical Professor in Psychiatry at the Yale University School of Medicine. His research interests include the etiology and treatment of adolescent violence and risk behaviors. He is also a private practitioner and consultant. He can be contacted at <david.tate@yale.edu>.

ANGELA M. WOLF is a senior researcher at the National Council on Crime and Delinquency and is the director of NCCD's Women and Justice Center. Her research interests include violence against women and children, as well as interventions for high-risk youth. She can be contacted at <awolf@SF.NCCD-CRC.ORG>.

Juvenile Delinquency

RICHARD E. REDDING, NAOMI E. SEVIN GOLDSTEIN,
AND KIRK HEILBRUN

Juvenile Delinquency
Past and Present

Youth offending and other antisocial behaviors are a great concern in contemporary society. How such concern is manifested, whether through law, policy, legal decisions about individuals, or the decisions of schools or families about adolescents, has significant implications for liberty, public safety, and accountability—important cornerstones of the kind of society in which we would like to raise our children. Too often, however, decisions about youthful offending and other antisocial behavior are made in the absence of good information, when such information is not sought or not readily available or is outweighed by competing political considerations.

It is our belief that good decision making requires good information. We have asked a number of researchers and scholars prominently associated with important questions in this area to describe what information is available and to critically analyze its implications for policy and practice. In the process, we offer our own description of the important aspects of these questions (in the present chapter) and, in the final chapter, our conclusions about the broader implications of the discussion and analyses in each of the earlier chapters.

Scope of the Book

This book considers 13 of the most important issues in juvenile delinquency and youth antisocial behavior. Each chapter addresses one such issue. In approximately the order in which they occur conceptually and sequentially in the juvenile justice system, these include (a) prevention, (b) school violence, (c) juvenile offending, (d) the mental health needs of juveniles, (e) risk factors and intervention outcomes derived through meta-analyses, (f) mental health and rehabilitative services, (g) diversion, (h) competencies, (i) the assessment of risk and treatment needs and amenability, (j) legal decision making, (k) community-based interventions, (l) residential interventions, and (m) the training of legal professionals in assessing juveniles. Our major goal is to provide a comprehensive description of what is currently known in these areas, with an emphasis on knowledge informed by empirical research. These chapters should interest researchers, policy-makers, and administrators seeking guidance in designing relevant research, formulating or amending policy on juvenile delinquent youth, or designing programs that are consistent with what is supported by empirical research. They should also interest students and trainees focusing on juvenile justice. This is not a "how to" book, however; it does not provide explicit or direct guidance for forensic clinicians seeking to evaluate juveniles or provide a specific kind of intervention.

Juvenile law and policy are important aspects of this book. Two of the most frequently recurring influences related to law and policy in the juvenile area are treatment/rehabilitation needs and amenability, and public safety. These considerations have guided the presentation of substantive content in chapters covering different areas.

We value a public health perspective on juvenile offending and adolescent antisocial behavior. Accordingly, these chapters describe available epidemiologic data and focus on risk factors and protective factors whenever possible. In discussing juvenile offending and adolescent antisocial behavior, the book addresses prevention and risk reduction by focusing on risk factors and protective factors that are legally relevant, empirically supported, and/or conceptually appropriate for the promotion of these goals.

Three broad areas are considered: prevention, assessment, and intervention. This discussion is guided by legal relevance, empirical and conceptual support, ethics, and standards of practice. Recommendations for reform are made when indicated.

The Juvenile Justice System: Overview and History

The landscape of juvenile justice changed dramatically in the latter part of the 20th century. There have been changes in the nature of juvenile offending; in the legal system's response to delinquent behavior; in our scientific understanding of the causes, prevention, and treatment of delinquency; and in service delivery and treatment programs for juvenile offenders.

The seriousness of juvenile crime has captured public attention. Despite recent encouraging trends, the juvenile crime rate, particularly for violent crime, remains higher than it was at mid-century and higher than those of other industrialized nations (Garbarino, 1999), though crime rates overall have risen worldwide during the last half of the 20th century (Rutter, Giller, & Hagell, 1998). Among African American and Hispanic male adolescents, homicide is the leading cause of death, and 100,000 children bring weapons to school every day in the United States (Hoffman & Summers, 2001). Rising rates of juvenile violence appear to be a worldwide phenomenon in industrialized nations. Potential explanations for the increase vary from country to country and include drug trafficking, breakdown of the family, political upheaval, and increased gang activity (Hoffman & Summers, 2001). In the United States, important contributing factors were the guns and violence accompanying the increase in neighborhood drug markets and the introduction of crack cocaine during the 1980s (Redding, 1997), along with juveniles' increased access to firearms (Blumstein, 2001). Other likely causes include family disintegration and inadequate parental supervision, violence in the media and video games, and an apparent increase in juvenile mental health problems (see Redding, 2002a). Most juvenile crime, however, is not violent crime; most juvenile offenders commit property offenses (Hoffman & Summers, 2001).

While it is true that the juvenile homicide rate more than doubled in the United States between 1985 and 1993, it has now dropped to pre-1985 levels and there is no discernible pattern of sustained increase for any other offense (Butts & Travis, 2002; Snyder, 2001; Zimring, 1998). Since 1993, there has been a decrease in the overall crime rate (Blumstein, 2001) that is attributable to substantial decreases in juvenile crime (including the key index crimes of homicide, aggravated assault, rape, and robbery) and a huge decrease in the number of juveniles arrested for homicide, probably due to the decline in the crack cocaine market and tougher antifirearms laws and policing programs (Butts & Travis, 2002; Zimring, 1998). The drop in the juvenile homicide rate parallels a decrease in juvenile arrest rates for weapons possession, leading Blumstein to conclude that "the growth in homicide committed by young people was more attributable to the weapons they used than to the emergence of inadequately socialized cohorts of 'superpredators' as some observers claimed" (2001, p. 14). In sum, juvenile crime rates are now roughly comparable to what they were in 1980, except for the large but brief increase in juvenile homicide rates in the late 1980s (Blumstein, 2001).

But the nature of juvenile offending *has* changed from years ago, when we did not have the problem with serious and violent juvenile crime that exists today. When the juvenile court was established at the turn of the 20th century, serious and violent juvenile crime was relatively rare, and the new court was established primarily to handle relatively minor offenses and status offenses (Redding, 1997). Moreover, while crime by girls was almost unheard of in the early 1900s, the rate of female juvenile crime (including violent crime) has increased substantially since 1980 (Snyder, 2001), though the reasons for that increase are unclear. Nonetheless, juvenile crime remains an overwhelmingly male phenomenon, often associated with antisocial peer groups or drugs (Hoffman & Summers, 2001).

In response to rising juvenile crime rates in the 1980s and early 1990s and the perception by legislators and policy-makers that the public wanted more punitive responses to juvenile crime, states as well as the federal government enacted laws designed to "get tough" on juvenile crime. There was a growing consensus among policy-makers that the juvenile court is too lenient, that rehabilitation is not effective or that serious juvenile offenders are beyond rehabilitation and must be incarcerated to ensure community safety, and that juvenile offenders are culpable for their crimes, as are adults (Redding, 1997). This also was the apparent consensus of the public, with voters passing state propositions allowing greater numbers of juveniles to be tried as adults (Beresford, 2000). Lawmakers could point to polls such as a 1993 Gallup Poll (see also Mears, 2001), which found that 73% of respondents were in favor of trying violent juveniles as adults, or to statements by influential public officials like Los Angeles County District Attorney Gil Garcetti, who said, "We need to throw out our entire juvenile justice system" (see Redding, 1997). Alfred Regnery, Administrator of the Office of Juvenile Justice and Delinquency Prevention in the Reagan administration, argued that juvenile offenders were "getting away with murder"—that juvenile offenders "are criminals who happen to be young, not children who happen to commit crimes"—and that rehabilitation was a "folly" ("Virtually no successful juvenile programs . . . rely on rehabilitation") (Regnery, 1985, pp. 65, 67). Congressman Bill McCollum, a key sponsor of the Juvenile Crime Control Bill that permits 13-year-olds to be tried as adults in federal court, concluded that " in America today, no population poses a greater threat to public safety than juvenile criminals" (see Lacayo & Donnelly, 1997).

The "get tough" approach was fueled by high-profile cases of violent juvenile crime and persistent news reports of violence in the schools. Georgia governor Zell Miller was quoted in the *New York Times* as saying that juvenile offenders "are not the Cleaver kids soaping up some windows. These are middle school kids conspiring to hurt their teachers, teenagers shooting people and committing rapes, young thugs running gangs and terrorizing neighborhoods, and showing no remorse when they get caught" (see Welch, Fenwick, & Roberts, 1997, p. 484). The press coverage of the juvenile violence "epidemic" reached a crescendo in 1994, when *Time* magazine ran the cover story "So Young to Kill, So Young to Die: The Short Violent life of 'Yummy' Sandifer." Eleven-year-old "Yummy," who had been arrested repeatedly, was shot by members of a rival gang after he shot a 14-year-old girl while attempting to kill rival gang members (Gibbs, 1994). The recent school shooting incidents in Pearl, Mississippi, and Jonesboro, Arkansas, and the mass school shooting at Columbine High School in Colorado have made an indelible mark on public consciousness (see Redding & Shalf, 2001).

Perhaps in large part due to media sensationalism, the public continues to believe that violent juvenile crime is rising and out of control (Shepherd, 1999). This "moral panic" is part of an alarmist reaction to crime generally (Welch et al., 1997). Based on the projected growth in the juvenile population during the early 21st century, some predicted a coming storm of youth violence (see Welch et al., 1997) and a wave of young "superpredators" (DiIulio, 1995). But as Zimring (1998) detailed in his historical analysis of juvenile crime in America, past generations have also seen juvenile crime wave scares. Consider the popular press reviews on the jacket of the 1954 book *Teen-Age Gangs* (Kramer & Karr, 1954): "A startling and sickening story of the unbelievable ferocity of juvenile delinquency. . . ."; "One of America's greatest perils . . . a problem that has authorities alarmed and baffled."

The reality is that juvenile crime rates have declined, high-profile incidents of violent juvenile crime are not representative of juvenile crime generally, and the public does not appear to favor abandoning the rehabilitative ideal of juvenile justice in favor of punitive responses to juvenile offenders. According to recent polls, about 58 to 65% of Americans favor trying violent juvenile offenders as adults (see The American Enterprise, 2001). But surveys also show that most still believe in the efficacy of the juvenile justice system and want it strengthened, favor early intervention and prevention programs along with rehabilitation over punishment for juvenile offenders, would reserve incarceration only for the most serious and violent offenders, want juvenile offenders tried as adults to receive rehabilitative treatment, and strongly disagree with the confinement of juveniles with adults (Moon, Sundt, Cullen, & Wright, 2000; Schiraldi & Soler, 1998; Shepherd, 1996). Sixty-three percent of the public favors rehabilitation as the main goal for juvenile correctional centers, while only 19% favors punishment (Moon et al., 2000). Polls that do report high public support for punitive policies typically ask omnibus questions about juvenile crime (for example, asking respondents if they favor "getting tough on juvenile offenders" or "punishing violent juvenile offenders as adults"—see The American Enterprise, 2001). More sophisticated surveys asking questions that provide respondents with more information about particular cases or options (e.g., the background of a particular offender, sentencing options, or rehabilitative programs available) find much less support for punitive policies for juveniles as well as adults (see Stalans & Henry, 1994). While the public favors incarceration for the serious and violent offenders who most threaten public safety, they do not favor wholesale imprisonment (particularly for young, nonviolent, and first-time offenders) but rather favor expending community and correctional resources on prevention, rehabilitation, and employment programs (Sundt, 1999). Similar results have been found in the public opinion polls of other industrialized nations (see Sessar, 1999).

The shifting landscape of juvenile crime and public opinion has produced a corresponding shift in the legal response to juvenile delinquency. Rooted in the emergence of the progressive "child savers" movement at the turn of the 20th century and the notion of the state intervening as beneficent parent in the child's best interest, the first juvenile court was created in Cook County, Illinois, in 1899 (Fox, 1970). The progressives viewed children as more malleable and more amenable to rehabilitation than adults and believed that they were not solely responsible for their criminal conduct, which was thought to be due to poverty and parental neglect. The juvenile court's focus was not on punishment but on identifying the underlying causes of the delinquent behavior and fashioning an individualized rehabilitative program for each juvenile by meting out individualized, nonstigmatizing, therapeutic dispositions. The goal was "To get away from the notion that the child is to be dealt with as a criminal. . . . The problem for determination by the judge is not, Has this boy or girl committed a specific wrong, but What is he, how has he become what he is, and what had best be done in his interest. . . . The child who must be brought into court should . . . be made to feel that he is the object of care and solicitude" (Mack, 1909, p. 109).

The juvenile was to be treated as an individual, with mental health and social workers providing a scientific assessment of each child's needs followed by individualized rehabilitative treatment, with children kept in their homes and communities whenever possible (see Burgess, 1923; U.S. Department of Labor, 1922). Because the court was designed to be informal and nonadversarial, there were few due process protections afforded and judges had broad adjudicatory and dispositional authority.

By 1925, 48 states had established separate juvenile justice systems (Coalition for Juvenile Justice, 1998). Yet even the early juvenile court did not live up to its ideals; in 1922 only 7% of juvenile courts had a mental health clinic (U.S. Department of Labor, 1922). Consider Judge Hoffman's comments before the first Conference on Juvenile Court Standards, sponsored by the U.S. Children's Bureau, held in 1922:

> It was the evident purpose of the founders of the first juvenile courts to save, to redeem, and to protect every delinquent child to the benefit of himself and of society and the State. . . . After two decades this exalted conception and great law—has not been realized in its fullness. . . . Children whom it was intended to take out of the pale of the criminal law and save by all the means that education, religion, science, and medicine could command have been subjected to treatment and conditions but little different from those of the last century. . . . Why have the juvenile courts failed to provide the machinery necessary for the redemption of offending children? Is the cause of this default inherent in the juvenile-court law, or is it to be found in administration? (U.S. Department of Labor, 1922, pp. 14, 15)

As Justice Abe Fortas noted, the reality of juvenile court was that "the child receives the worst of both worlds . . . he gets neither the protection afforded to adults, nor the solicitous care and regenerative treatment postulated for children" (*In re Gault*, 1967, p. 18). The informal nature of juvenile court meant that juveniles received far fewer procedural and due process protections than adult defendants, it not being uncommon (even today) for juvenile court judges to adjudicate a juvenile "delinquent" without sufficient evidence of guilt to ensure juvenile court jurisdiction for the delivery of services (see Guggenheim & Hertz, 1998). At the same time, rehabilitative services often were not forthcoming, with juvenile offenders frequently incarcerated for indeterminate periods in the state "training schools" that were de facto juvenile prisons (Fox, 1970).

Recognizing the need for greater due process protections in the juvenile court, the landmark U.S. Supreme Court cases *In re Gault* (1967) and *In re Winship* (1970) established, except for the right to trial by jury, full due process protections in the juvenile court.[1] *Gault*-era juvenile justice reforms helped ensure that juvenile dispositions would be based on the offense rather than the judges' perceptions of a juvenile's treatment needs, while also ensuring that juvenile dispositions would be shorter and more rehabilitative than those of adults

---

1. Fifteen-year-old Gerald Gault was adjudicated delinquent for making an obscene phone call and committed to an institution, where he remained for 6 years. The penalty for an adult convicted of the same offense would have been a small fine or imprisonment for not more than 2 months. At the adjudicatory hearing in juvenile court, Gault was not afforded the rights to counsel or to confront his accuser.

(Scott, 2000). Even today, however, juvenile court proceedings often lack full due process (Redding, 2002b).

Policy-makers and the public also began to question, just as Judge Hoffman had in 1922, why juvenile courts were failing to rehabilitate youthful offenders. In the midst of the Supreme Court's extending due process protections to juveniles, the President's Commission on Law Enforcement and Administration of Justice (1967) reported that the juvenile justice system was ineffective in rehabilitating offenders and in reducing recidivism. Many felt that juvenile courts and sanctions should be less lenient. A 1994 poll found that a third of juvenile court judges thought that the juvenile justice system was too lenient (Sherman, 1994). The early juvenile courts handled relatively minor offenses, but by the 1930s they became courts of original jurisdiction for all juvenile offenders below the age of majority (Redding, 1997). The juvenile justice reforms during the last two decades, however, have returned more of the serious or violent juvenile offenders to the criminal court. Legislatures across the country enacted laws to remove these offenders from juvenile court jurisdiction, and sweeping changes were made in juvenile delinquency laws to diminish the use of rehabilitation while increasing the use of punishment. Some states changed the purpose clause in their juvenile code to make accountability or punishment, rather than rehabilitation, the primary goal (Szymasnki, 1997). The most notable change was states' revision of their transfer laws to expand the type of offenses and offenders eligible for transfer from the juvenile court for trial and sentencing in the criminal court. Changes also occurred at the federal level with the passage of the Violent Crime Control and Law Enforcement Act of 1994, which allowed the transfer of 13-year-olds who committed crimes with firearms on federal property. States also eliminated or restricted juvenile court confidentiality laws and expanded the decision-making authority of prosecutors (Torbet & Szymanski, 1998).

Along with the changes in state and federal law have come new calls for wholesale reform of the juvenile justice system. Some have proposed abolishing the juvenile court and processing all offenders in criminal court, which would provide reduced or rehabilitative sentences for juveniles (Feld, 1997). This is unlikely to occur. Rather, current reforms are aimed at integrating accountability or punishment with treatment and rehabilitation (see Tate & Redding, ch. 7 in this volume). The reforms proposed by the Office of Juvenile Justice and Delinquency Prevention under the Comprehensive Strategy for Serious, Violent, and Chronic Juvenile Offenders (Wilson & Howell, 1995) include a comprehensive assessment of each juvenile who enters the system, early and immediate intervention, the use of multiple interventions to address multiple risk factors, service integration across the juvenile justice, mental health, and social service systems, a system of graduated sanctions (immediate, intermediate, and secure corrections) that increase with the severity of offending, and intensive aftercare. A separate juvenile court is likely to remain, but there is a growing convergence between the juvenile and criminal justice systems that avoids the problems engendered by a "binary, either/or juvenile versus adult" (Feld, 1993, p. 419) justice system. About half the states have enhanced the sentencing authority of the juvenile court by allowing it to impose limited adult sentences or extend its sentencing authority into early adulthood (Redding & Howell, 2000). This "adultification" of the juvenile court has made forensic topics such as adjudicative competence (Redding & Frost, 2002) and the insanity defense, which previously were irrelevant in juvenile court, key issues of concern in the modern juvenile court. In addition, specialty courts (e.g., drug court, gun court, mental health court, teen court) are being established to address particular offense types and offenders as part of an ongoing effort to develop a comprehensive prevention and treatment program within juvenile justice (Merlo & Benekos, 2000).

Such reforms recognize that "the kid is a criminal and the criminal is a kid" (Feld, 1999, p. 19). Historically, juvenile justice policy has vacillated between two different views of juvenile offenders—that they are youth in need who require beneficence and a therapeutic response or criminals requiring punishment and deterrence (Bernard, 1992). The progressives who founded the juvenile court had a romanticized image of juvenile offenders as wayward but innocent youth, while modern conservative reformers have an incorrect image of offenders as fully culpable, "little adult" criminals. Both are inaccurate and harmful to public policy (Scott, 2000). Reasonable juvenile justice policy should not view juvenile offenders either as children or adults, but rather, as adolescents who are in "a transitional stage of development that requires a developmentally based approach to juvenile justice." Public safety and juvenile offenders are better served "if policy makers recognize that young offenders are neither innocent children nor mature adults" (Scott, 2000, p. 589). Paradigms that adopt balanced policies by requiring accountability from juvenile offenders while also promoting rehabilitation represent the best chance to establish reasonable juvenile justice policy that is effective, balanced, responsive to public concern, and consistent with the reality of juvenile offending and offenders. Such balanced approaches are now the explicit basis of some states' juvenile justice systems. For example, the Pennsylvania Juvenile Justice Act's (1999) "balanced approach" includes supervisory and rehabilitative programs that serve the goals of community protection, accountability, and competency development.

But until fairly recently, the view that rehabilitation was ineffective dominated the criminal and juvenile justice fields, particularly after Martinson's (1974) seminal review of program evaluations in juvenile and criminal justice systems concluded that "Nothing works." It became widely cited in the literature, with the "Nothing works" refrain often repeated among politicians and policy-makers. Since Martinson's review, tremendous progress has made in the treatment and rehabilitation of juvenile offenders, so that we now can say unequivocally that the "Nothing works" view is no longer tenable. Effective programs are now available for rehabilitating offenders in the juvenile justice system, even serious and violent offenders. Lipsey and Wilson (1998) conducted a meta-analysis of all 200 evaluations of treatment programs serving adjudicated serious or violent offenders. The average program reduced recidivism by about 12% over the control groups, slightly larger that the 10% recidivism reduction found in an earlier review of 400 programs for juvenile offenders generally (Lipsey, 1995).

We now have an understanding of "what works" (Henggeler, 1996). The success of recent programs is due in large part to our enhanced understanding of the risk factors and developmental pathways for delinquency, forming the basis for more sophisticated and scientifically based intervention programs. There still is no "magic bullet" cure for delinquency, but significant advances have been made in the last two decades in our understanding of the characteristics of effective intervention and treatment programs. There are a variety of reasons many programs are ineffective, but common reasons are that they address only one or two risk factors or fail to address the most important risk factors for delinquency, are not individualized to the child, are based on an unproven theory, are improperly implemented or fail to maintain program quality, do not hold service providers accountable for outcomes, or are of insufficient duration (Corbett & Petersilia, 1994; Hollin, 1999; Lipsey & Wilson, 1998).

While the components of successful programs differ, most are based on a recognition that effective treatment of juvenile delinquency requires an individualized and family-centered intervention that ameliorates the multiple risk factors contributing to antisocial behavior while strengthening protective factors, in a comprehensive and integrated manner. Although successful intervention programs generally target multiple risk factors and thus deliver a variety of treatment services, research has shown which specific treatments are generally the most effective: cognitive-behavioral programs emphasizing social skills and problem-solving training, behavioral programs, parent management training (for children under age 13), and functional family therapy (Lipsey & Wilson, 1998; Redding, 2000).

Effective programs target risk factors at the level of the individual child, family, peer group, school, and neighborhood. While a large number of risk factors for delinquency have been identified that differ somewhat across age groups and type of delinquency (see Office of Juvenile Justice and Delinquency Prevention, 1998), certain risk factors are particularly significant in adolescence but are also amenable to treatment. These significant risk factors at the child level include substance abuse, mental health problems, impulsivity, and poor social problem-solving skills. Low parental warmth, poor parental supervision, and ineffective or harsh discipline practices are significant factors at the family level. At the school level, risk factors include untreated learning disabilities, low academic achievement, alienation from school, and truancy. At the peer-group level, they include association with delinquent peers and gang membership. Exposure to violence and drug dealing and access to firearms are among the significant risk factors at the community level.

Many of the risk factors existing at the child, peer, and school levels can in turn be traced to problems within the family. "There is no single cause of youth violence, but when there is a common factor that cuts across different causes, it is usually some kind of family dysfunction" (Steinberg, 1999, quoted in Mendel, 2000, p. 14). Causal modeling studies of delinquency suggest that family dysfunction (e.g., ineffective or harsh discipline, poor parental supervision) and school problems (e.g., academic failure, truancy) often lead to association with delinquent peers, which in turn leads to delinquency. Juveniles typically commit crimes in groups (Zimring, 1981), and association with delinquent peers is one of the best predictors of delinquency (Patterson, Forgatch, Yoerger, & Stoolmiller, 1998).

The most effective treatments target the set of delinquency risk factors described above. Such treatments may also serve to prevent or treat other adolescent problem behaviors, the risk factors for which overlap substantially with those for delinquency (see Howell, 1997). One of the best available treatments is multisystemic therapy (MST), developed by Henggeler and colleagues at the Medical College of South Carolina (Henggeler, Schoenwald, Borduin, Rowlands, & Cunningham, 1998). MST simultaneously and intensely intervenes in the key risk factors for a particular child. In particular, MST aims to improve parental discipline practices and family relations, diminish a juvenile's association with delinquent peers while increasing his association with prosocial peers and participation in positive recreational activities, and improve school performance. It involves parents as active participants and leaves them with the skills to deal with problem behaviors when treatment ends, which are key ingredients in the program's demonstrated effectiveness with treatment-resistant or "difficult" families. Rigorous outcome studies have been conducted on MST, comparing it with traditional treatment approaches (e.g., individual therapy, traditional case management, family therapy) for inner-city offenders, violent sex offenders, chronic offenders, substance-abusing offenders, and violent and chronic juvenile offenders. All have shown substantial reductions in recidivism beyond those achieved through traditional programs. Previous programs often failed because they addressed only one or two risk factors (Henggeler, 1989), thus leading to Martinson's famous conclusion that "Nothing works." The single-versus-multiple-treatment effect can be seen in a study comparing MST to traditional treatment for serious juvenile offenders at risk for institutional placement. One 5-year posttreatment survival analysis on the effects of MST with serious and violent juvenile offenders showed a 25% recidivism rate for those completing MST, a 50% recidivism rate for those who dropped out of MST after a limited course of treatment, a 65% recidivism rate for those who completed traditional treatment, and an 80% recidivism rate for those who dropped out of traditional treatment or refused treatment (Henggeler et al., 1998). These findings illustrate that while traditional treatment targeting one or two risk factors has some effect on reducing recidivism, MST targeting multiple risk factors has a substantial effect, with even a limited course of MST treatment being more efficacious than a completed course of traditional treatment.

Even the most effective programs, however, do not work with all juvenile offenders. The most successful experimental trials of two of the most effective treatments currently available—MST and functional family therapy—produced recidivism reductions in about 70% of participants. While this result is very impressive, particularly in comparison with other programs, much remains to be achieved in our understanding of how to prevent and treat juvenile delinquency, particularly among children who begin exhibiting behavioral problems at an early age that are likely due in large part to genetic, neurological, and temperamental problems, such as attention-deficit/hyperactivity disorder (ADHD), frontal lobe dysfunction, impulsivity, and low IQ (see Moeller, 2001). Children with comorbid conduct disorder and ADHD are at particular risk for delinquency and the later development of antisocial personality disorder (Lexcen & Redding, 2002). Recent years have seen a resurgence in the biological and individual differences theories of delinquency that were popular in the early part of the last century. For example, a growing body of research suggests a link between neurological deficits such as frontal lobe dysfunction and delinquency, with a very high percentage of juvenile offenders showing signs of brain dysfunction or neurological abnormality (Pallone & Hennessy, 1998). In addition, chronic exposure to violence and early childhood trauma is a source of *softer* neurological abnormalities in juvenile offenders (see Garbarino, 1999). Recent research also suggests the existence of psychopathy in adolescence, an important area for continued research (see Lynam, 1996; Seagrave & Grisso, 2002).

Indeed, the role of mental health problems as risk factors for delinquency is increasingly being recognized, with the mental health needs of juvenile offenders now a popular area for research and program development in juvenile justice. Epidemiological studies show that levels of adolescent psychopathology have increased in recent years, particularly depression and behavioral problems (Rutter et al., 1998). Studies show particularly high rates of mental disorders among juvenile offenders. One study of detained youth found that 9% had severe mental health needs requiring immediate treatment (Policy Design Team, 1994). Many juvenile offenders have multiple mental health problems, 15 to 20% have a serious mental illness (Cocozza & Skowyra, 2000), and a much larger percentage (up to 80%, in some studies) experience some mental health problem requiring mental health services. High rates of substance abuse as well as physical and sexual abuse are also found in this population.

Several studies, however, suggest that many juvenile court judges give little weight to mental health factors in fashioning dispositions, but rather focus on the seriousness of the offense and the juvenile's offending history (see Campbell & Schmidt, 2000). This indicates that more needs to be done to educate judges and juvenile justice personnel about the role of mental disorders as risk factors for delinquency and their amenability to treatment. Additionally, substantial barriers continue to exist in the delivery of mental health services within the juvenile justice system (see Tate & Redding, ch. 7 in this volume). Integrated programs are crucial for effective service delivery, particularly since there is a substantial overlap between youth with mental health problems and those with juvenile court involvement (see Tate & Redding, ch. 7 in this volume). A promising development is the establishment of community assessment centers, which provide a single entry point for juveniles (referred by juvenile justice, schools, social agencies, or parents) in need of mental health and other services and a centralized process for screening, assessment, and referral (Dembo & Brown, 1994).

In particular, prevention and early intervention in offender careers is critical for reducing recidivism (see DeMatteo & Marczyk, ch. 2 in this volume), as indicated by recent research on delinquent careers and the developmental pathways to delinquency. Most adult offenders began their criminal careers in childhood, often at a young age (Moffitt, 1993). The approximately 4% of juvenile offenders whose offending is serious, violent, and chronic (Snyder, 1998) tend to be multiple-problem youth who exhibit behavioral and other problems in early childhood, with an early onset of criminality perhaps the most robust predictor (Loeber & LeBlanc, 1990). The behavioral and temperamental markers for the development of disruptive behavior disorders can now be detected as early as age 3 (Rutter et al., 1998), and early intervention programs (such as the Perry Preschool Program) have proven effective in long-term reductions in delinquent behavior later in life (see DeMatteo & Marczyk, ch. 2 in this volume).

To be sure, delinquent behavior (particularly of the nonviolent variety) is a normal part of growing up for adolescent males (Moffitt, 1993), most of whom desist by the time they reach adulthood. Most offenders do not require punitive action to desist, which may have the undesired effect of delaying desistence and promoting life-course criminality (Scott, 2000). A small number of repeat offenders (about 8 to 10%) are responsible for most of the serious or violent offenses committed (between 60 and 80%) by juveniles, and they are the offenders most likely to become the *career criminals* (Tracy, Wolfgang, & Figlio, 1990). Sentencing reforms should be structured to have maximum impact on these life-course-persistent and most dangerous offenders (Loeber, Farrington, & Waschbusch, 1998). Additionally, a good fit should be achieved between the position of delinquents along the pathways toward life-course-persistent offenders' careers and sanctions, which are graduated in concert with progression toward life-course persistence. As offenders progress in a graduated sanctions system, interventions must become more structured and intensive. Community-based programs generally are more effective (and much less expensive), even for serious and violent offenders, with incarceration appearing only to increase recidivism (see Redding & Mrozoski, ch. 11 in this volume). But a small percentage of offenders who are chronic, severe, or violent offenders will require incarceration to ensure community safety. These residential programs should provide rehabilitative services and be linked to community programs by way of comprehensive aftercare services (see Redding & Mrozoski, ch. 11 in this volume).

Life-course-persistent offenders can be distinguished from adolescence-limited offenders, who desist from offending after adolescence. Five factors are associated with life-course offending: early age of onset, active offending during adolescence, offense specialization, offense seriousness, and offense escalation (Moffitt, 1993). Because the distinction between life-course-persistent and adolescent-limited offenders is critical for structuring juvenile sentencing policy and determining individual dispositions, the development of better tools for predicting life-course persistence is an important agenda item for future research.

Empirical research on the causes and correlates of delinquency and on effective prevention and rehabilitation programs can substantially inform juvenile justice policy and practice, as the contributors to this volume demonstrate. Media sensationalism and public sentiment as measured by opinion polls must not be the driving force behind reform. Legislators may embrace punitive reforms having popular, commonsense appeal that do not withstand empirical scrutiny in terms of their effectiveness in preventing youth crime or reducing recidivism. The most persuasive arguments to policy-makers may be the cost-benefit analyses showing the huge cost of juvenile crime to victims, offenders, and society in comparison to the cost effectiveness of successful prevention and treatment programs (see Schweinhart & Weikart, 1980). For example, economic analyses of MST show that it produces a net savings to taxpayers of about $22,000 per child, when comparing its cost to that of juvenile crime (Washington State Institute of Public Policy, 1998). At the same time, juvenile justice advocates and professionals must recognize the reality of juvenile crime, which remains a serious social problem, as well as the reality of juvenile offenders, who are not merely innocent children. Sanctions and intervention programs must require accountability from offenders as well.

References

The American Enterprise Institute for Public Policy Research. (2001, June). Parents, juveniles, and justice. *The American Enterprise, 62*.

Beresford, L. (2000). Is lowering the age at which juveniles can be transferred to adult criminal court the answer to juvenile crime? A state-by-state assessment. *San Diego Law Review, 37*, 783–851.

Bernard, T. (1992). *The cycle of juvenile justice.* New York: Oxford University Press.

Blumstein, A. (2001). *Why is crime falling—or is it?* Washington, DC: U.S. Department of Justice, National Institute of Justice (NCJ 187007).

Burgess, E. W. (1923). The study of the delinquent as a person. *American Journal of Sociology, 28*(6), 657–680.

Butts, J., & Travis, J. (2002, March). *The rise and fall of American youth violence: 1980 to 2000.* Washington, DC: Urban Institute, Justice Policy Center.

Campbell, M. A., & Schmidt, F. (2000). Comparison of mental health and legal factors in the disposition outcome of young offenders. *Criminal Justice and Behavior, 27*, 688–715.

Coalition for Juvenile Justice. (1998). *A celebration or a wake? The juvenile court after 100 years.* Washington, DC: Author.

Cocozza, J. J., & Skowyra, K. R. (2000). Youth with mental health disorders: Issues and emerging responses. *Juvenile Justice, 7*(1), 3–13.

Corbett, R. P., & Petersilia, J. (1994). What works with juvenile offenders: A synthesis of the literature and experience. *Federal Probation, 58*(4), 63–67.

Dembo, R., & Brown, R. (1994). The Hillsborough County juvenile assessment center. *Journal of Child and Adolescent Substance Abuse, 3*, 25–43.

DiIulio, J. J. (1995, November 27). The coming of the super-predators. *The Weekly Standard*, 23–28.

Feld, B. C. (1993). Juvenile (in)justice and the criminal court alternative. *Crime and Delinquency, 39*, 403–424.

Feld, B. C. (1997). Abolish the juvenile court: Youthfulness, criminal responsibility and sentencing policy. *Journal of Criminal Law and Criminology, 88*, 68–136.

Feld, B. C. (1999). The honest politician's guide to juvenile justice in the twenty-first century. *Annals of the American Academy of Political and Social Science, 564*, 10–27.

Fox, S. (1970). Juvenile justice reform: An historical perspective. *Stanford Law Review, 22*, 1187–1239.

Garbarino, J. (1999). *Lost boys: Why our sons turn violent and how we can save them.* New York: Free Press.

Gibbs, N. R. (1994, September 19). Murder in miniature. *Time*, 54–60.

Guggenheim, M., & Hertz, R. (1998). Reflections on judges, juries, and justice: Ensuring the fairness of juvenile delinquency trials. *Wake Forest Law Review*, 33, 553–593.

Henggeler, S. W. (1989). *Delinquency in adolescence*. Newbury Park, CA: Sage.

Henggeler, S. W. (1996). Treatment of violent juvenile offenders—we have the knowledge: Comment on Gorman-Smith et al. *Journal of Family Psychology*, 10(2), 137–141.

Henggeler, S. W., Schoenwald, S. K., Borduin, C. M., Rowlands, M. D., & Cunningham, P. B. (1998). *Multisystemic treatment of antisocial behavior in children and adolescents*. New York: Guilford Press.

Hoffman, A. M., & Summers, R. W. (Eds.). (2001). *Teen violence: A global view*. Westport, CT: Greenwood Press.

Hollin, C. R. (1999). Treatment programs for offenders: Meta-analysis, "what works," and beyond. *International Journal of Law and Psychiatry*, 22, 361–372.

Howell, J. (1997). *Juvenile justice and youth violence*. Thousand Oaks, CA: Sage.

In re Gault, 387 U.S. 1 (1967).

In re Winship, 397 U.S. 358 (1970).

Kramer, D., & Karr, M. (1954). *Teen-age gangs*. New York: Henry Holt.

Lacayo, R., & Donnelly, S. B. (1997, July 21). Teen crime: Congress wants to crack down on juvenile offenders. But is throwing teens into adult court—and adult prisons— the best way? *Time*, 26.

Lexcen, F., & Redding, R. E. (2002, November/December). Mental health needs of juvenile offenders. *Juvenile Correctional Mental Health Report*, 3(1), 1, 2, 8–16.

Lipsey, M. W. (1995). What do we learn from 400 research studies on the effectiveness of treatment with juvenile delinquents? In J. McGuire (Ed.), *What works? Reducing reoffending* (pp. 313–345). New York: Wiley.

Lipsey, M. W., & Wilson, D. B. (1998). Effective interventions with serious juvenile offenders: A synthesis of research. In R. Loeber & D. Farrington (Eds.), *Serious and violent juvenile offenders: Risk factors and successful interventions* (pp. 313–345). Thousand Oaks, CA: Sage.

Loeber, R., Farrington, D. P., & Waschbusch, D. A. (1998). Serious and violent juvenile offenders. In R. Loeber & D. P. Farrington (Eds.), *Serious and violent juvenile offenders: Risk factors and successful interventions*. Thousand Oaks, CA: Sage.

Loeber, R., & LeBlanc, M. (1990). Towards a developmental criminology. In M. Tonry & N. Morris (Eds.), *Crime and justice: A review of research* (Vol. 12, pp. 375–473). Chicago: University of Chicago Press.

Lynam, D. (1996). Early identification of chronic offenders: Who is the fledgling psychopath? *Psychological Bulletin*, 120, 209–234.

Mack, J. W. (1909). The juvenile court. *Harvard Law Review*, 23, 104–122.

Martinson, R. (1974). What works? Questions and answers about prison reform. *The Public Interest*, 35, 22–54.

Mears, D. (2001). Getting tougher with juvenile offenders. *Criminal Justice and Behavior*, 82, 206–226.

Mendel, R. A. (2000). *Less hype, more help: Reducing juvenile crime, what works—and what doesn't*. Washington, DC: American Youth Policy Forum.

Merlo, A. V., & Benekos, P. J. (2000). *What's wrong with the criminal justice system: Ideology, politics, and the media*. Cincinnati, OH: Anderson.

Moeller, T. (2001). *Youth aggression and violence: A psychological approach*. Mahwah, NJ: Erlbaum.

Moffitt, T. E. (1993). Adolescence-limited and life-course-persistent antisocial behavior: A developmental taxonomy. *Psychological Review*, 100, 674–701.

Moon, M. M., Sundt, J. L., Cullen, F. T., & Wright, J. P. (2000). Is child saving dead? Public support for juvenile rehabilitation. *Crime and Delinquency, 46,* 38–60.

Office of Juvenile Justice and Delinquency Prevention, U.S. Department of Justice. (1998, May). *Serious and violent juvenile offenders.* Washington, DC: U.S. Department of Justice.

Pallone, J., & Hennessy, J. (1998, September/October). Brain dysfunction and criminal violence. *Society,* 21–27.

Patterson, G. R., Forgatch, M. S., Yoerger, K., & Stoolmiller, M. (1998). Variables that initiate and maintain an early-onset trajectory for juvenile offending. *Development and Psychopathology, 10,* 531–547.

Pennsylvania Juvenile Justice Act. 42 PA. CONS. STAT. ANN. Sect. 6301.

Policy Design Team. (1994). *Mental health needs of youth in Virginia's juvenile detention centers.* Richmond, VA: Virginia Department of Criminal Justice Services.

President's Commission on Law Enforcement and Administration of Justice. (1967). *Task force report: Juvenile delinquency and youth crime* (cited in Howell, J. [1997], *Juvenile justice and youth violence,* Thousand Oaks, CA: Sage).

Redding, R. E. (1997). Juveniles transferred to criminal court: Legal reform proposals based on social science research. *Utah Law Review, 1997,* 709–797.

Redding, R. E. (2000). Characteristics of effective treatments and interventions for juvenile offenders. *Juvenile justice fact sheet.* Charlottesville, VA: University of Virginia, Institute of Law, Psychiatry and Public Policy.

Redding, R. E. (2002a). Rehabilitating the souls of violent boys. *Contemporary Psychology, 47,* 286–289.

Redding, R. E. (2002b). Using juvenile adjudications for sentence enhancement under the Federal Sentencing Guidelines. Is it sound policy? *Virginia Journal of Social Policy and the Law, 10,* 231–260.

Redding, R. E., & Frost, L. E. (2002). Adjudicative competence in the modern juvenile court. *Virginia Journal of Social Policy and the Law, 9,* 353–410.

Redding, R. E., & Howell, J. C. (2000). Blended sentencing in American juvenile courts. In J. Fagan & F. E. Zimring (Eds.), *The changing borders of juvenile justice: Transfer of adolescents to the criminal court* (pp. 145–179). Chicago: University of Chicago Press.

Redding, R. E., & Shalf, S. M. (2001). The legal context of school violence: The effectiveness of federal, state, and local law enforcement efforts to reduce gun violence in schools. *Law and Policy, 23,* 297–343.

Regnery, A. S. (1985). Getting away with murder: Why the juvenile justice system needs an overhaul. *Policy Review, 34,* 65–68.

Rutter, M., Giller, H., & Hagell, A. (1998). *Antisocial behavior by young people.* Cambridge: Cambridge University Press.

Schiraldi, V., & Soler, M. (1998). The will of the people? The public's opinion of the violent and repeat juvenile offender act of 1997. *Crime and Delinquency, 44,* 590–601.

Schweinhart, L. J., & Weikart, D. P. (1980). *Young children grow up: The effects of the Perry Preschool study through age twenty-seven.* Ypsilanti, MI: High/Scope Press.

Scott, E. S. (2000). The legal construction of adolescence. *Hofstra Law Review, 29,* 547–598.

Seagrave, D., & Grisso, T. (2002). Adolescent development and the measurement of juvenile psychopathy. *Law and Human Behavior, 26,* 219–239.

Sessar, K. (1999). Punitive attitudes of the public: Reality and myth. In G. Bazemore & L. Walgrave (Eds.), *Restorative juvenile justice: Repairing the harm of youth crime* (pp. 287–304). Monsey, NY: Criminal Justice Press.

Shepherd, R. E. (1996, Spring). What does the public really want? *Criminal Justice*, 51–52.

Shepherd, R. E. (1999). Film at eleven: The news media and juvenile crime. *Quinnipiac Law Review, 18*, 687–700.

Sherman, R. (1994, August 8). Juvenile judges say: Time to get tough. *National Law Journal*, 1.

Snyder, H. N. (1998). Serious, violent, and chronic juvenile offenders—an assessment of the extent of and trends in officially recognized serious criminal behavior in a delinquent population. In R. Loeber & D. P. Farrington (Eds.), *Serious and violent offenders: Risk factors and successful interventions* (pp. 428–444). Thousand Oaks, CA: Sage.

Snyder, H. N. (2001, December). *Juvenile offenders and victims*. U.S. Department of Justice, Office of Juvenile Justice and Delinquency Prevention.

Stalans, L. J., & Henry, G. T. (1994). Societal views of justice for adolescents accused of murder. *Law and Human Behavior, 18*, 675–696.

Sundt, J. L. (1999). Is there room for change? A review of public attitudes toward crime control and alternatives to incarceration. *Southern Illinois University Law Journal, 23*, 519–537.

Szymanski, L. A. (1997). Juvenile delinquency code purpose clauses. *Juvenile and Family Law Digest, 29*, 1822.

Torbet, P., & Szymanski, L. (1998). *State legislative responses to violent juvenile crime: 1996–97 update*. U.S. Justice Department, Office of Juvenile Justice and Delinquency Prevention. Washington, DC: Author.

Tracy, P. E., Wolfgang, M. E., & Figlio, R. M. (1990). *Delinquency careers in two birth cohorts*. New York: Plenum.

U.S. Department of Labor, Children's Bureau. (1922). *Proceedings of the conference on juvenile-court standards* (Bureau Publication No. 97). Washington, DC: Author.

Violent Crime Control and Law Enforcement Act of 1994. 42 U.S.C.A. Sect. 13701, Ch. 136 (1995).

Washington State Institute of Public Policy. (1998). *Watching the bottom line: Cost-effective interventions for reducing crime in Washington*. Olympia, WA: Author.

Welch, M., Fenwick, M., & Roberts, M. (1997). Primary definitions of crime and moral panic: A content analysis of experts' quotes in feature newspaper articles on crime. *Journal of Research in Crime and Delinquency, 34*, 474–494.

Wilson, J. J., & Howell, J. C. (1995). *Comprehensive strategy for serious, violent, and chronic juvenile offenders*. Washington, DC: U.S. Department of Justice, Office of Juvenile Justice and Delinquency Prevention.

Zimring, F. E. (1981). Kids, groups and crime: Some implications of a well-known secret. *Journal of Criminal Law and Criminology, 72*, 867–88.

Zimring, F. E. (1998). *American youth violence*. New York: Oxford University Press.

2

DAVID DeMATTEO AND GEOFFREY MARCZYK

Risk Factors, Protective Factors, and the Prevention of Antisocial Behavior Among Juveniles

In recent years, youth violence has become a significant concern in almost every sector of society. Several recent high-visibility violent crimes committed by juveniles have served to focus the attention of researchers, policy-makers, the judiciary, and the media on the prevalence and deleterious effects of youth violence. Although recent statistics suggest that the arrest rate for juveniles is at its lowest point since the mid-1980s (Snyder, 2002), there are still a significant number of juveniles who come into contact with the criminal justice system. For example, in 2000, approximately 2.4 million juveniles were arrested, which is around 10% of the entire juvenile population in the United States (Federal Bureau of Investigation [FBI], 2000; Snyder, 2002).

A particularly salient concern is the number of violent offenses committed by those under the age of 18. From 1989 to 1994, the arrest rate for juveniles who committed violent offenses increased by 62% (Bureau of Justice Statistics [BJS], 1998; Office of Juvenile Justice and Delinquency Prevention [OJJDP], 1999a). After peaking in 1994, the juvenile arrest rate for violent offenses began to decline, and that trend continued for several years (Snyder, 2002). By 1997, the rate of juvenile arrests for violent offenses was at its lowest level in approximately 10 years (BJS, 1998; FBI, 1994; OJJDP, 1999a). Recently released statistics from the OJJDP (U.S. Department of Justice) indicate that from 1994 to 2000, the juvenile arrest rate for violent offenses dropped by 41% to its lowest rate since the mid-1980s (Snyder, 2002). In addition, in 2000 the juvenile arrest rate for murder dropped 74% from its peak level in 1993 to its lowest level since the 1960s (Snyder, 2002).

Although these trends in juvenile offending appear encouraging, criminal justice statistics suggest that a fairly significant proportion of juveniles continue to engage in criminal and often violent behavior (Snyder, 2000, 2002). In 2000, for example, juveniles accounted for 17% of all arrests and 16% of all violent crime arrests, including 9% of murder arrests, 14% of aggravated assault arrests, 16% of forcible rape arrests, 19% of sex offenses, 24% of weapons arrests, 25% of robbery arrests, and 53% of arson arrests (Snyder, 2002). Also, of the 2.4 million juveniles arrested in 2000, approximately 100,000 were arrested for serious violent crimes, such as robbery, forcible rape, aggravated assault, and homicide (Snyder, 2002). In addition to examining arrest statistics, which is the primary means of measuring youth violence, it is instructive to examine self-reports of youth violence. Recently released self-report statistics indicate that the proportion of juveniles who engage in nonfatal violent behavior has not declined since the peak years in the mid-1990s (Department of Health and Human Services [DHHS], 2001). These statistics are particularly troubling given recent estimates that the number of teens (ages 14–17) will increase by 20% in the year 2005 (Fox, 1996).

These multiple sources of data in the aggregate suggest that youth violence is a continuing and devastating national problem. In response to the growing concern over youth violence, a number of researchers have begun to examine the factors that may be contributing to the commission of criminal and violent offenses by juveniles. The combined results of several long-term research studies suggest that there are multiple influences that likely contribute to juvenile offending, including increased access to firearms, higher levels of gang involvement, adverse social conditions, and victimization (American Bar Association, 1993; American Psychological Association, 1993; Handler, 1993; Howell, Krisberg, & Jones, 1995; OJJDP, 1999a).

A particularly promising line of research pertains to the relationship between risk factors and protective factors and juvenile offending. Recent empirical research suggests that serious, violent, and chronic offending by juveniles may be directly related to the presence of multiple risk factors (Hawkins et al., 2000; Loeber, Farrington, Stouthamer-Loeber, Moffitt, & Caspi, 1998; see also Cottle, Lee, & Heilbrun, 2001). By contrast, research suggests that the presence of multiple protective factors may reduce the likelihood of antisocial behavior among juveniles (Hanna, 2001; Werner, 1993, 2000). Accordingly, the accurate identification of risk factors and protective factors among juveniles has become a high priority in a variety of policy, correctional, and treatment contexts.

In this chapter, we review the recent theoretical and empirical literature regarding risk factors and protective factors among juvenile offenders. We highlight the distinction between static and dynamic factors, particularly the implications that they have for the development, implementation, and effectiveness of intervention strategies. This chapter includes a discussion of the current trends in the treatment of juvenile offenders, with a particular emphasis on empirically tested "best-practice" intervention approaches. We conclude by discussing directions for future research in the area of juvenile offending.

Risk and Protective Factors

Although the definition of "risk factors" often differs depending on the context (e.g., clinical/treatment vs. correctional), we define risk factors broadly as external or internal influences or conditions that are associated with or predictive of a negative outcome (such as delinquency or antisocial behavior). While research suggests that some risk factors are merely *correlated* with a negative outcome, other risk factors are *causally related* to a negative outcome. Focusing on risk factors that have an established causal relationship to antisocial behavior has proven valuable in developing effective intervention strategies for juvenile offenders, which will be discussed in later sections of this chapter. When viewed as a whole, the most recent research suggests that the more risk factors a juvenile has, the greater the likelihood that the juvenile will engage in antisocial behavior (Hawkins et al., 2000; Loeber et al., 1998; see also Hanna, 2001).

During the past several years, the concept of protective factors has been a subject of considerable interest to researchers (e.g., Carson & Butcher, 1992; Grisso, 1998; Hanna, 2001; Hoge & Andrews, 1996; Kashani, Jones, Bumby, & Thomas, 1999; Stoiber & Good, 1998). However, despite substantial advances in the understanding of protective factors, researchers have been unable to reach a consensus regarding the definition of protective factors. For example, some define protective factors as merely the absence of risk factors, while others define protective factors as influences that moderate or buffer risk and thereby decrease the likelihood of a negative outcome (Jessor, Van Den Bos, Vanderryn, Costa, & Turbin, 1995). In this chapter, we define protective factors more generally as external or internal influences or conditions that decrease the likelihood of a negative outcome or enhance the likelihood of a positive outcome. As with the risk factors, recent research suggests that the more protective factors that a juvenile has, the less likely it is that the juvenile will engage in serious antisocial behavior (Grisso, 1998; Werner, 1993, 2000).

Another topic of much debate is the manner by which protective factors achieve their risk-reducing influence (e.g., Clayton, Leukefeld, Donohew, Bardo, & Harrington, 1995; Hoge, Andrews, & Leschied, 1996). The results of separate lines of research suggest that protective factors may reduce the likelihood of a negative outcome in two ways. First, protective factors may reduce the negative effects of risk factors by interacting with and moderating the risk factors (Clayton et al., 1995). Second, protective factors may exert an independent influence on the negative outcome, regardless of whether risk factors are present (Hoge et al., 1996). Regardless of the particular mechanism of action, risk factors are consistently associated with a decreased risk of antisocial behavior among juveniles.

In the past several years, researchers have identified numerous risk and protective factors that are related to juvenile offending. These risk and protective factors cover a wide variety of psychological, medical, biological, behavioral, and social domains at several different levels of functioning, including the individual, family, and community levels (Carson & Butcher, 1992; Chase-Lansdale, Wakschlag, & Brooks-Gunn, 1995; Hawkins et al., 2000; Kashani et al., 1999; Melton, Petrila, Poythress, & Slobogin, 1997; Plutchik, 1995). In addition to identifying a significant number of risk and protective factors, researchers have developed several different approaches for the broad classification of risk and protective factors. Therefore, before addressing specific risk and protective factors, we discuss the major classification approaches that have been developed.

Classification of Risk and Protective Factors

A key distinction is generally made between static and dynamic risk factors (Andrews & Bonta, 1998). Static risk factors are unmodifiable, and they typically include historical variables (e.g., age at first offense and number of prior arrests) and demographic variables (e.g., gender and race). Although, by definition, static risk factors are not amenable to intervention, they have considerable predictive utility, which makes them useful in the evaluation of long-term recidivism potential (Andrews & Bonta, 1998). By contrast, dynamic risk factors are modifiable, and they include such variables as access to weapons, substance abuse, delinquent peers, and certain psychiatric disorders. Because dynamic risk factors are amenable to direct interventions, the most effective intervention strategies for juvenile offenders focus on eliminating (or ameliorating the effects of) dynamic risk factors. Intervention efforts focused on changeable, risk-relevant characteristics can effectively reduce the juvenile offender's overall level of risk, as is discussed in later sections of this chapter (see Heilbrun, 1997).

Some researchers have also noted a distinction between criminological and clinical risk factors (e.g., Monahan et al., 2001; see Wessely & Taylor, 1991). The criminological risk factors are those factors that have been identified in the criminal justice literature as having a relationship to antisocial behavior, such as prior criminality, negative childhood experiences, and an impoverished neighborhood. The clinical risk factors are those factors that have been identified by treatment providers as having a relationship to antisocial behavior, such as psychotic symptoms, anger, and psychopathy. Although there is some overlap between these two categories of risk factors, this classification scheme promotes a multidisciplinary approach to risk assessment and intervention.

A more specific classification approach divides risk and protective factors into categories that are derived from a multidimensional psychosocial framework (e.g., Kashani et al., 1999). For example, risk factors and protective factors are often classified as personal/dispositional (e.g., age, gender), historical (e.g., arrest history, years of education), contextual (e.g., homelessness, social support), and clinical (e.g., psychiatric diagnosis, problem-solving ability) (Monahan et al., 2001). This multilevel, domain-focused classification framework often serves as the basis for the development of comprehensive preventive and intervention strategies for at-risk adolescents.

A comparable multilevel classification approach is based on the ecological model, and it divides risk and protective factors into individual, family, community, and environmental factors (see Bronfenbrenner, 1979). The ecological model is a public health perspective for reducing and preventing disease, illness, and injury (Garbarino, 1985). The underlying premise of the ecological model is that an individual functions within a complex and interrelated network of contexts that exert an independent influence on risk level. Therefore, instead of focusing solely on the individual, the ecological model considers the individual in the context of the surrounding environment.

A similar classification scheme was used in a recent report on youth violence by the U.S. Department of Health and Human Services (DHHS, 2001), which divides risk factors for youth violence into five categories: individual, family, school, peer group, and community. Citing a lack of reliable research regarding protective factors, the DHHS report discusses only *proposed* protective factors in four categories: individual, family, school, and peer group. As with the classification schemes developed based on the ecological model, the DHHS classification approach is based on the premise that risk and protective factors do not operate in isolation. Rather, individuals' risk levels are produced by a complex interaction between their unique characteristics and multiple external influences (DHHS, 2001).

Examination of Specific Risk and Protective Factors

Over the past several years, researchers and clinicians have identified numerous factors that are correlated with or predictive of antisocial behavior among juveniles. In the sections that follow, we discuss several of the risk and protective factors that have been identified in the most recent empirical and theoretical literature. We have structured our discussion of risk and protective factors by grouping them according to the categories delineated in the multidimensional psychosocial classification approach. Accordingly, we discuss risk and protective factors at each of the following levels: individual, family, school, peer, and environmental (community/neighborhood).

INDIVIDUAL FACTORS

Most of the research regarding risk factors for antisocial behavior among juveniles has focused on individual-level factors that are associated with or predictive of antisocial behavior. Before discussing these risk factors, however, two cautions are necessary. First, because the appropriateness of behavior can vary greatly with age, it is important to consider individual-level risk factors within the juvenile's developmental framework. Second, it is important to remember that individual-level risk factors rarely, if ever, operate alone. Rather, these risk factors operate within the context of the juvenile's larger environment, and it is the interaction between individual-level risk factors and the juvenile's environment that produces varying levels of risk for antisocial behavior.

Researchers have identified a core set of individual-level risk factors that are associated with juvenile criminality and recidivism. Some of the more salient risk factors include a history of early aggression, age at first adjudication, number of prior arrests, and number of out-of-home placements or institutional commitments (Cornell, Peterson, & Richards, 1999; Farrington & Hawkins, 1991; Flannery & Williams, 1999; Heilbrun, 1997, 1999; OJJDP, 1999a; Tolan, 1987). These static risk factors have a demonstrated relationship to juvenile offending, and their predictive utility has been firmly established (Hawkins et al., 2000).

Another risk factor that has received considerable support as a predictor of juvenile offending is substance abuse (Elliott, Huizinga, & Ageton, 1985; OJJDP, 1999a), which is generally considered the most powerful dynamic individual risk factor for juvenile offending. The majority of juvenile offenders have a history of

alcohol and drug abuse, and about 50% of incarcerated adolescents report having used drugs or alcohol at the time they committed the offense for which they
are incarcerated (Bilchik, 1999). Although recent research suggests that substance abuse is a strong predictor of juvenile delinquency and recidivism, the
predictive utility of substance abuse as a risk factor for antisocial behavior
decreases with age (DHHS, 2001). For example, substance abuse at age 9 is a
stronger predictor of antisocial behavior than substance abuse at age 14 (DHHS,
2001). It should be noted, however, that the relationship between drug use and
antisocial behavior among juveniles is not entirely clear. For example, there is
evidence that drug use contributes to *continued* antisocial behavior as opposed
to the *onset* of antisocial behavior, so findings in this area should be interpreted
with caution (DHHS, 2001).

A related risk factor is drug dealing, which is predictive of specific forms of
antisocial and violent behavior, such as possession of a weapon, automobile
theft, and fraud (Loeber et al., 1998). As with drug use, however, it is difficult to
interpret the relationship between juvenile violence and drug dealing because
each is a risk factor for the other (Loeber et al., 1998). Nevertheless, because substance abuse and drug dealing are dynamic risk factors, they are often the focus
of intervention strategies aimed at preventing or reducing juvenile offending in
general and violence in particular.

The Pittsburgh Youth Study, a large-scale longitudinal study of 1,517 urban
adolescents, identified several individual-level static and dynamic risk factors for
juvenile delinquency, including high impulsivity, low IQ, and specific personality traits (Loeber et al., 1998). There was a significant positive correlation
between two types of impulsivity—cognitive and behavioral—and delinquent
behavior, with behavioral impulsivity (e.g., restlessness, poor behavioral controls) being a particularly strong correlate of delinquent behavior. There was a
significant negative correlation between IQ scores and delinquent behavior.
Specifically, when compared to nondelinquent youth, self-reported delinquent
youth scored an average of eight points lower on the Wechsler Intelligence Scale
for Children, revised edition (WISC-R). Finally, with respect to personality
traits, higher levels of delinquent behavior were associated with greater negative
emotionality (e.g., anger, fear) and less personal constraint (e.g., thrill-seeking
behavior) (Loeber et al., 1998).

In a recent meta-analysis sponsored by the OJJDP, researchers examined
66 studies of juvenile violence in an attempt to identify common risk factors
(Hawkins et al., 2000). The meta-analysis identified several individual-level risk
factors across medical, physiological, and psychological domains. The psychological variables included early initiation of violent behavior; hyperactivity, concentration problems, restlessness, and risk taking; aggressiveness; involvement
in other forms of antisocial behavior; and beliefs and attitudes favorable to deviant or antisocial behavior (Hawkins et al., 2000). Although the predictive utility
of these risk factors varies according to the age and developmental level of the
juvenile, each risk factor was consistently correlated with a higher likelihood of
violent behavior.

The results of the OJJDP meta-analysis revealed that early onset of violent behavior, which is a commonly identified static risk factor across studies, is a particularly strong correlate of more serious and chronic juvenile violence (Hawkins et al., 2000). Similarly, the meta-analysis indicated that involvement in other forms of antisocial activity, such as theft, selling drugs, and destruction of property, was also consistently associated with a greater risk of violence among male juveniles. The meta-analysis revealed that early aggressive behavior (as opposed to actual violent behavior) was predictive of juvenile violence, which is consistent with the observation that antisocial behavior often begins with early aggressive behavior and culminates in serious violent behavior. The meta-analysis reflected a consistent correlation between antisocial behavior and hyperactivity, concentration problems, restlessness, and risk taking. For example, in one study analyzed in the meta-analysis, boys with restlessness and concentration problems were five times more likely to be arrested for violent behavior than boys without those characteristics (Klinteberg, Andersson, Magnusson, & Stattin, 1993). Finally, the OJJDP meta-analysis revealed that antisocial beliefs and attitudes, attitudes favorable to violence, and hostility toward the police are correlated with subsequent violent behavior among male juveniles (Hawkins et al., 2000). These dynamic risk factors have consistently been associated with violent behavior among juveniles.

There has also been some recent interest in the relationship between psychiatric diagnoses and juvenile antisocial behavior. Although more research is needed, some researchers have noted a positive correlation between certain psychiatric disorders and juvenile antisocial behavior (e.g., Kashani et al., 1999). For example, Kashani et al. (1999) concluded that juveniles who appear in juvenile justice and forensic psychiatric settings often meet the *Diagnostic and Statistical Manual of Mental Disorders (DSM-IV)* (American Psychiatric Association, 1994) diagnostic criteria for conduct disorder, parent-child relationship disorder, attention-deficit/hyperactivity disorder (ADHD), or a depressive disorder. With respect to conduct disorder, the physical aggression component appears to be the strongest predictor of aggressive behavior among juveniles (DHHS, 2001). Researchers have also noted, however, that most psychiatric disorders that have been linked to juvenile aggression, such as ADHD, anxiety disorders, and depressive disorders, are *indirectly* related to juvenile offending (DHHS, 2001). For example, it is likely that these disorders reflect emotional and behavioral problems that may lead to the development of risk factors in other psychosocial domains (e.g., poor family relations, low educational achievement), and it is the development of these additional risk factors that is primarily responsible for an increased risk for juvenile offending.

There has also been some recent interest regarding individual-level protective factors. Several researchers have found that intelligence/education serves as a protective factor for most juveniles who are at high risk for engaging in antisocial behavior (e.g., Carson & Butcher, 1992; Hoge & Andrews, 1996; see Kandel et al., 1988). For example, Kandel et al. (1988) found that high-risk individuals often do not become involved in antisocial behavior because of the positive reinforcement that education provides. According to Carson and Butcher (1992), these high-risk individuals may not be engaging in antisocial behavior because they are focusing their time and energy on more socially acceptable behaviors, such as their academic performance. It is also possible that having a high IQ could increase the likelihood that an adolescent will benefit from the resulting educational opportunities that may be presented (DHHS, 2001).

According to the DHHS (2001) report, there is only one individual-level protective factor that exerts a significant buffering effect on risk factors for juvenile violence—an intolerant attitude toward deviant behavior. This protective factor likely reflects a commitment to social norms and disapproval of behaviors that violate social norms. This protective factor may also decrease the probability that a juvenile will associate with delinquent peers, which would further reduce the likelihood of engaging in antisocial behavior. The DHHS (2001) report cites four other individual-level factors that may buffer the risk of antisocial behavior or general delinquency, but that have not been shown to moderate violence—high IQ, being female, strong social orientation, and perceived disapproval by peers of antisocial behavior.

There are several other individual-level protective factors that fall under the general category of personality/psychological variables, such as sociability, positive temperament, the ability to seek social support, and acting in a reflective (not impulsive) manner (Hanna, 2001). Resilient adolescents typically utilize flexible coping strategies, and their cognitive style is characterized by flexibility and reflection (Hanna, 2001). Having a sense of mastery over one's environment may also be associated with a decreased risk for antisocial behavior. The ability to view situations from multiple perspectives is an important component in the development of empathy, which may reduce the likelihood of antisocial behavior. The acquisition of various skill sets, such as problem solving, conflict resolution, anger management, and critical thinking, may also function to reduce the likelihood of juvenile antisocial behavior. In fact, these skills and related cognitive and behavioral strategies often form the cornerstone of intervention programs for at-risk juveniles. Finally, there is some empirical evidence that the presence of certain internalizing disorders, such as nervousness and anxiety, may have a modest negative correlation with juvenile violence (Hawkins et al., 2000; Mitchell & Rosa, 1979).

FAMILY FACTORS

Several studies have examined the relationship between family risk factors and antisocial behavior among juveniles (e.g., DHHS, 2001; Hawkins et al., 2000; Hoge et al., 1996; Loeber et al., 1998; see also Flannery & Williams, 1999; Patterson, 1982; Patterson, DeBaryshe, & Ramsey, 1989; Patterson & Dishion, 1985). Key family risk factors for antisocial behavior among juveniles include child abuse/neglect; low levels of parental involvement; high levels of hostility, conflict, and aggression within the family; parental criminality; family conflict; inadequate parental supervision; early parental loss; and emotional deprivation (Carson & Butcher, 1992; Greenacre, 1945; Kumpfer & Alvarado, 2003; Melton et al., 1997; see also Grisso, 1998; Monahan et al., 2001). The recent OJJDP meta-analysis identified several family-related risk factors that have an established relationship to juvenile offending, including such factors as antisocial parents, poor family management practices, child maltreatment, low levels of parental involvement, and parent-child separation (Hawkins et al., 2000).

The family-related risk factors with perhaps the strongest predictive utility for juvenile antisocial behavior are intrafamilial violence (Dembo et al., 2000; Kashani & Allan, 1998), poor parental supervision (Hawkins et al., 2000; Loeber et al., 1998), and antisocial parents (DHHS, 2001). In several studies, these three risk factors are consistently associated with future antisocial behavior among juveniles (e.g., Hawkins et al., 2000). Juveniles who are exposed to spousal abuse and/or child abuse engage in higher levels of violent behavior than juveniles from families with less violence. Widom (1989), for example, found that abused or neglected children were 38% more likely to be arrested for a violent offense than children who had not been abused or neglected. Also, poor parental supervision and parental antisocial behavior are associated with an increased likelihood of delinquent and antisocial behavior among juveniles. Specifically, adolescents whose parents engage in criminal behavior are twice as likely to be involved in serious delinquent behavior as adolescents without antisocial parents (Bilchik, 1999).

Hoge et al. (1996) examined several family risk factors in a sample of 338 youth between the ages of 12 and 17. Based on prior research, Hoge et al. (1996) identified three family risk factors for inclusion in their study: family relationship problems, parenting problems, and parental problems. The results of the study indicated that higher levels of family relationship problems and parental problems were significantly associated with higher levels of reoffending among their sample of youth (Hoge et al., 1996).

A great deal of research has been conducted regarding the development of aggressive behavior among juveniles (e.g., Huizinga, Esbensen, & Weiher, 1991; Patterson, 1982; Patterson et al., 1989; Patterson & Dishion, 1985; Thornberry, Huizinga, & Loeber, 1995). According to Patterson's (1982) "coercive family process" model, aggressive behavior among adolescents develops as the result of imitation of the parents and parental reinforcement. Specifically, Patterson contends that (a) aggressive children tend to imitate aggressive parents and (b) parents of aggressive children often reinforce the aggression by responding with attention or approval. Another element of Patterson's model is the role of parental supervision in the development of aggressive behavior among adolescents. Patterson suggests that aggression among adolescents results from poor parental supervision, inconsistent directives (i.e., not related to the adolescent's behavior), and harsh physical punishment (see Patterson, 1982). The causal model developed by Huizinga and colleagues (1991) suggests that there are multiple developmental pathways that lead to delinquent behavior among juveniles. According to Huizinga et al. (1991), delinquency should be viewed as a multidetermined phenomenon, and intervention approaches should address multiple risk factors. Finally, a large-scale longitudinal study by Thornberry and colleagues (1995), conducted as part of the Program of Research on the Causes and Correlates of Delinquency, similarly identified multiple pathways—involving the interaction of risk factors—leading to the development of aggressive behavior among juveniles.

Several researchers have concluded that the positive influence of an individual's family is a protective factor for some high-risk individuals (e.g., Carson & Butcher, 1992; Kumpfer & Alvarado, 2003; Melton et al., 1997; Thornberry et al., 1995). Accordingly, the absence of significant family disturbances is often cited as a protective factor with respect to the likelihood of engaging in antisocial behavior (Hoge & Andrews, 1996; Melton et al., 1997). Recent research also suggests that enhancing the warmth of family relationships, providing nonaggressive role models, establishing a strong attachment between parents and child, increasing parental monitoring of children's behavior, and providing clear and consistent norms for behavior can assist in preventing high-risk juveniles from engaging in antisocial behavior (Melton et al., 1997). Finally, Thornberry et al.'s (1995) longitudinal research identified high levels of parental supervision and strong parent-child attachment as being related to resilience among adolescents.

One of the strongest protective factors against juvenile violence is the establishment of a close relationship with at least one supportive adult (Hanna, 2001; Hawkins et al., 2000; Werner, 2000). Research suggests that the unconditional acceptance of a child by an adult caregiver may be the most important factor contributing to the resiliency of a child despite the presence of multiple risk factors (Werner, 2000). This protective factor is generally effective regardless of whether the adult caregiver is a parent, teacher, or even a volunteer, which may account for the popularity and effectiveness of some juvenile mentoring programs (e.g., Big Brothers/Big Sisters of America).

SCHOOL-RELATED FACTORS

There are several risk factors related to academic performance/achievement and the school environment that appear to contribute to delinquent and violent behavior among juveniles (Hanna, 2001; Hawkins et al., 2000). Factors such as low academic achievement, poor academic performance, low commitment to school, and failing to complete school are associated with delinquent and violent behavior among juveniles (Hinshaw, 1992). Even factors such as school overcrowding can be associated with increased aggression among the students (Kashani et al., 1999).

The OJJDP meta-analysis identified academic failure, frequent absences, withdrawal from school, multiple school transitions, and delinquent peers as school-related factors that are associated with juvenile delinquency and violence (Hawkins et al., 2000). For example, poor academic achievement, particularly poor performance in elementary school, has consistently predicted delinquent and violent behavior among juveniles, although this relationship is typically stronger for females (Hawkins et al., 2000). The relationship between truancy and juvenile delinquency is also firmly established. In a 1989 study, Farrington found that high truancy rates between the ages of 12 and 14 were associated with higher rates of violence in adolescence and adulthood. Although frequent school transitions were found to be associated with juvenile violence in the

OJJDP meta-analysis (Hawkins et al., 2000), this finding must be interpreted with caution because school transitions may be reflective of other factors that are associated with violence among juveniles, such as poor family relations. This is an example of multiple factors from different psychosocial domains interacting to increase a given risk level.

Several researchers have concluded that school-related factors can effectively reduce the level of risk for certain at-risk adolescents. For example, educational achievement is often cited as a protective factor for most high-risk juveniles (e.g., Carson & Butcher, 1992; Hoge & Andrews, 1996; Kandel et al., 1988). In addition, commitment to school was cited in the DHHS (2001) report as being a factor that significantly buffers the effects of risk factors. Research suggests that adolescents who are committed to school engage in less antisocial behavior, perhaps out of concern that antisocial behavior would jeopardize their educational potential (Jessor et al., 1995). It is also likely that participation in school-related extracurricular activities (e.g., sports, academic clubs) reduces the likelihood of antisocial behavior. Participation in structured extracurricular activities may achieve a risk-reducing effect in several ways, such as by providing adolescents with a sense of achievement and taking up free time that may otherwise be occupied with antisocial activities.

PEER-RELATED FACTORS

During adolescence, the influence of the peer group often becomes paramount over the influence of the family. Accordingly, peer-related risk factors take on particular importance during the teen years, and these risk factors are often regarded as the most potent risk factors among adolescents. Research has consistently demonstrated that adolescents with negative peer relations tend to engage in higher levels of delinquent and antisocial behavior (Hawkins et al., 2000). Also, juveniles who are socially isolated or withdrawn (e.g., low involvement in traditional social activities) are at an increased risk for engaging in violent behavior (DHHS, 2001).

Associating with delinquent youth, whether they are siblings or peers, is also related to increased juvenile offending. For example, Farrington (1989) found that the presence of delinquent siblings was predictive of violent behavior among juveniles. Similarly, the presence of delinquent peers, particularly during adolescence, has been associated with increased antisocial behavior (Moffitt, 1993). In a study that examined the relationship between peer risk factors and antisocial behavior, researchers found that exposure to deviant peers was significantly correlated with the subsequent initiation of delinquent behaviors (Keenan, Loeber, Zhang, Stouthamer-Loeber, & van Kammen, 1995). Some researchers have asserted that adolescents with delinquent peers are 10 times more likely to be involved in serious delinquent behavior than adolescents without delinquent peers (e.g., Bilchik, 1999). In related research, gang membership was more predictive of antisocial behavior than the presence of delinquent peers (Battin, Hill, Abbott, Catalano, & Hawkins, 1998; DHHS, 2001).

The positive effect of peers on antisocial behavior is a much-debated topic, and research in this area has demonstrated mixed results. Some researchers contend that associating with prosocial peers reduces the likelihood of antisocial behavior among juveniles (e.g., Jessor et al., 1995), but this conclusion is not universally accepted (DHHS, 2001). The OJJDP meta-analysis noted that adolescents associating with peers who disapproved of delinquent behavior were less likely themselves to report a history of delinquent behaviors (Hawkins et al., 2000). Other studies have not found a clear relationship between prosocial peers and the prevention or reduction of antisocial behavior among juveniles (DHHS, 2001).

ENVIRONMENTAL FACTORS

Environmental influence is a broad category of risk factors that includes living arrangements and cultural, community, and neighborhood variables. In recent years, researchers have emphasized the effects of environmental factors in causing or facilitating antisocial behavior among juveniles. One of the most heavily researched of these environmental risk factors is socioeconomic status. Several studies have found that being raised in a low-income neighborhood is predictive of self-reported violence and convictions for violent offenses among juveniles (Farrington, 1989; Henry, Avshalom, Moffitt, & Silva, 1996). In the OJJDP meta-analysis, for example, researchers noted that self-reported felony assault and robbery were twice as common in juveniles raised in poverty as among juveniles raised in a middle-class environment (Hawkins et al., 2000).

In the Pittsburgh Youth Study (Loeber et al., 1998), researchers considered the relationship between several socioeconomic factors and delinquency. They found that the strongest correlate of delinquent behavior among their sample involved being in a family that receives public financial assistance. Other socioeconomic correlates of delinquent behavior included a small house, an unemployed father, and a poorly educated mother (Loeber et al., 1998). Finally, living in a high-crime and low-socioeconomic-status neighborhood (defined by census data or mother's self-report) doubled the rate of delinquent behaviors among the juveniles in the sample (Loeber et al., 1998). Although the relationship between low socioeconomic status and delinquent behaviors is not entirely clear, it is conceivable that adolescents who are raised in a low socioeconomic neighborhood may have less access to structured activities and healthy school environments, which have been found to reduce the risk of delinquent behavior among juveniles.

Other researchers have suggested that repeated exposure to violence, whether media-based violence or that observed in the home or community, may contribute to aggressive behavior and attitudes among juveniles (American Psychological Association, 1993; Centerwall, 1992; Dawson & Reiter, 1998; Flannery & Williams, 1999; Kashani et al., 1999). Some have speculated that witnessing violence may desensitize adolescents to the effects of violence (Dawson & Reiter, 1998), which may reduce their inhibitions for committing violent acts. Another theory is that repeated exposure to violence may reinforce the perception that violence is a normative behavior and an appropriate problem-solving strategy. These theories received some empirical support from Bandura's well-known behavioral experiments, in which he demonstrated that social learning plays an important role in the perpetuation of violent behavior when children witness a violent episode (Bandura, Ross, & Ross, 1961). More recently, researchers noted that there is a positive correlation between exposure to community violence and the frequency of violent behavior among juveniles (Farrell & Bruce, 1997).

Surprisingly, there has been little research in the area of environmental protective factors. As previously noted, the DHHS (2001) report did not identify any protective factors in this category. Nevertheless, there are certain environmental factors that may serve a protective function, particularly for at-risk adolescents. One particularly important protective factor is a strong community infrastructure. Among other benefits, having a well-developed community infrastructure provides adolescents with opportunities to participate in structured activities, which has a documented risk-reducing effect. A strong community infrastructure also produces a sense of community cohesion, which may further reduce the likelihood of antisocial behavior. In a recent study, for example, social cohesion was associated with reduced levels of violence among juveniles (Sampson, Raudenbush, & Earls, 1997).

As the preceding sections illustrate, there are numerous risk factors across multiple psychosocial domains and there may also be some protective factors. The interaction of these individual, family, school, peer, and environmental risk and protective factors contributes to the juvenile's overall level of risk; there is no single combination of risk and protective factors that has been shown to infallibly predict or prevent antisocial behavior. Despite a substantial body of research, the process by which these risk and protective factors affect violence among juveniles is not well understood. As noted previously, however, the multiple risk and protective factors that have been identified in recent years serve as the basis for intervention strategies aimed at preventing or reducing antisocial behavior among juveniles. The following section discusses the current trends in intervention strategies for juvenile offenders.

Intervention Strategies for Juvenile Offenders

Before discussing specific intervention strategies for juvenile offenders, however, it is important to make some general comments about the existing research in this area. Much of this research is affected by two methodological concerns, which may be contributing to the often contradictory findings (see Mulvey, Arthur, & Reppucci, 1993). The first methodological concern is the lack of a uniform definition of delinquency. Because delinquency is often the primary outcome variable, the definition used in research studies is directly relevant to the observed effectiveness of the intervention being examined. Differing operational definitions of delinquency make it difficult to compare the effectiveness of interventions across studies. The second methodological concern is the lack of specificity regarding the mechanisms that link specific risk factors and intervention strategies to decreases in juvenile offending. A well-developed intervention strategy should be grounded upon an understanding of the relationship among risk factors, the intervention, and the resulting decrease in delinquent behavior (Hawkins & Nederhood, 1987). Unfortunately, research in this area does not routinely address these issues and, as a result, it is often difficult to determine the reasons that a particular intervention failed or succeeded.

Despite these methodological concerns, researchers have identified several effective intervention strategies for juveniles. A review of the recent literature suggests that certain prevention and treatment programs can be effective with both adolescents from the general population and high-risk adolescents with multiple risk factors (DHHS, 2001). Rather than discussing the effectiveness of specific treatment programs that have been developed, we discuss the prevention and treatment of juvenile offending more broadly. We first consider the prevention and treatment of juvenile offending borrowing from a public health perspective. Following that, we discuss the general characteristics of intervention strategies that have proven effective in the prevention and treatment of juvenile offending.

Public Health Perspective: Levels of Intervention

According to the public health model, the prevention and treatment of juvenile offending can occur at primary, secondary, and tertiary levels (Flannery & Williams, 1999; see also Caplan, 1964; Mulvey et al., 1993). In short, primary interventions attempt to reduce the incidence of violence before it begins, secondary interventions attempt to reduce the prevalence of existing violence, and tertiary interventions attempt to prevent the reoccurrence of violence. These levels of intervention provide a structured mechanism for identifying the types of intervention efforts that can be used at various stages in the development of youth violence (e.g., prior to the onset of violence, after some violence has occurred). As noted by Mulvey et al. (1993), this typology of levels is best viewed as a way of systematically categorizing the types of intervention strategies that are available at each stage in the development of youth violence. In the following sections, we discuss each of these levels of intervention.

PRIMARY INTERVENTION STRATEGIES

The focus of primary prevention strategies is to keep violence from occurring. As such, the thrust of these prevention strategies is to identify adolescents who may be at high risk for engaging in youth violence and then to address their needs *before* the violence occurs. Therefore, the effectiveness of primary prevention strategies often lies in recognizing existing static and dynamic risk factors across each of the psychosocial domains previously discussed and then either ameliorating the harmful effects of those risk factors or promoting the development of protective factors (Mulvey et al., 1993). In contrast with secondary intervention strategies, which target high-risk *individuals*, the target of primary prevention strategies is high-risk *populations*.

Primary intervention strategies can be accurately characterized as prevention efforts, because these intervention strategies are utilized *before* violence occurs. Because the focus of these strategies is on the *prevention* of youth violence, as opposed to the *treatment* of youth violence after it has occurred, primary intervention strategies typically occur at broad levels, such as the family, school, and community. These system-level, broad-based intervention efforts are effective in part because they can easily reach a large number of high-risk adolescents. Each locus for primary prevention efforts—family, school, and community—is briefly discussed in the sections that follow.

FAMILY-BASED APPROACHES. Family-based intervention efforts have become the centerpiece of many youth violence prevention programs. Given the potential negative influence of family-level risk factors, targeting families appears to be an effective way of preventing violence among high-risk adolescents (see Kumpfer & Alvarado, 2003). According to Mulvey et al. (1993), family-based intervention efforts can generally be classified as either parent-focused or family-supportive. Parent-focused intervention efforts may include assisting parents to recognize warning signs for youth violence and/or training parents to effectively manage any behavioral problems that may occur. Rather than being used as stand-alone strategies, these techniques are often used in collaboration with other intervention strategies, such as community- or school-based intervention efforts. These interventions, which are voluntary and typically offered without charge, are often made available to all parents within a particular school, school district, or community. One example of a parent-focused intervention is the teaching of child management skills to the parents of children who display behavioral problems in school. Although parent-focused approaches have shown some success, the most common research finding is that parents of high-risk youth tend to discontinue the training at rates that may exceed 50% (see Mulvey et al., 1993). With such high attrition rates, particularly among families with the greatest need for these services, it is unlikely that parent-focused approaches will be a reliable mechanism for preventing youth violence.

Family-supportive intervention efforts seek to provide needed social support services to families, particularly families from economically disadvantaged backgrounds. These social services may include child care, medical assistance, counseling, and assistance from other social service agencies (Mulvey et al., 1993). These social service intervention efforts have the benefit of being comprehensive in scope, which may help to reduce risk factors across several psychosocial domains. Family-supportive intervention efforts have achieved mixed results in studies of their efficacy and effectiveness, and there has not been an evaluation of the long-term effects of family-supportive interventions with respect to delinquency and antisocial behavior (see Mulvey et al., 1993).

SCHOOL-BASED APPROACHES. School is another common environment in which primary prevention strategies are often employed. As with family-based intervention efforts, school-based intervention strategies may be particularly effective because there are many risk factors for violence that are school- or academic-related, such as low academic achievement, poor academic performance, low commitment to school, withdrawal from school, school overcrowding, frequent absences, multiple school transitions, and delinquent peers (Hawkins et al., 2000; Hinshaw, 1992; Kashani et al., 1999). Some examples of school-based violence prevention efforts include preschool programs (e.g., Project Head Start), social skills training (e.g., cognitive-behavioral therapy), and broad-based social interventions that are designed to alter the school environment (Mulvey et al., 1993; see also Greenberg et al., 2003; Loeber & Farrington, 1998a).

Preschool programs, such as Project Head Start and the Perry Preschool Project, attempt to prevent the development of academic problems among children from economically disadvantaged backgrounds. An integral component of these programs is the concomitant provision of a diverse array of social services, which may have the effect of reducing existing barriers to learning. Studies of these preschool programs have produced mixed results, and there is not overwhelming evidence that these programs can produce long-lasting effects with respect to the subsequent development of delinquent behavior (Mulvey et al., 1993; see Loeber & Farrington, 1998a).

Social skills training, which is often provided in the school setting to small groups of children, helps at-risk youth to develop techniques for creating (or maintaining) positive social relationships with family members, peers, and teachers. Some studies have found that social skills training can produce short-term behavioral improvements, but there have been few studies that have evaluated the long-term effectiveness of these approaches in terms of preventing anti-social behavior among youth. As a result, it is difficult to draw firm conclusions about the effectiveness of these approaches.

An alternative school-based approach, often termed social process intervention (see Mulvey et al., 1993), seeks to improve problem-solving skills and promote greater individual involvement among students by modifying some of the social/environmental mediators that can be found in the school environment (Gauce, Comer, & Schwartz, 1987). These approaches generally involve changing school procedures, and examples include (a) changing teaching practices to promote bonding among students with learning difficulties, (b) facilitating the transition from elementary school to junior high school, (c) improving perceptions of school safety, and (d) providing the opportunity for greater community involvement among students (see Mulvey et al., 1993). Many of these approaches have shown some success in terms of outcome variables that are related to academic achievement (e.g., improving school behavior, reducing withdrawal rates), but these approaches have not been evaluated with specific reference to preventing or reducing delinquent behavior among adolescents.

COMMUNITY-BASED APPROACHES. The final category of primary prevention efforts is community-based preventive approaches, which include intervention strategies such as increasing community organization and making constructive activities available to adolescents. Instituting community organizations, such as Neighborhood Watch, is a common approach for fostering community organization, increasing community cohesion, and increasing community involvement, but there are mixed results regarding the effectiveness of these programs in terms of preventing youth violence. By contrast, recreational organizations, such as the Police Athletic League and the Boys' Club, have been shown to be associated with lower levels of delinquent behavior (e.g., Segrave & Chu, 1978). Not surprisingly, participation in a structured activity has been shown to be an effective protective factor with respect to youth violence. Although youth recreation programs appear to be a promising approach for preventing youth violence, we are unaware of any systematic, empirical investigations of the effectiveness of these programs with specific reference to youth violence.

To summarize, there is some evidence that primary prevention strategies may be effective in preventing youth offending among high-risk adolescents, but many of the studies evaluating these approaches have produced mixed results. Research also suggests that these strategies may be less effective with high-risk adolescents who have multiple risk factors, which is the segment of the population most in need of these primary prevention efforts (see Mulvey et al., 1993). Finally, it is clear that primary prevention strategies need to be systematically evaluated more thoroughly before we can draw any firm conclusions regarding their effectiveness in terms of preventing youth violence.

SECONDARY INTERVENTION STRATEGIES

Secondary prevention strategies target adolescents who have been identified as being at risk for engaging in antisocial behavior, usually through some contact with the police or a juvenile court (Flannery & Williams, 1999). In contrast to primary intervention strategies, which target high-risk *populations* before violence occurs, secondary intervention strategies are typically more narrowly focused and aimed at adolescents who have either had contact with the juvenile justice system or demonstrated behavioral problems in a school setting. The main purpose of these strategies is to identify risk factors, typically at the individual, family, and school levels, and provide social and clinical services that will reduce the likelihood that at-risk adolescents will engage in serious antisocial behavior. Therefore, the success of secondary intervention strategies partially lies in understanding the risk factors that distinguish between juveniles who exhibit short-term behavioral problems and juveniles who are likely to engage in serious and chronic offending.

The clinical focus of secondary intervention strategies is on modifying existing behavioral problems before they culminate in serious antisocial behavior. Many of the approaches utilized in primary prevention schemes, such as parent-focused and community-based interventions, can also be used as secondary intervention strategies. As previously noted, the distinction between primary and secondary intervention strategies lies more in the targets of the interventions (i.e., high-risk populations vs. high-risk individuals) rather than in the content of the interventions. Some of the more common secondary intervention strategies include diversion programs, alternative and vocational education, family therapy, and skills training (see Mulvey et al., 1993). Diversion programs, for example, typically divert offending adolescents from the juvenile justice system into community- or school-based treatment programs. The diversion approach is premised on the belief that involvement in the juvenile justice system can be harmful and that the provision of treatment and social services may be more effective in reducing further delinquent behavior. Another secondary intervention strategy is alternative and vocational education programs, which provide job-related and educational training to adolescents with behavioral problems who have performed poorly in mainstream classroom settings. Finally, the family therapy and skills training approach is based on the idea that interventions aimed at the adolescent's family, rather than simply at the adolescent, may be an effective way to reduce the delinquent behavior of the adolescent (see Kumpfer & Alvarado, 2003). In fact, Kumpfer and Alvarado (2003) concluded that the three most effective family-focused secondary intervention strategies for reducing behavioral problems among adolescents are behavioral parent training, family skills training, and family therapy.

Research suggests that many of these secondary intervention approaches effectively reduce rates of antisocial behavior among adolescents. According to Davidson and Redner (1988), diversion programs with well-defined and well-implemented interventions that include a variety of strategies to change behavior have produced promising results in terms of reducing antisocial behavior. In a review of secondary intervention programs, Kazdin (1996) noted that certain family-, school-, and community-based intervention programs were effective in reducing the number of psychosocial risk factors associated with antisocial behavior among at-risk youth. Additionally, in a recent meta-analysis of 165 studies of school-based prevention efforts, Wilson, Gottfredson, and Najaka (2001) concluded that environmentally focused interventions, such as schoolwide discipline management programs, are particularly effective in reducing delinquent behavior. As with the primary prevention approaches, however, the research regarding secondary intervention approaches has occasionally produced mixed results. Nevertheless, the demonstrated success of some of these approaches, such as diversion programs, school-based programs, and vocational programs, counsels in favor of further study, particularly with respect to long-term effects and recidivism.

TERTIARY INTERVENTION STRATEGIES

Finally, tertiary intervention strategies are aimed at adolescents who have already engaged in antisocial behavior and who may already have been adjudicated delinquent through formal court proceedings (Flannery & Williams, 1999). As such, these intervention efforts are typically characterized as treatment rather than prevention, and the recipients of these efforts are often chronic and serious juvenile offenders. The goal of these tertiary intervention strategies is to minimize the impact of existing risk factors and foster the development of protective factors, which may reduce the likelihood that the at-risk adolescent will engage in future acts of antisocial behavior.

Tertiary intervention strategies include both inpatient treatment (i.e., institutional, residential) and community-based treatment (see Mulvey et al., 1993), and the field is divided regarding which approach should be used with juveniles who engage in serious and chronic violent behavior. According to Mulvey et al. (1993), part of the debate centers around whether juvenile justice should be focused on retribution or rehabilitation. Those who favor the retribution role of juvenile justice assert that juveniles should be held accountable for their actions, punished accordingly, and segregated from society. Any treatment that they receive must therefore be provided in an institutional setting (e.g., juvenile detention center, wilderness program). By contrast, those who favor rehabilitation assert that providing community-based treatment may be a more effective way to rehabilitate these youth. The results of at least one meta-analysis suggested that violent youth may benefit the most from shorter stays in institutional settings and increased involvement with community services (Wooldredge, 1988). For a summary of research describing interventions in other settings, see the chapters in this volume on institutional and community interventions.

Characteristics of Effective Intervention Strategies

The public health model serves as a useful way to classify the various intervention approaches that have been developed in recent years to prevent and reduce juvenile offending. With the public health model in mind, we now turn to three general characteristics of effective prevention and treatment strategies: (a) comprehensive and individualized assessment; (b) simultaneous focus on risk factors and protective factors, with a particular emphasis on dynamic risk factors; and (c) a coordinated, multipronged, multitargeted treatment approach (see Weissberg, Kumpfer, & Seligman, 2003, for a brief summary of prevention and intervention strategies that are effective for adolescents).

A successful prevention and treatment program will be based on a comprehensive and individualized assessment of the juvenile's risk and protective factors across each psychosocial domain and at each level of functioning (DHHS, 2001; OJJDP, 1999b). In a recent review of the literature, Nation and colleagues (2003) concluded that effective prevention programs for adolescents must be multiproblem-focused (e.g., family, neighborhood, school, and peers). Furthermore, effective intervention strategies, whether they are directed at reducing juvenile offending or reducing the effects of a mental health disorder, should be based on a proper assessment of individuals and their environment. A comprehensive and individualized assessment will help to identify the juvenile's strengths (i.e., protective factors) and deficits (i.e., risk factors), which will help to ensure that a particular intervention program is an appropriate fit for the juvenile.

An effective intervention strategy will also have a simultaneous focus on risk and protective factors. The overall goal is to eliminate or ameliorate the effects of risk factors and strengthen existing protective factors or foster the development of new protective factors. Although static risk factors are not amenable to direct intervention efforts, an effective prevention and treatment program will nonetheless identify the static risk factors. This is particularly important because of the demonstrated predictive utility (in terms of juvenile offending) of certain static risk factors. Effective intervention efforts will be multifocused on dynamic risk factors, such as substance abuse, access to weapons, impulse-control problems, and psychiatric disorders. Such interventions will also attempt to strengthen existing protective factors or create new protective factors, such as commitment to school, flexible coping strategies, exposure to a positive role model, and participation in a structured activity.

Finally, effective juvenile prevention and treatment programs should take a coordinated, multipronged, multitargeted approach by addressing multiple risk and protective factors across multiple settings (e.g., Kumpfer & Alvarado, 2003; Nation et al., 2003; Redding, 2000a; see Weissberg et al., 2003). This approach is based on the ecological model discussed previously, which views the juvenile as functioning within a complex and interrelated network of contexts that exert an independent influence on the overall risk level (see Zigler, Taussig, & Black, 1992). This multipronged and multitargeted approach ensures a comprehensive response to the juvenile's needs. By addressing multiple psychosocial risk and protective factors across several levels of functioning, the intervention becomes a more integrated component of the juvenile's daily life, which increases the chances of a favorable outcome in the form of lowered risk of antisocial behavior (e.g., Henggeler, 1991; Schoenwald, Ward, Henggeler, Rowland, & Brondine, 2000; see also Lipsey & Williams, 1998; Loeber & Farrington, 1998b, 2001).

One example of a treatment strategy that takes a multifaceted approach to delinquent behavior is multisystemic therapy (MST; e.g., Henggeler, 1991; Henggeler & Borduin, 1990; Henggeler, Schoenwald, Borduin, Rowland, & Cunningham, 1998; see also Lipsey & Williams, 1998; Loeber & Farrington, 1998b, 2001; Redding, 2000a). MST is a multimodal treatment approach that targets the adolescent's family, peer, and school networks (see Redding, 2000a). The MST approach views the development of delinquent behavior as resulting from the relationship and interplay between the adolescent and the larger environment in which the adolescent is embedded (Henggeler, 1991). The results of several studies suggest that MST is a promising intervention for, among other things, reducing behavioral problems among at-risk adolescents (e.g., Borduin, Henggeler, Blaske, & Stein, 1990; Mann, Borduin, Henggeler, & Blaske, 1990; Schoenwald et al., 2000). Some researchers regard MST as the only treatment approach that results in both short- and long-term reductions in violent behavior among serious and chronic juvenile offenders (e.g., Tate, Reppucci, & Mulvey, 1995). Although MST is costly and requires a great number of resources, it is generally less expensive than incarcerating a juvenile (see Redding, 2000b).

Future Research

There are several avenues for future research in this area. More research is needed to identify specific dynamic risk factors that have a causal relationship to juvenile offending, which would facilitate the development of tailored and effective intervention strategies. Additional research is also needed in the area of protective factors. In addition to identifying additional protective factors in each psychosocial domain, it is essential that we obtain a better understanding of the role of protective factors in the prevention and reduction of juvenile offending. Research regarding the mechanism of action of protective factors would be particularly valuable. Future research should take a broad-based approach that views the juvenile as functioning within a large and interconnected network of contexts. With respect to existing intervention strategies, future research should be focused on obtaining a better understanding of which components are effective for which adolescents. This will perhaps enable treatment providers to tailor intervention strategies to the specific needs and strengths of each adolescent. Another important empirical question is whether intervention efforts should be specifically targeted at high-risk adolescents or whether they should be more broad-based in application. Finally, more research is needed regarding the most effective and efficient ways to implement the empirically supported intervention strategies.

Although juvenile violence is a continuing national concern, recent research regarding the role of risk and protective factors in the assessment and treatment of juvenile offending is encouraging. Researchers have identified numerous psychosocial risk and protective factors that can be found in multiple aspects of an adolescent's life. Many of these risk factors are strongly associated with or predictive of antisocial behavior, and several protective factors have been shown to reduce the likelihood of continued offending among juveniles. As this chapter illustrates, comprehensive, multipronged, multitargeted interventions based on empirically derived risk and protective factors show great promise in reducing the frequency of violent offending in juveniles. As more research is conducted, it will become increasingly important to bridge the gap between science and practice by integrating empirically supported intervention strategies into existing or newly developed prevention and treatment programs for adolescents.

References

American Bar Association. (1993). *America's children at risk: A national agenda for legal action.* Report of the ABA Presidential Working Group on the Unmet Legal Needs of Children and Their Families. Washington, DC: Author.

American Psychiatric Association. (1994). *Diagnostic and statistical manual of mental disorders* (4th ed.). Washington, DC: Author.

American Psychological Association. (1993). *Summary report of the American Psychological Association Commission on Violence and Youth* (Vol. 1). Washington, DC: Author.

Andrews, D. A., & Bonta, J. (1998). *The psychology of criminal conduct* (2nd ed.). Cincinnati, OH: Anderson.

Bandura, A., Ross, D., & Ross, S. (1961). Transmission of aggression through imitation of aggressive models. *Journal of Abnormal and Social Psychology, 63,* 575–583.

Battin, S. R., Hill, K. G., Abbott, R. D., Catalano, R. F., & Hawkins, J. D. (1998). The contribution of gang membership to delinquency beyond delinquent friends. *Criminology, 36,* 93–115.

Bilchik, S. (1999, December). Opening remarks (summary of proceedings). National Assembly: Drugs, Alcohol Abuse, and the Criminal Offender, Washington, DC.

Borduin, C. M., Henggeler, S. W., Blaske, D. M., & Stein, R. (1990). Multisystemic treatment of adolescent sexual offenders. *International Journal of Offender Therapy and Comparative Criminology, 34*, 105–113.

Bronfenbrenner, U. (1979). *The ecology of human development: Experiments by nature and design.* Cambridge, MA: Harvard University Press.

Bureau of Justice Statistics. (1998). 1973–1997 National Crime Victimization Survey data (Web site data files). Washington, DC: Author.

Caplan, G. (1964). *Principles of preventive psychiatry.* New York: Basic Books.

Carson, R. C., & Butcher, J. N. (1992). *Abnormal psychology and modern life* (9th ed.). New York: HarperCollins.

Centerwall, B. S. (1992). Television and violence: The scale of the problem and where to go from here. *Journal of the American Medical Association, 267*, 3059–3063.

Chase-Lansdale, P. L., Wakschlag, L. S., & Brooks-Gunn, J. (1995). A psychological perspective on the development of caring in children and youth: The role of the family. *Journal of Adolescence, 18*, 515–556.

Clayton, R. R., Leukefeld, C. G., Donohew, L., Bardo, M., & Harrington, N. G. (1995). Risk and protective factors: A brief review. *Drugs and Society, 8*, 7–14.

Cornell, D. G., Peterson, C., & Richards, H. (1999). Anger as a predictor of aggression among incarcerated adolescents. *Journal of Consulting and Clinical Psychology, 67*, 108–115.

Cottle, C. C., Lee, R. J., & Heilbrun, K. (2001). The prediction of criminal recidivism in juveniles: A meta-analysis. *Criminal Justice and Behavior, 28*, 367–394.

Davidson, W. S., & Redner, R. (1988). The prevention of juvenile delinquency: Diversion from the juvenile justice system. In R. H. Price, E. L. Cowen, R. P. Lorion, & J. Ramos-McKay (Eds.), *Fourteen ounces of prevention: A casebook for practitioners* (pp. 123–137). Washington, DC: American Psychological Association.

Dawson, D., & Reiter, J. (1998, September). Juvenile violence overview: An introduction to the available literature. *American Academy of Psychiatry and the Law Newsletter, 23*, 10–11.

Dembo, R., Wothke, W., Shemwell, M., Pacheco, K., Seeberger, W., Rollie, M., et al. (2000). A structural model of the influence of family problems and child abuse factors on serious delinquency among youths processed at a juvenile assessment center. *Journal of Child and Adolescent Substance Abuse, 10*, 17–31.

Department of Health and Human Services. (2001). *Youth violence: A report of the surgeon general.* Rockville, MD: Author.

Elliott, D. S., Huizinga, D., & Ageton, S. S. (1985). *Explaining delinquency and drug use.* Thousand Oaks, CA: Sage.

Farrell, A. D., & Bruce, S. E. (1997). Impact of exposure to community violence on violent behavior and emotional distress among urban adolescents. *Journal of Clinical Child Psychology, 26*, 2–14.

Farrington, D. P. (1989). Early predictors of adolescent aggression and adult violence. *Violence and Victims, 4*, 79–100.

Farrington, D. P., & Hawkins, D. (1991). Predicting participation, early onset and later persistence in officially recorded offending. *Criminal Behavior and Mental Health, 1*, 1–33.

Federal Bureau of Investigation. (1994). *Uniform crime reports, 1993.* Washington, DC: Author.

Federal Bureau of Investigation. (2000). *Crime in the United States, 2000.* Washington, DC: Author.

Flannery, D. J., & Williams, L. (1999). Effective youth violence prevention. In T. Gullotta & S. J. McElhaney (Eds.), *Violence in homes and communities: Prevention, intervention, and treatment.* Thousand Oaks, CA: Sage.

Fox, J. A. (1996). *Trends in juvenile violence: A report to the United States Attorney General on current and future rates of juvenile offending.* Washington, DC: Bureau of Justice Statistics.

Garbarino, J. (1985). *Adolescent development: An ecological perspective.* Columbus, OH: Merrill.

Gauce, A. M., Comer, J. P., & Schwartz, D. (1987). Long term effects of a systems-oriented school prevention program. *American Journal of Orthopsychiatry, 57,* 127–131.

Greenacre, P. (1945). Conscience in the psychopath. *American Journal of Orthopsychiatry, 15,* 495–509.

Greenberg, M. T., Weissberg, R. P., O-Brien, M. U., Zins, J. E., Fredericks, L., Resnik, H., et al. (2003). Enhancing school-based prevention and youth development through coordinated social, emotional, and academic learning. *American Psychologist, 58,* 466–474.

Grisso, T. (1998). *Forensic evaluation of juveniles.* Sarasota, FL: Professional Resource Press.

Handler, J. F. (1993). *Losing generations: Adolescents in high-risk settings.* Washington, DC: National Academy Press.

Hanna, A. (2001, June). *Risk and protective factors for delinquency.* Presentation to the Virginia Juvenile Justice and Delinquency Prevention Advisory Committee, Richmond, VA.

Hawkins, J. D., Herrenkohl, T. I., Farrington, D. P., Brewer, D., Catalano, R. F., Harachi, T. W., et al. (2000). *Predictors of youth violence.* Juvenile Justice Bulletin. Washington, DC: U. S. Department of Justice, Office of Justice Programs, Office of Juvenile Justice and Delinquency Prevention.

Hawkins, J. D., & Nederhood, B. (1987). *Handbook for evaluating drug and alcohol prevention programs: Staff/team evaluation of prevention programs (STEPP)* (DHHS Publication No. ADM 87-1512). Washington, DC: U.S. Government Printing Office.

Heilbrun, K. (1997). Prediction versus management models relevant to risk assessment: The importance of legal decision-making context. *Law and Human Behavior, 21,* 347–359.

Heilbrun, K. (1999). *Basic and advanced issues in risk assessment: Approaches, populations, communications, and decision-making.* Workshop presented for the OMHSAS Clinical Staff, Department of Public Welfare, Commonwealth of Pennsylvania.

Henggeler, S. W. (1991). Multidimensional causal models of delinquent behavior and their implications of treatment. In R. Cohen & A. W. Siegel (Eds.), *Context and development* (pp. 211–231). Hillsdale, NJ: Erlbaum.

Henggeler, S. W., & Borduin, C. M. (1990). *Family therapy and beyond: A multisystemic approach to treating the behavior problems of children and adolescents.* Pacific Grove, CA: Brooks/Cole.

Henggeler, S. W., Schoenwald, S. K., Borduin, C. M., Rowland, M. D., & Cunningham, P. B. (1998). *Multisystemic treatment of antisocial behavior in children and adolescents.* New York: Guilford Press.

Henry, B., Avshalom, C., Moffitt, T. E., & Silva, P. A. (1996). Temperamental and familial predictors of violent and non-violent criminal convictions. *Developmental Psychology, 32,* 614–623.

Hinshaw, S. P. (1992). Externalizing behavior problems and academic underachievement in childhood and adolescence: Causal relationships and underlying mechanisms. *Psychological Bulletin, 111*, 127–155.

Hoge, R. D., & Andrews, D. A. (1996). *Assessing the youthful offender: Issues and techniques.* New York: Plenum.

Hoge, R. D., Andrews, D. A., & Leschied, A. W. (1996). An investigation of risk and protective factors in a sample of youthful offenders. *Journal of Child Psychology and Psychiatry, 37*, 419–424.

Howell, J. C., Krisberg, B., & Jones, M. J. (1995). Trends in juvenile crime and youth violence. In J. C. Howell, B. Krisberg, J. D. Hawkins, & J. J. Wilson (Eds.), *A sourcebook: Serious, violent, and chronic juvenile offenders* (pp. 1–30). Thousand Oaks, CA: Sage.

Huizinga, D., Esbensen, F., & Weiher, A. W. (1991). Are there multiple paths to delinquency? *Journal of Criminal Law and Criminology, 82*, 83–118.

Jessor, R., Van Den Bos, J., Vanderryn, J., Costa, F. M., & Turbin, M. S. (1995). Protective factors in adolescent problem behavior: Moderator effects and developmental change. *Developmental Psychology, 31*, 923–933.

Kandel, E., Mednick, S. A., Kirkegaard-Sorensen, L., Hutchings, B., Knop, J., Rosenberg, R., et al. (1988). IQ as a protective factor for subjects at high risk for antisocial behavior. *Journal of Consulting and Clinical Psychology, 56*, 224–226.

Kashani, J. H., & Allan, W. D. (1998). *The impact of family violence on children and adolescents.* Thousand Oaks, CA: Sage.

Kashani, J. H., Jones, M. R., Bumby, K. M., & Thomas, L. A. (1999). Youth violence: Psychosocial risk factors, treatment, prevention, and recommendations. *Journal of Emotional and Behavioral Disorders, 7*, 200–210.

Kazdin, A. E. (1996). *Conduct disorders in childhood and adolescence* (2nd ed.). Thousand Oaks, CA: Sage.

Keenan, K., Loeber, R., Zhang, Q., Stouthamer-Loeber, M., & van Kammen, W. B. (1995). The influence of deviant peers on the development of boys' disruptive and delinquency behavior: A temporal analysis. *Development and Psychopathology, 7*, 715–726.

Klinteberg, B. A., Andersson, T., Magnusson, D., & Stattin, H. (1993). Hyperactive behavior in childhood as related to subsequent alcohol problems and violent offending: A longitudinal study of male subjects. *Personality and Individual Differences, 15*, 381–388.

Kumpfer, K. L., & Alvarado, R. (2003). Family-strengthening approaches for the prevention of youth problem behaviors. *American Psychologist, 58*, 457–465.

Lipsey, M. W., & Williams, D. B. (1998). Effective intervention for serious juvenile offenders: A synthesis of research. In R. Loeber & D. P. Farrington (Eds.), *Serious and violent juvenile offenders: Risk factors and successful interventions* (pp. 313–345). Thousand Oaks, CA: Sage.

Loeber, R., & Farrington, D. P. (1998a). Never too early, never too late: Risk factors and successful interventions for serious and violent juvenile offenders. *Studies on Crime and Crime Prevention, 7*, 7–30.

Loeber, R., & Farrington, D. P. (Eds.). (1998b). *Serious and violent juvenile offenders: Risk factors and successful interventions.* Thousand Oaks, CA: Sage.

Loeber, R., & Farrington, D. P. (Eds.). (2001). *Child delinquents: Development, intervention, and service needs.* Thousand Oaks, CA: Sage.

Loeber, R., Farrington, D. P., Stouthamer-Loeber, M., Moffitt, T. E., & Caspi, A. (1998). The development of male offending: Key findings from the first decade of the Pittsburgh youth study. *Studies on Crime and Crime Prevention, 7*, 141–171.

Mann, B. J., Borduin, C. M., Henggeler, S. W., & Blaske, D. M. (1990). An investigation of systemic conceptualizations of parent-child coalitions and symptom change. *Journal of Consulting and Clinical Psychology, 58*, 336–344.

Melton, G. B., Petrila, J., Poythress, N. G., & Slobogin, C. (1997). *Psychological evaluations for the courts: A handbook for mental health professionals and lawyers* (2nd ed.). New York: Guilford Press.

Mitchell, S., & Rosa, P. (1979). Boyhood behavior problems as precursors of criminality: A fifteen-year follow-up study. *Journal of Child Psychology and Psychiatry, 22*, 19–33.

Moffitt, T. E. (1993). Adolescent-limited and life-course-persistent antisocial behavior: A developmental taxonomy. *Psychological Review, 100*, 674–701.

Monahan, J., Steadman, H. J., Silver, E., Appelbaum, P. S., Robbins, P. C., Mulvey, E. P., et al. (2001). *Rethinking risk assessment: The MacArthur study of mental disorder and violence.* New York: Oxford University Press.

Mulvey, E. P., Arthur, M. W., & Reppucci, N. D. (1993). The prevention and treatment of juvenile delinquency: A review of the research. *Clinical Psychology Review, 13*, 133–167.

Nation, M., Crusto, C., Wandersman, A., Kumpfer, K. L., Seybolt, D., Morrissey-Kane, E., et al. (2003). What works in prevention: Principles of effective prevention programs. *American Psychologist, 58*, 449–456.

Office of Juvenile Justice and Delinquency Prevention. (1999a). *Juvenile offenders and victims: 1999 national report.* Washington, DC: Author.

Office of Juvenile Justice and Delinquency Prevention. (1999b). *OJJDP research: Making a difference for juveniles.* Washington, DC: Author.

Patterson, G. R. (1982). *Coercive family process.* Eugene, OR: Castalia.

Patterson, G. R., DeBaryshe, B. D., & Ramsey, E. (1989). A developmental perspective on antisocial behavior. *American Psychologist, 44*, 329–335.

Patterson, G. R., & Dishion, T. J. (1985). Contributions of families and peers to delinquency. *Criminology, 23*, 63–79.

Plutchik, R. (1995). Outward and inward directed aggressiveness: The interaction between violence and suicidality. *Pharmacopsychiatry, 28*, 47–57.

Redding, R. E. (2000a). Characteristics of effective treatments and interventions for juvenile offenders. *Juvenile justice fact sheet.* Charlottesville: University of Virginia, Institute of Law, Psychiatry, and Public Policy.

Redding, R. E. (2000b). Graduated and community-based sanctions of juvenile offenders. *Juvenile justice fact sheet.* Charlottesville: University of Virginia, Institute of Law, Psychiatry, and Public Policy.

Sampson, R. J., Raudenbush, S. W., & Earls, F. (1997). Neighborhoods and violent crime: A multilevel study of collective efficacy. *Science, 277*, 918–924.

Schoenwald, S., Ward, D., Henggeler, S., Rowland, M., & Brondine, M. (2000). Multisystemic therapy versus hospitalization for crisis stabilization of youth: Placement outcomes 4 months post-referral. *Mental Health Services Research, 2*, 3–12.

Segrave, J. O., & Chu, D. B. (1978). Athletics and juvenile delinquency. *Review of Sports and Leisure, 3*, 1–24.

Snyder, H. N. (2000). *Juvenile arrests 1999.* Washington, DC: Office of Juvenile Justice and Delinquency Prevention.

Snyder, H. N. (2002). *Juvenile arrests 2000.* Washington, DC: Office of Juvenile Justice and Delinquency Prevention.

Stoiber, K. C., & Good, B. (1998). Risk and resilience factors linked to problem behavior among urban, culturally diverse adolescents. *The School Psychology Review, 27*, 380–397.

Tate, D. C., Reppucci, N. D., & Mulvey, E. P. (1995). Violent juvenile delinquents: Treatment effectiveness and implications of future action. *American Psychologist, 50,* 777–781.

Thornberry, T. P., Huizinga, D., & Loeber, R. (1995). The prevention of serious delinquency and violence: Implications from the program of research on the causes and correlates of delinquency. In J. C. Howell, B. Krisberg, J. D. Hawkins, & J. J. Wilson (Eds.), *A sourcebook: Serious, violent, and chronic juvenile offenders* (pp. 213–237). Thousand Oaks, CA: Sage.

Tolan, P. H. (1987). Implications of age of onset for delinquency risk. *Journal of Abnormal Child Psychology, 15,* 47–65.

Weissberg, R. P., Kumpfer, K. L., & Seligman, M. E. P. (2003). Prevention that works for children and youth: An introduction. *American Psychologist, 58,* 425–432.

Werner, E. (1993). Risk, resilience, and recovery: Perspectives from the Kauai longitudinal study. *Development and Psychopathology, 5,* 503–515.

Werner, E. (2000). Protective factors and individual resilience. In J. Shonkoff & S. Meisels (Eds.), *Handbook of early childhood intervention* (2nd ed.). Cambridge: Cambridge University Press.

Wessely, S., & Taylor, P. (1991). Madness and crime: Criminology versus psychiatry. *Criminal Behaviour and Mental Health, 1,* 193–228.

Widom, C. S. (1989). The cycle of violence. *Science, 244,* 160–166.

Wilson, D. B., Gottfredson, D. C., & Najaka, S. S. (2001). School-based prevention of problem behaviors: A meta-analysis. *Journal of Quantitative Criminology, 17,* 247–272.

Wooldredge, J. D. (1988). Differentiating the effects of juvenile court sentences on eliminating recidivism. *Journal of Research in Crime and Delinquency, 25,* 264–300.

Zigler, E., Taussig, C., & Black, K. (1992). Early childhood intervention: A promising preventative for juvenile delinquency. *American Psychologist, 47,* 997–1006

3

DEWEY G. CORNELL

School Violence
Fears Versus Facts

What is school violence? In the 1990s the term "school violence" became associated with frightening images of terrified children running from a school building where their classmates had been shot. Highly publicized school shootings brought nationwide attention to little-known places such as Pearl, Mississippi; Paducah, Kentucky; Jonesboro, Arkansas; and Springfield, Oregon. In 1999, Columbine High School became the best-known high school in America because two boys went on a shooting rampage, killing 12 students and a teacher before they killed themselves. Live, nationwide television coverage of the Columbine tragedy began during the incident, while students were still hiding in the school and police were attempting to locate the shooters. In the following weeks and months the American public was exposed to numerous images of bloody victims and interviews with traumatized, grief-stricken survivors. As new aspects of the story came to light, the shooters appeared on the covers of *Time* (May 3, 1999; December 20, 1999) and other national magazines. More than three years after the shooting, crime scene photos still made the cover of the *National Enquirer* (June 4, 2002); four years later, filmmaker and social critic Michael Moore released a widely acclaimed, Oscar-winning documentary, *Bowling for Columbine*, which used the incident as the basis for searing social commentary on the violent aspects of American culture.

High-profile school shootings focused attention on the important issue of school safety, but generated fears that skewed public perceptions and dramatically altered school discipline policy and practice (Mulvey & Cauffman, 2001). Anxious school administrators increased security measures, hired a new kind of police officer known as a "school resource officer," and implemented strict zero tolerance policies. At a national level, both the Federal Bureau of Investigation (FBI) and the Secret Service conducted studies of school shootings (O'Toole, 2000; Vossekuil, Fein, Reddy, Borum, & Modzeleski, 2002). The U.S. Department of Education distributed "warning signs" guidebooks to schools giving advice on identifying potentially violent students (Dwyer, Osher, & Warger, 1998),

45

and the U.S. Surgeon General (2001) released a major report on youth violence. Nevertheless, is there good cause to speak of "school violence" as though violence at school were a special form of juvenile crime or as if schools were especially dangerous places? An analysis of the available evidence suggests that the risk of violent crime at school has been greatly exaggerated, but that less serious forms of juvenile aggression, such as bullying and fighting, are more pervasive in schools and deserve greater attention.

School Homicides

Homicides committed by students at school are exceedingly rare events within a population of more than 53 million students attending 119,000 public and private schools in the United States (U.S. Department of Education, 2002). According to case reports compiled by the National School Safety Center (2003), 116 persons were murdered by students at school in 93 incidents that took place between the 1992–1993 and the 2001–2002 school years.[1] Considering that 93 incidents occurred over 10 years, the annual probability of a school experiencing a student-perpetrated homicide is .0000781, or about 1 in 12,800. Likewise, the numbers of students who commit homicide at school is miniscule compared to the overall number of juvenile homicides; from 1992 through 2001, a total of 19,830 juveniles were arrested for homicide in the United States (FBI, 1993–2002).

Contrary to public perception, the number of student-perpetrated homicides at school did not soar in the 1990s and actually declined following the 1997–1998 school year; there were two cases in 2000–2001, and only one case in 2001–2002 (National School Safety Center, 2003; U.S. Surgeon General, 2001). There was a series of highly publicized cases beginning in 1997, raising the possibility that media attention stimulated copycat behavior among a small group of students. In each of these cases, one or more students engaged in a deliberate, planned shooting rampage that resulted in multiple injuries and fatalities. The two perpetrators of the shooting at Columbine High School stated on a videotape made before the shooting that they were inspired by previous shooters and wished to outdo them and achieve even greater notoriety (*Time*, December 20, 1999).

---

1. The National School Safety Center (2003) compiles an inclusive list of "school-associated violent deaths" based on news media reports of homicides that are in any way linked to schools. Their report includes suicides and accidental deaths, as well as homicides that took place near school or on school property when school was not in session. The report also includes homicides committed by persons other than students, such as the murder of a teacher by an estranged husband. For the purposes of this chapter, I counted only homicides committed by students and included cases that occurred at school during regular school hours or while students were traveling to or from school. The National School Safety Center report is online at www.nssc1.org.

Profiling

One of the more controversial responses to the school shootings has been the effort to *profile* seemingly dangerous students before they engage in violence. The U.S. Department of Education and the Department of Justice disseminated to every public school in the nation a series of "warning signs" for identifying potentially violent youth (Dwyer et al., 1998). The American Psychological Association (1999) released a warning-signs pamphlet, and the National School Safety Center (NSSC, 1998) published a Checklist of Characteristics of Youth Who Have Caused School-Associated Violent Deaths. Other state and national organizations have released their own checklists and warning signs (Sewell & Mendelsohn, 2000).

Warning-signs checklists tend to contain very general criteria that cast a broad net in identifying potentially violent youth. The 16 warning signs in the federal government's guide (Dwyer et al., 1998) include such items as " history of discipline problems," "drug use and alcohol use," "feelings of being picked on and persecuted," and "excessive feelings of rejection." The American Psychological Association's (1999) warning-signs pamphlet sounds an ominous note with the statement, "If you see these immediate warning signs, violence is a serious possibility." The list of "immediate warning signs" includes "increase in risk-taking behavior," "increase in use of drugs or alcohol," "significant vandalism or property damage," and "loss of temper on a daily basis." Most school authorities could identify students in their schools who appear to meet these signs.

Similarly, the National School Safety Center (1998) promulgated a 20-item "Checklist of Characteristics of Youth Who Have Caused School-Associated Violent Deaths." This checklist includes some very general items, such as "has been previously truant, suspended, or expelled from school," "has little or no supervision from parents or a caring adult," and "tends to blame others for difficulties she or he causes." The items on such checklists may well describe the small group of youth who committed school shootings, but this does not make them useful, specific indicators of violence. Because the base rate for severe violence is low, checklists of student characteristics will invariably lead to the false-positive identification of a very large number of students who will not be violent (Sewell & Mendelsohn, 2000).

The warning-signs lists are not without some scientific basis at the item level. For each item, there are studies that support its link with violent behavior; for example, alcohol and drug use is a well-known correlate of delinquency and violence. Certainly some of the items, such as losing one's temper on a daily basis or committing acts of vandalism, are by themselves cause for concern and merit intervention. Some of the lists, for example, the federal warning-signs list (Dwyer et al., 1998), were developed in consultation with a panel of experts and contain good general advice. However, there is a lack of supporting evidence on the compilation of even the federal warning-signs items into a checklist and an accompanying lack of research determining how such checklists should be employed.

The authors of the federal government's warning-signs document (Dwyer et al., 1998) recognized the potential problems of a warning-signs approach. They cautioned, "Unfortunately, *there is a real danger that early warning signs will be misinterpreted*" (Dwyer et al., 1998, p. 7). These authors urged school authorities to refrain from using the warning signs as a basis for punishing students or excluding them from school. They expressed concerns that the warning signs could be used without regard to the student's situational or developmental context. They warned against acting on the basis of stereotypes or overreacting to single signs. Despite multiple admonitions about their potential for misuse, it remains unclear how the warning signs should be used and by what criteria school authorities should take action. In the years since the federal warning signs were disseminated, there does not appear to have been any follow-up research on their validity or more generally on their use by school authorities and their impact on students. The warning signs were presented again in a follow-up action guide for schools (Dwyer & Osher, 2000). The action guide contains thoughtful advice and recommendations for school authorities and gives many examples of strategies, interventions, and programs designed to prevent student violence, but does not provide new information about the warning signs.

In 1999 the FBI's National Center for the Analysis of Violent Crime, a group with unsurpassed expertise in the use of criminal profiling, convened a conference on school shootings. The FBI report firmly rejected the application of profiling to school shootings, concluding:

> One response to the pressure for action may be an effort to identify the next shooter by developing a "profile" of the typical school shooter. This may sound like a reasonable preventive measure, but in practice, trying to draw up a catalogue or "checklist" of warning signs to detect a potential school shooter can be shortsighted, even dangerous. Such lists, publicized by the media, can end up unfairly labeling many nonviolent students as potentially dangerous or even lethal. In fact, a great many adolescents who will never commit violent acts will show some of the behaviors or personality traits included on the list. (O'Toole, 2000, pp. 2, 3)

Zero Tolerance

In contrast to profiling, the zero tolerance approach ignores student characteristics and instead focuses entirely on whether the student committed an absolutely forbidden act, such as bringing a weapon to school. Anxious educators turned to zero tolerance policies as a simple, albeit draconian, response to student threats of violence that relieved them of the need to exercise judgment and make reasoned decisions in response to student infractions. "Zero tolerance" refers to the practice of automatic expulsion of students for violations of school safety rules. Skiba and Peterson (1999) traced the emergence of zero tolerance policies to drug abatement efforts of the U.S. Navy and U.S. Customs Service. The notion of absolute sanctions against drug use in the military became a model for schools that was applied to violence as well as drug use.

In 1994, the Gun-Free Schools Act required that any school division receiving funds under the Elementary and Secondary Education Act expel for 1 calendar year any student found to be in possession of a firearm at school. Although the law permitted local school districts to modify the expulsion on a case-by-case basis, this provision was frequently overlooked in favor of less flexible policies that mandated automatic expulsion for any infraction (Tebo, 2000). In addition, many schools expanded zero tolerance well beyond the arena of firearms to include other weapons and even objects that were not weapons. For example, the prohibition of weapons in many school divisions often included toy weapons and objects that appeared to be weapons. In one case, a 10-year-old boy was expelled from elementary school because he brought to school a 1-in. plastic toy pistol that was an accessory to his G.I. Joe action figure. The boy discovered he had the tiny toy in his pocket when he checked to see if he had his lunch money (*Seattle Times*, January 8, 1997). Skiba and Peterson (1999; see also Skiba & Knesting, 2001) documented numerous cases of excessive punishment, which they referred to as "the dark side of zero tolerance." Among the examples they cited:

- A 5-year-old in California was expelled after he found a razor blade at his bus stop, carried it to school, and gave it to his teacher
- A 9-year-old in Ohio was suspended for having a 1-in. knife in a manicure kit
- A 12-year-old in Rhode Island was suspended for bringing a toy gun to school
- A 17-year-old in Chicago was arrested and subsequently expelled for shooting a paper clip with a rubber band

How common are such cases? There are many cases reported in the news media across the country (Skiba & Knesting, 2001), and organizations such as the American Bar Association (Tebo, 2000), The Advancement Project and the Civil Rights Project of Harvard University (2000), the Justice Policy Institute (Brooks, Schiraldi, & Ziedenberg, 2000), and the Rutherford Institute (Whitehead, 2001) have expressed concern that this is a nationwide problem, but no study has documented just how frequently inappropriate suspensions and expulsions occur. Such data would be hard to collect because it requires making a judgment about the facts and circumstances surrounding individual cases. Nonetheless, suspensions and expulsions are a frequent event in American schools, affecting millions of students. For example, during the 2001–2002 school year there were 187,928 suspensions and 1,022 expulsions in Virginia, a state with more than 1.1 million students enrolled in 1,929 public schools (Virginia Department of Education, 2003).

The federal government requires all states to document their compliance with the Gun-Free Schools Act by reporting the number of students expelled for bringing a firearm to school (U.S. Department of Education, 2002). During the 1999–2000 school year, 2,837 students were expelled for bringing a firearm to school. Sixty percent of these expulsions were for handguns, 10% were for rifles or shotguns, and the remaining 30% were for other types of firearms, such as bombs and starter pistols. The federal government does not require states to report student expulsions for knives or other weapons and specifically excludes toy guns and pellet guns from the definition of firearms.

A 2000 report by the Advancement Project and The Civil Rights Project of Harvard University (*Opportunities Suspended: The Devastating Consequences of Zero Tolerance and School Discipline Policies*) pointed out that zero tolerance policies were originally intended to apply only to serious criminal behavior involving firearms or illegal drugs, but have been expanded to cover many more types of behavior and circumstances: "Zero Tolerance has become a philosophy that has permeated our schools; it employs a brutally strict disciplinary model that embraces harsh punishment over education" (p. 3). The report raised concern that zero tolerance policies were resulting in high levels of suspension and expulsion of minority students. In 1998, more than 3.1 million students were suspended from school; although African American children represent 17% of the public school enrollment, they constituted 32% of the out-of-school suspensions.

An article in the *American Bar Association Journal* (Tebo, 2000) sharply criticized zero tolerance policies as making "zero sense." Tebo contended that the central problem with zero tolerance policies is that all threats of violence are treated as equally dangerous and deserving of the same consequences. For example, Ohio state law requires every school district to have a zero tolerance policy that makes no exceptions (Tebo, 2000). These kinds of policies provide no latitude for school authorities to consider the seriousness of the threat or degree of risk posed by the student's behavior. Tebo (2000) described cases in which Ohio schools imposed severe consequences on students whom they recognized did not pose a danger to others, such as a student suspended for displaying a school election poster that contained humorous threatening language in parody of a popular movie. A Pennsylvania court overturned one school's expulsion of a seventh-grade student who inadvertently brought his Swiss Army knife to school, but in almost all cases the courts have been unwilling to interfere with zero tolerance practices in schools (Tebo, 2000). In 2001 the American Bar Association passed a resolution condemning zero tolerance: " . . . [T]he ABA opposes, in principle, 'zero tolerance' policies that have a discriminatory effect, or mandate either expulsion or referral of students to juvenile or criminal court, without regard to the circumstances or nature of the offense or the student's history." More generally, Mulvey and Cauffman (2001) criticized zero tolerance policies as creating a harsh and unreasonable school environment that is inconsistent with the goal of establishing the atmosphere of trust and open communication which they believe is critical to working effectively with high-risk students.

Threat Assessment

A key finding from the FBI study of school shootings was that in almost every case the student shooter communicated his intentions to peers days or weeks in advance of the crime. Had these intentions been reported to authorities, it would have been possible to investigate the threat and prevent the shootings. In support of this conclusion, the FBI found other cases in which school shootings were prevented because students did report a classmate's threats to authorities. These observations led the FBI researchers to conclude: "Although the risk of an actual shooting incident at any one school is very low, threats of violence are potentially a problem at any school. Once a threat is made, having a fair, rational, and standardized method of evaluating and responding to threats is critically important" (O'Toole, 2000, p. 1). The FBI report recognized that "all threats are not created equal" (p. 5) and that each threat must be carefully investigated to determine what danger the student poses to others. Students who make threats differ in their motivation and capacity, as well as their intention, to carry out a violent act.

The FBI report advised schools to institute a threat management system that would provide a standard procedure for evaluating threats and responding with appropriate interventions and risk reduction strategies based on the seriousness of the threat (O'Toole, 2000). This process is called *threat assessment*. Threat assessment was developed by the U.S. Secret Service based on studies of persons who attacked or threatened to attack public officials (Fein & Vossekuil, 1998, 1999; Fein, Vossekuil, & Holden, 1995). Reddy and colleagues (2001) advocated the application of threat assessment to schools and in 2002, a joint report of the U.S. Secret Service and Department of Education recommended that schools train threat assessment teams to respond to student threats of violence (Fein et al., 2002).

Threat assessment has the potential to overcome many of the limitations of both profiling and zero tolerance policies. Unlike profiling, threat assessment does not rely on checklists of student characteristics; instead an assessment is conducted only when a student has made a threat. Threat assessment involves the examination of specific behaviors directly linked to committing a violent act. Has the student made a statement of intent to harm someone? Has the student made specific plans to carry out the act? Has the student attempted to recruit accomplices or invited an audience to observe the violence? More general student characteristics that are described in typical profile checklists play a secondary or tertiary role in evaluating the potential for violence.

In contrast to zero tolerance, threat assessment places heavy emphasis on the context and meaning of the student's threat. The school's response to a threat is based on the danger posed by the student, so that possession of a toy gun or a small pocketknife would not be treated in the same way as possession of a handgun or a switchblade. Moreover, a student who accidentally brought a weapon to school would receive different consequences than a student who brought a weapon to school after voicing intent to harm someone. In short, the principle of "one size fits all" that characterizes zero tolerance does not apply to threat assessment.

Threat assessment is not a simple procedure. When a student engages in threatening behavior, how do school authorities determine what a student intended to do? There is no formula or prescription to replace the need for informed judgment based on a careful investigation of the circumstances and precipitants of the threat. Threat assessment in schools can be guided by six principles that apply to cases in which a person carries out an act of violence against a specific victim or target (Fein et al., 2002). These six principles are reviewed briefly below.

The first principle of threat assessment is that a targeted act of violence is not a spontaneous, unpredictable event, but the result of a deliberate and detectable process. Students who commit serious acts of violence do not suddenly "snap" and begin shooting at random; their behavior is preceded by days or weeks of thought and planning (Vossekuil et al., 2002). This form of violence can be prevented if enough is known about the student's preparatory behavior.

Second, threat assessment must include investigation of situational factors and the broader context of the threat. Students who commit serious acts of violence may be distressed by family conflicts or other problems not directly associated with the threat. There may be factors in the student's setting that encourage violence or discourage more appropriate ways of resolving problems. Several of the school shooters, for instance, were encouraged by antisocial peers to carry out their attacks. Also, characteristics or behaviors of the intended victim must be considered. The intended victim may be perceived by the student as provocative, abusive, or otherwise deserving of attack.

Third, school authorities investigating a threat must adopt a critical and skeptical mind-set. They must be fair-minded and willing to accept or reject hypotheses based on a careful analysis of all available facts. They must resist pressure to conclude that a student is dangerous based on rumors or unverified allegations.

The fourth principle is that conclusions must be based on objective facts and behaviors, rather than on inferred traits or student characteristics. School authorities cannot make judgments based on a hypothetical profile of the violent student. Instead, they must seek out specific evidence that the student is planning or threatening to commit an act of violence.

The fifth principle is that information should be gathered from multiple sources within and outside the school system. School authorities should seek cooperation with law enforcement and social service agencies, mental health providers, religious organizations, and other community groups. This principle requires schools to look beyond their own boundaries rather than function as a closed and isolated system.

The final principle is that threat assessment is ultimately concerned with whether the student *poses* a threat, not whether the student has *made* a threat. Any student can make a threat, but relatively few will engage in behavior that indicates planning and preparation to carry out the threat. Threat assessment attempts to identify those students who have the intent and means to carry out the threat. Moreover, threat assessment does not end when a student is found to have made a serious threat; rather, it aims to determine what should be done about the threat to reduce the risk that it will be carried out.

A zero tolerance approach to threats would simply suspend or expel students who made threats of violence. The argument might be made that schools should err on the safe side by removing from school any student who makes a violent threat. Such an approach is based on the assumption that student threats are rare and that the consequences would be slight, but there is evidence to the contrary. For example, Virginia state discipline records (Virginia Department of Education, 2003) indicate that threats are a common disciplinary problem. In the 2001–2002 school year there were 7,760 assaults against students or staff, but also 10,626 threats.

The threats that come to the attention of school authorities represent only a fraction of the total number of threats that occur among students. Singer and Flannery (2000) reviewed survey results for 9,487 students in grades 3–12 who were asked, "How often in the past year did you threaten to hurt someone?" They found that over half of the boys and more than one third of the girls reported making at least one threat in the past year. Similarly, a survey of more than 8,000 middle and high school students (Cornell & Loper, 1996, 1998) found that students frequently reported being threatened with violence. Approximately one third of the boys and nearly one quarter of the girls reported that someone had threatened to hurt them at school in the preceding 30 days (Cornell & Loper, 1996). Students who report being threatened are also more likely to report carrying a weapon for protection at school (Marsh & Cornell, 2001; Singer & Flannery, 2000).

Field Testing of Student Threat Assessment

Student threat assessment is a new approach that has not been extensively studied. The literature on threat assessment advises schools on what principles to follow, but not how to put them into practice. To bridge the gap between principle and practice, Cornell and colleagues (in press) developed and field-tested practical guidelines for schools to follow in responding to student threats of violence. Although the design of this study did not include a comparison group of schools not using threat assessment guidelines, the results of this field testing provided supportive evidence for the viability of student threat assessment.

Threat assessment teams from 35 schools participated in the field-testing project over the course of a full school year. The teams followed a seven-step decision tree described in a detailed set of guidelines (Cornell, 2001). Teams consisted of a principal or assistant principal, a school resource officer, a school psychologist, and a school counselor for each school. The leader of the threat assessment team is the school staff member responsible for handling student discipline, usually the principal or assistant principal. When threats are reported to the team leader, he or she conducts a preliminary assessment or triage to determine the seriousness of the threat. Other team members become involved if the threat is determined to be serious.

In order to capture the fundamental difference between less serious threats that are readily resolved and threats that constitute a continuing danger to others, the threat assessment guidelines distinguish between *transient* and *substantive* threats. Transient threats are defined as behaviors that could be readily identified as expressions of anger or frustration, or perhaps inappropriate attempts at humor, that dissipate in a short period of time when the student has time to reflect on the meaning of what he or she has said. The most important feature of a transient threat is that the student does not have a sustained intention to harm someone. Transient threats might merit a disciplinary consequence, but there is no need to take protective action to prevent a future act of violence because the threat is short-lived. Transient threats are resolved with an explanation and apology by the student.

Threats that cannot be readily identified as transient are classified as substantive threats. Substantive threats are serious in the sense that they represent a sustained intent to harm someone beyond the immediate incident or argument where the threat was made. Substantive threats may be identified by several features that are regarded as *presumptive, but not absolute,* indicators, derived from the FBI report (O'Toole, 2000). Among these factors are whether the threat has specific plausible details, such as a specific victim, time, place, and method of assault; whether the threat has been repeated over time or related to multiple persons; whether the student has accomplices, or has attempted to recruit accomplices; and whether there is evidence of planning or intent to carry out the threat, such as a weapon, bomb materials, or a written plan.

When a student has made a substantive threat to kill or seriously injure someone, a behavior that would constitute a felonious assault, the threat is regarded as very serious and requires a full-scale safety evaluation and follow-up plan involving the entire threat assessment team. In brief, the team goals in these cases are first to protect potential victims and second to identify the reasons for the student's threatening behavior. Accordingly, the school resource officer investigates the threat from a law enforcement perspective and takes legally appropriate action. The school psychologist conducts a mental health assessment of the student to determine if the student requires emergency mental health services and to identify factors that have contributed to the student's threatening behavior. The team then develops a plan for the student that might involve alternative school placement or, in some cases, a return to school under specific conditions identified by the team.

During the 2001–2002 school year, researchers gathered data on 188 student threats of violence that came to the attention of school authorities (Cornell et al., in press). Seventy percent of the threats were classified as transient and 30% were deemed substantive. The substantive threats included just 8% (16 threats) that were classified as very serious and required a comprehensive assessment and follow-up plan. In contrast to a zero tolerance approach, a threat assessment approach permitted school authorities to make clear distinctions among different types of threats and to respond without severe consequences for most students (Cornell et al., 2003). Among the 132 students who made transient threats, 37% were suspended from school, and among the 55 who made substantive threats, 80% received a school suspension. Only 3 students were expelled from school, all in association with a substantive threat. Based on follow-up interviews with school principals, the threats were satisfactorily resolved and the students who made the threats engaged in few subsequent acts of violence. Approximately 17% of the students engaged in some form of aggressive act, such as a fight or assault, during the remainder of the school year, but *none* of the students carried out their threat of violence against their intended victims. These findings support the need for more extensive, controlled studies to investigate the potential value of threat assessment in preventing student acts of violence.

Threat assessment arose as a response to the perceived risk of homicide in schools, but other forms of violence must be considered as well. Many, if not most, student threats are threats to strike or injure someone without intent to kill. Even stated threats to kill are often hyperbole and unlikely to result in a fatality. As a result, evaluation of student threats must take into account the likelihood of violent outcomes less than homicide. In the remainder of this chapter, attention turns to the broader range of aggressive and violent behaviors in school settings and how schools have responded to them.

School Crime

Although school homicides are rare, other school-based crimes are more common. According to a nationally representative survey of principals, 10% of all public schools reported at least one serious violent crime to law enforcement in 1996–1997 (DeVoe et al., 2002). Serious violent crimes included murder, rape or other types of sexual battery, suicide, assault with a weapon, and robbery. Another 47% of schools reported a less serious crime, such as an assault without a weapon, theft/larceny, or vandalism. Altogether, 57% of U.S. public schools experienced at least one crime serious enough to contact the police. Police-reported crimes occurred less often in elementary schools (45% reported a crime) and with approximately equal frequency in middle schools (74%) and high schools (77%). Serious violent crime was reported by more city schools (17%) than schools in urban fringe (11%), rural (8%), or town (5%) locations. Crimes were included in the survey if they occurred on school property, on school buses, at school athletic events, or at any place holding a school-sponsored event.

The most common crimes reported to police were an assault without a weapon, followed by theft/larceny and vandalism, all of which occurred in more than half of high schools, nearly half of middle schools, and fewer than one third of elementary schools (DeVoe et al., 2002). Assault with a weapon occurred in fewer than 15% of middle and high schools and only 2% of elementary schools. Robbery and rape or sexual battery were reported in fewer than 10% of middle and high schools and barely 1% of elementary schools.

The national survey of school principals also generated rates of violent crime per 1,000 students. In general, rates for elementary school are low, but rise abruptly in middle school and increase only slightly in high school. For elementary school students, the rate of serious violent crime was 0.1 per 1,000, for middle school the rate increased to 0.9 per 1,000, and for high school the rate was 1.0 per 1,000. The rates for less serious violent crime were 3, 15, and 17 per 1,000, respectively (DeVoe et al., 2002).

There are some obvious limitations to the survey of school principals. Many crimes might go undetected by school authorities, and principals do not report to law enforcement many less serious crimes, such as thefts and simple assaults. Because the principal survey was conducted only once, there is no way to determine trends in school crimes reported to police.

Student Reports of Crime

An alternative approach is to survey students about their experiences as victims of crime. Data from the well-known annual National Crime Victimization Study (NCVS) include surveys of students aged 12 through 18 (Bureau of Justice Statistics, 2000). The NCVS data indicate much higher rates of school crime than the principal survey, although precise comparisons are not possible because the surveys employ different survey methods, use different definitions of crime, and break down the data in different ways. Despite these limitations, it is provocative to observe that the NCVS rate of serious violent crime was 7 per 1,000 students for boys and 2 per 1,000 students for girls, compared to just 1 per 1,000 students in the principal survey. For theft/larceny, students in the NCVS reported a rate for 45 crimes per 1,000 for girls and 47 per 1,000 for boys, whereas the principals reported a rate of approximately 2.3 to 3.2 crimes per 1,000 students. Evidently, students experience far more crime than is reported to law enforcement authorities. The underreporting of crime to law enforcement is a well-recognized problem in the general community, not just in schools. According to a large-scale, nationally representative study based on the NCVS from 1992 through 2000, only about one half of all violent crimes, and only one third of property crimes, are reported to law enforcement (Hart & Rennison, 2003).

The NCVS survey is most useful in comparing the rate of crimes in different settings and in identifying trends over time. Although students aged 12 through 18 report disturbing levels of crime victimization at school, they report much higher rates of serious violent crimes outside of school (2000 data reported in DeVoe et al., 2002). For boys, the rate of serious violent crime outside of school (17 per 1,000) is more than double the rate at school (7 per 1,000) and for girls, the rate difference is also substantial (10 vs. 2 per 1,000). For theft and non-serious violent crime combined, the rates are similar at school (80 per 1,000 for boys and 62 per 1,000 for girls) and outside of school (84 per 1,000 for boys and 63 per 1,000 for girls).

The NCVS data also indicate a general decline in crime victimization at school (DeVoe et al., 2002). The 6-month victimization rate for violent crime and theft declined from 10 per 1,000 in 1995 to 8 per 1,000 in 1999 and 6 per 1,000 in 2001. One area where victimization did not decline is bullying. From 1999 to 2001, the percentage of students who reported being bullied at school during the past 6 months rose from 5 to 8%.

The Youth Risk Behavior Surveillance Survey (YRBS) is the most widely used student self-report instrument used in schools to measure high-risk behavior and was administered in at least 34 states in 2001(Grunbaum et al., 2002). Repeated administrations of the YRBS since 1993 suggest general decline in both physical fights and weapon possession at school (see review by Furlong, Morrison, Austin, Huh-Kim, & Skager, 2001b).

Sources of Error in School Crime Reporting

The study of violence in schools has been plagued by numerous sources of error and even overt attempts at misinformation. One particular example is especially instructive because it demonstrates public susceptibility to false information that casts public schools in a negative light. A widely publicized survey of "top problems of public schools in 1940" listed items such as talking, chewing gum, and running in the halls. The list was a stark contrast with an accompanying list of 1980s school problems that included drug abuse, pregnancy, suicide, assault, and other serious problems. In the 1980s and 1990s the two lists were widely cited by educational authorities and political pundits such as William Bennett, Rush Limbaugh, Carl Rowan, and George Will. The lists appeared in national news magazines, such as *Time* and *Newsweek*, and newspapers, such as the *New York Times* and the *Wall Street Journal*; they were cited in numerous speeches and were aired on CBS News (O'Neill, 1994).

A skeptical professor at Yale University, Barry O'Neill, investigated the origins of the lists, in the process collecting over 250 different versions and eventually tracing them to T. Cullen Davis of Fort Worth, Texas (O'Neill, 1994). Mr. Davis was a wealthy oil businessman and born-again Christian who in 1982 constructed the lists as part of an effort to attack public education and then shared them with like-minded fundamentalists, who assisted in their dissemination. Asked how he arrived at the lists, Mr. Cullen told Professor O'Neill, "They weren't done from a scientific survey. How did I know what the offenses in the schools were in 1940? I was there. How do I know what they are now? I read the newspapers" (O'Neill, 1994, p. 48).[2]

Even objective, scientifically credible efforts to assess violence in school are vulnerable to error, misinterpretation, and exaggeration. When a national study reports that 17% of U.S. high school students have carried a weapon such as a gun, knife, or club in the past 30 days (DeVoe et al., 2002; Grunbaum et al., 2002), the results might seem startling until one considers that they could include students who carried a pocketknife while camping or a firearm while hunting, among many other legitimate reasons for weapon carrying. A broadly worded question does not necessarily identify students who have engaged in a criminally dangerous or high-risk behavior.

Another potential problem is the time frame for student recall of events. Morrison and Furlong (2002) reported results from a study comparing two versions of the California School Climate and Safety Survey, one version inquiring about victim experiences in the past 30 days and the other version asking about the same experiences in the past year. Surprisingly, on many items the students

2. Most troubling is that even though the lists were exposed as a hoax in 1994, they continue to be cited as factual. At a 2001 state school safety conference, I heard an official from the U.S. Department of Education begin her keynote address by presenting the same lists, unaware that they were fabricated.

asked about events in the past 30 days reported *more* victim experiences than the students asked to report victim experiences for an entire year. Such findings cast reasonable doubt on the credibility and accuracy of student recall of victim experiences.

Although the YRBS is widely used and well regarded (Grunbaum et al., 2002), there is relatively little published research on its reliability and validity, its constructs are measured with single items, and there are no validity scales to detect exaggerated or random responding (Furlong et al., 2001b; Morrison & Furlong, 2002). Furlong, Bates, and Smith (2001a) identified a group of YRBS respondents who claimed to have carried a weapon to school 6 or more times in the past month (the most extreme response). While this might be a credible response in some cases, a large proportion of these students gave other extreme responses, such as exercising vigorously 7 days per week and participating in three or more sports teams. Furlong et al. (2001a) concluded that a group of students gave extreme responses to survey questions regardless of item content.

A study of test-retest reliability for the YRBS for a 2-week period found only modest stability in items assessing violence-related behaviors (Brener et al., 2002). For example, κ coefficients, an index of agreement corrected for chance, were .58 for carrying a weapon versus not carrying a weapon on school property in the past 30 days, .41 for being threatened or injured with a weapon on school property in the past 12 months, and .64 for being in a physical fight on school property in the past 12 months. Because these events are salient enough that memory should not be a limiting factor in student recall, some other source(s) of error must account for the inconsistency in student reports. One limitation of a 2-week reliability assessment is that some of the questions focus on substantially different time periods (e.g., the past 30 days starting on dates 2 weeks apart), so that real differences in behavior (e.g., a student carried a weapon to school during one 30-day period but not the other) would decrease the reliability estimate.

A more salient question is whether students are accurate when they claim to have carried a gun or other weapon to school. Almost all research on student weapon possession relies on unverified, anonymous self-report, which may tempt some students to exaggerate their behavior. According to YRBS data aggregated from 34 states (Grunbaum et al., 2002), approximately 6.2% of students in grades 9–12 reported "carrying a weapon on school property" in the past 30 days. An important question is how many of these weapons were guns.

Estimates of the prevalence of guns in schools vary widely (Redding & Shalf, 2001). In their survey of 6th-, 8th-, and 10th-grade students in Illinois public schools, Williams, Mulhall, Reis, and DeVille (2002) found that 266 of 21,679 students (1.2%) reported carrying a handgun to school in the past year. Even this small percentage would indicate a large number of handguns in schools if it reflected true national trends. In their review of the literature, Redding and Shalf (2001) found even larger estimates. They cited one authority's assertion that 135,000 students carry guns to school every day and another equally frightening contention that in urban high schools there is likely to be at least one gun in every classroom. Certainly it is difficult to formulate school safety policy without accurate, credible information about the nature and extent of the problem. Compare the huge estimates of gun carrying at school with the relatively small numbers of students who are caught with guns at school each year. If there were 135,000 students carrying a gun to school for each of the 180 days in a typical school year, that would mean 24.3 million occasions when a student brought a gun to school, but fewer than 3,000 cases—a hundredth of 1%—in which the student was caught (U.S. Department of Education, 2002).

The use of validity screening procedures can substantially reduce estimates of the prevalence of student involvement in high-risk behavior such as fights, drug use, and gangs. In a survey of 10,909 middle and high school students, Cornell and Loper (1998) found that one fourth of the surveys failed to meet validity screening criteria that included detection of students who omitted demographic information, marked a series of items all in the same way, and gave inappropriate answers to validity questions (e.g., answering "No" to "I am telling the truth on this survey"). The deletion of invalid self-report surveys reduced the estimated 30-day prevalence of fighting at school from 28.7 to 19.2%. Similarly, the estimated prevalence of self-reported drug use at school dropped from 25.1 to 14.8%, gang membership dropped from 8.4 to 5.2%, and carrying a knife at school dropped from 18.4 to 7.7%. Nevertheless, even the best screening procedures are unlikely to identify all false reports. The question of weapon carrying at school cannot be definitively answered using student self-report alone and will require more extensive research than has been undertaken to date.

Bullying

Bullying is perhaps the most pervasive form of interpersonal violence in schools, although it encompasses behavior that ranges from criminal assault to mere social insult. Bullying typically is defined as the use of one's strength or status to injure, threaten, or humiliate another person. Bullying can be physical (hitting and threatening to hit), verbal (teasing and name-calling), or social (spreading rumors and inducing others to reject or ignore someone), but does not include arguments or fights between two students of about the same strength or size (Olweus, 1993). The breadth of definition and range in severity of bullying make it difficult to formulate specific policies and practices, and it generates controversy about the seriousness of bullying and whether it constitutes a law enforcement issue. Adults sometimes ignore bullying or dismiss it as little more than an unpleasant rite of passage in childhood (Craig, Pepler, & Atlas, 2000; Olweus, 1993; Unnever & Cornell, 2003).

Bullying became a national concern in the United States after the news media reported, and studies by the FBI (O'Toole, 2000) and Secret Service (Vossekuil et al., 2002) confirmed, that many of the high-profile school shootings were motivated by students seeking revenge for bullying. In recent years, national and worldwide interest in bullying has increased dramatically. Large-scale bullying intervention programs have been undertaken in Canada, Japan, Norway, and Great Britain, among other countries (Smith & Brain, 2000).

A recent national study (Nansel et al., 2001) found that 29.9% of U.S. students are involved in bullying as a bully (13.0%), a victim (10.6%) or both a bully and a victim (6.3%). In middle schools, bullying is so common that students appear to share a normative set of beliefs that accept and help maintain it. A study of 2,472 students in six middle schools found that, in most cases, students believed that neither their classmates nor their teachers would intervene to stop bullying (Unnever & Cornell, 2003), and as a result many middle school students fail to seek help when they are bullied (Unnever & Cornell, in press).

School bullying has both immediate and long-term detrimental effects. Victimization due to bullying is correlated with student absenteeism (Rigby, 1996), poorer academic achievement (Nolin, Davies, & Chandler, 1996), social isolation (Slee & Rigby, 1992), and internalizing problems such as depression, anxiety, and poorer psychosocial adjustment (Nansel et al., 2001; Olweus, 1979; Sourander, Helstela, Helenius, & Piha, 2000). Craig (1998) reported that physical, verbal, and social forms of bullying were predictive of victim anxiety. In a 1-year longitudinal study of kindergarten students, Kochenderfer and Ladd (1996) found that peer victimization was a precursor, rather than a consequence, of school maladjustment.

Sourander et al. (2000) found that students who were repeatedly victimized in elementary school reported higher levels of internalizing problems at age 16. Likewise, longitudinal research suggests that many of the negative effects associated with childhood victimization (e.g., low self-esteem, depression, social isolation) continue into adulthood (Olweus, 1993; Rigby, 1996).

Our understanding of bullying is built upon the seminal work of Dan Olweus, a Norwegian researcher who undertook a nationwide bullying prevention effort in Norway after a series of highly publicized suicides by middle school boys who had been bullied by their classmates (Olweus, 1991, 1993). Olweus found that a schoolwide intervention program could dramatically reduce bullying (Olweus, 1991, 1994; Olweus & Limber, 2000). Although current research findings are not conclusive, an effective bullying prevention program is believed to include a whole-school approach that includes (a) a schoolwide campaign to raise awareness of bullying and to communicate school policies that oppose bullying and support peaceful conflict resolution, (b) a classroom curriculum that teaches strategies for responding to bullying, and (c) counseling for students identified as bullies or victims (Olweus & Limber, 2000). There are several intervention and curriculum programs designed to reduce bullying in schools (e.g., Garrity, Jens, Porter, Sager, & Short-Camilli, 1994; Hoover & Oliver, 1996; Olweus & Limber, 2000). Given the popularity of antibullying programs, there is an urgent need for controlled studies in this area.

School Violence Prevention

There is solid evidence that school violence can be prevented or reduced with well-conceived and carefully implemented interventions. Wilson, Lipsey, and Derzon (2003) conducted a meta-analysis of school-based interventions that attempted to reduce aggressive behavior. They identified 221 studies of school-based interventions involving nearly 56,000 students. Each of these studies included pre–post assessment of at least one form of aggressive behavior broadly defined to include fighting, bullying, assault, conduct disorder, and acting out. These researchers found a wide range in program effectiveness, but calculated an average effect size of .25 for well-implemented demonstration programs. They estimated that an effect size of this magnitude would eliminate approximately half the incidents of fighting in a typical school year. Similarly, Wilson, Gottfredson, and Najaka (2001) found that school-based prevention programs were effective in reducing a variety of problem behaviors, such as substance use, conduct problems, and truancy, although effects varied widely across programs and some programs showed negative effects.

The most extensively studied programs are designed to enhance students' social competence (Wilson et al., 2003). A typical social competence program includes lesson plans for instructors to teach students how to resolve peer conflicts. Students are taught, often through role-playing and demonstration exercises, communication skills such as how to deflect criticism and assert their opinions in a nonprovocative manner. They are taught how to listen and respond respectfully to others. They are presented with typical peer situations in which they must resolve a conflict or cope with disappointment. Some programs include a cognitive-behavioral component in which students learn relaxation techniques, practice self-monitoring, or rehearse step-by-step procedures for thinking through problems. Peer mediation programs are also popular, but less frequently studied. Peer mediation programs involve teaching students how to resolve conflicts between peers. Typically, a small group of students are trained to serve as mediators for the student body. When two students have an argument or dispute, they bring their grievances to a pair of mediators who guide them through a standard procedure designed to facilitate a discussion to resolve the conflict.

What are the characteristics of the most effective programs? Not surprisingly, Wilson et al. (2003) found that quality of program implementation was critical. Schools that experienced problems in fully implementing a program experienced less success, and programs that were implemented as part of a demonstration project—where presumably great attention is given to program fidelity—were more successful than programs operating under routine conditions. Perhaps the most striking difference among programs was the apparent positive impact of researcher involvement in implementing a program. The evaluation of programs that were already implemented as routine practice showed relatively weak effectiveness, even if they were evaluated by outside researchers. This finding argues for greater attention to program fidelity in routine administration of school-based programs, particularly in light of studies on the quality of school-based prevention programs. In their survey of 3,691 school-based prevention programs, Gottfredson and Gottfredson (2001) found that typical prevention efforts are not well integrated into normal school operations and that the school staff members who implement these programs are in need of better training, support, and supervision.

Wilson et al. (2003) found that violence prevention programs were effective at all age levels, but larger effect sizes were achieved for preschool and high school interventions than for elementary and middle school interventions. There were no differences in program effectiveness associated with gender and ethnic composition of the samples. Both high- and low-risk students benefited from interventions, although as might be expected, the degree of improvement was greater in high-risk populations, where there would be greater room for change.

Programs delivered by teachers were most effective, followed by programs delivered by researchers, and then those delivered by laypersons. Programs that delivered more intensive services and provided more one-on-one attention demonstrated stronger effects. Wilson et al. (2003) next attempted to compare different types of programs, after controlling for differences due to study methodology, sample characteristics, and general program attributes, such as implementation quality and program intensity. An unexpected finding was that the relatively few demonstration programs that delivered academic services (such as tutoring and reading development) obtained the largest effect sizes. One intriguing hypothesis is that many students engage in aggressive behavior because of frustration over poor academic performance and that attention to their academic needs will pay dividends in good behavior. However, the two studies of routine academic programs yielded mixed evidence of effectiveness.

There were few consistent differences in the measured effectiveness of other types of programs; most programs were effective. Notably, social competence interventions have been the most frequently studied programs and stood out as demonstrating substantial effectiveness in most studies. Social competence training is designed to help students understand and resolve interpersonal conflicts and often involves the teaching of communication and negotiation skills. Peer mediation appeared to be effective, but there were few rigorous studies of this popular and widely used approach.

Conclusion

School violence is a serious and complex problem that has received a great deal of attention in the past decade. Public perceptions of school violence can be skewed by a few highly publicized, extreme cases, leading authorities to adopt dubious zero tolerance policies or to pursue questionable practices such as profiling. Threat assessment is a promising alternative that gives school authorities a more flexible, problem-solving approach to potentially violent students. The fear of school violence must be countered by a fact-based analysis of the problem and the adoption of empirically defensible methods of assessment, prevention, and intervention.

References

Advancement Project and the Civil Rights Project. (2000). *Opportunities suspended: The devastating consequences of zero tolerance and school discipline policies.* Boston: Harvard Civil Rights Project. Retrieved March 1, 2003, from http://www.law.harvard.edu/civilrights/conferences/ zero/zt_report2.htm

American Psychological Association. (1999). *Warning signs.* Washington, DC: Author

Brener, N. D., Kann, L., McManus, T., Kinchen, S. A., Sundberg, E. C., & Ross, J. G. (2002). Reliability of the 1999 Youth Risk Behavior Survey Questionnaire. *Journal of Adolescent Health, 31,* 336–342.

Brooks, K., Schiraldi, V., & Ziedenberg, J. (2000). *School house hype: Two years later.* Washington, DC: Justice Policy Institute.

Bureau of Justice Statistics. (2000). *National Crime Victimization Survey.* Washington, DC: U.S. Department of Justice.

Cornell, D. G. (2001). *Guidelines for responding to student threats of violence.* Charlottesville: University of Virginia.

Cornell, D. G., & Loper, A. B. (1996). *High risk behavior in Virginia schools: A survey of middle and high school students.* Charlottesville: University of Virginia, Curry School of Education.

Cornell, D. G., & Loper, A. B. (1998). Assessment of violence and other high-risk behaviors with a school survey. *School Psychology Review, 27,* 317–330.

Cornell, D. G., Sheras, P. L., Kaplan, S., Levy, A., McConville, D., McKnight, L., et al. (2003, August). Guidelines for responding to student threats of violence. Paper presented at the 111th Annual Convention of the American Psychological Association, Chicago.

Cornell, D. G., Sheras, P. L., Kaplan, S., Levy, A., McConville, D., McKnight, L., et al. (in press). Guidelines for responding to student threats of violence: Field test of a threat assessment approach. In M. J. Furlong, P. M. Kingery, & M. P. Bates (Eds.), *Appraisal and prediction of school violence: Context, issues, and methods.* Binghamton, NY: Haworth Press.

Craig, W. M. (1998). The relationship among bullying, victimization, depression, anxiety, and aggression in elementary school children. *Personality and Individual Differences, 24,* 123–130.

Craig, W. M., Pepler, D., & Atlas, R. (2000). Observations of bullying in the playground and in the classroom. *School Psychology International, 21,* 22–36.

DeVoe, J. F., Ruddy, S. A., Miller, A. K., Planty, M., Snyder, T. D., Duhart, D. T., et al. (2002). *Indicators of school crime and safety: 2002* (NCES 2003-009/NCJ196753). Washington, DC: U.S. Departments of Education and Justice.

Dwyer, K., & Osher, D. (2000). *Safeguarding our children: An action guide.* Washington, DC: U.S. Departments of Education and Justice, American Institutes for Research.

Dwyer, K., Osher, D., & Warger, C. (1998). *Early warning, timely response: A guide to safe schools.* Washington, DC: U.S. Department of Education.

Federal Bureau of Investigation. (1993–2002). *Uniform crime reports: Crime in the United States.* Washington, DC: U.S. Government Printing Office.

Fein, R. A., & Vossekuil, F. (1998). *Protective intelligence and threat assessment investigations: A guide for state and local law enforcement officials.* Washington, DC: U.S. Secret Service.

Fein, R. A., & Vossekuil, F. (1999). Assassination in the United States: An operational study of recent assassins, attackers, and near-lethal approachers. *Journal of Forensic Sciences, 44,* 321–333.

Fein, R. A., Vossekuil, F., & Holden, G. A. (1995). Threat assessment: An approach to prevent targeted violence. *National Institute of Justice: Research in action,* 1–7 (NCJ 155000). Retrieved August 12, 2004, from http://www.secretservice.gov/ntac.htm

Fein, R. A., Vossekuil, F., Pollack, W. S., Borum, R., Modzeleski, W., & Reddy, M. (2002). *Threat assessment in schools: A guide to managing threatening situations and to creat-*

ing safe school climates. Washington, DC: U.S. Secret Service and U.S. Department of Education.

Furlong, M. J., Bates, M. P., & Smith, D. C. (2001a, August). Low-risk but frequent school weapon possession: An invisible group. Paper presented at the annual meeting of the American Psychological Association, San Francisco.

Furlong, M. J., Morrison, G. M., Austin, G., Huh-Kim, J., & Skager, R. (2001b). Using student risk factors in school violence surveillance reports: Illustrative examples for enhances policy formation, implementation, and evaluation. *Law and Policy, 23,* 271–295.

Garrity, C., Jens, K., Porter, W., Sager, N., & Short-Camilli, C. (1994). *Bully-proofing your school*. Longmont, CO: Sopris West.

Gottfredson, D. C., & Gottfredson, G. D. (2001). Quality of school-based prevention programs: Results from a national survey. *Journal of Research in Crime and Delinquency, 39,* 3–35.

Grunbaum, J. A., Kann, L., Kinchen, S. A., Williams, B., Ross, J. G., Lowry, R., et al. (2002). Youth Risk Behavior Surveillance—United States 2001. *Morbidity and Mortality Weekly Report: Surveillance Summaries, 51,* 1–64.

Gun-Free Schools Act, Public Law 103-882, 20 U.S.C. § 8921 (1994) (See also Title XIV, Part F, Section 14601).

Hart, T. C., & Rennison, C. (2003). *Reporting crime to the police: 1992–2000* (NCJ-195710). Washington DC: Bureau of Justice Statistics.

Hoover, J. H., & Oliver, R. (1996). *The bullying prevention handbook: A guide for principals, teachers, and counselors*. Bloomington, IN: National Educational Service.

Kochenderfer, B. J., & Ladd, G. W. (1996). Peer victimization: Cause or consequence of school maladjustment? *Child Development, 67,* 1305–1317.

Marsh, T., & Cornell, D. (2001). The contribution of student experiences to understanding ethnic differences in high-risk behaviors at school. *Behavioral Disorders, 26,* 152–163.

Morrison, G., & Furlong, M. J. (2002, June). Understanding the turning points in students' school discipline histories. Paper presented at Safe Schools for the 21st Century, National Conference of the Hamilton Fish Institute, Monterey, CA.

Mulvey, E. P., & Cauffman, E. (2001). The inherent limits of predicting school violence. *American Psychologist, 56,* 797–802.

National School Safety Center. (1998). Checklist of characteristics of youth who have caused school-associated violent deaths. Westlake Village, CA. Retrieved January 29, 2003, from http://www.nssc1.org

National School Safety Center. (2003). School associated violent deaths. Westlake Village, CA. Retrieved January 29, 2003, from http://www.nssc1.org

Nansel, T. R., Overpeck, M., Pilla, R. S., Ruan, W. J., Simons-Morton, B., & Scheidt, P. (2001). Bullying behaviors among U.S. youth, prevalence and association with psychosocial adjustment. *Journal of the American Medical Association, 285,* 2094–2100.

Nolin, M. J., Davies, E., & Chandler, K. (1996). Student victimization at school. *Journal of School Health, 66,* 216–221.

Olweus, D. (1979). *Aggression in the schools*. New York: Wiley.

Olweus, D. (1991). Bully/victims problems among school children: Basic facts and effects of a school-based intervention program. In I. Rubin & D. Pepler (Eds.), *The development and treatment of childhood aggression* (pp. 411–447). Hillsdale, NJ: Erlbaum.

Olweus, D. (1993). *Bullying at school: What we know and what we can do*. Cambridge, MA: Blackwell.

Olweus, D. (1994). Bullying at school: Basic facts and effects of a school based intervention program. *Journal of Child Psychology and Psychiatry, 35,* 1171–1190.

Olweus, D. & Limber, S. (2000). *Blueprints for violence prevention: Book 9, bullying prevention program.* Institute of Behavioral Science, Regents of the University of Colorado. Golden, CO: Venture Publishing.

O'Neill, B. (1994, March 6). The history of a hoax. *The New York Times Magazine,* 46–49.

O'Toole, M. E. (2000). *The school shooter: A threat assessment perspective.* Quantico, VA: Federal Bureau of Investigation, National Center for the Analysis of Violent Crime.

Redding, R. E., & Shalf, S. M. (2001). The legal context of school violence: The effectiveness of federal, state, and local law enforcement efforts to reduce gun violence in schools. *Law and Policy, 23,* 297–343.

Reddy, M., Borum, R., Berglund, J., Vossekuil, B., Fein, R., & Modzeleski, W. (2001). Evaluating risk for targeted violence in schools: Comparing risk assessment, threat assessment, and other approaches. *Psychology in the Schools, 38,* 157–172.

Rigby, K. (1996). *Bullying in schools and what to do about it.* Melbourne, Victoria, Australia: The Australian Council for Educational Research Ltd.

Sewell, K. W., & Mendelsohn, M. (2000). Profiling potentially violent youth: Statistical and conceptual problems. *Children's Services: Social Policy, Research, and Practice, 3,* 147–169.

Singer, M. I., & Flannery, D. J. (2000). The relationship between children's threats of violence and violent behaviors. *Archives of Pediatric and Adolescence Medicine, 154,* 785–790.

Skiba, R., & Peterson, R. (1999, March). The dark side of zero tolerance: Can punishment lead to safe schools? *Phi Delta Kappan, 80,* 372–376, 381, 382.

Skiba, R. J., & Knesting, K. K. (2001). Zero tolerance, zero evidence: An analysis of school disciplinary practice. In R. J. Skiba & G. G. Noam (Eds.), *New directions for youth development: No. 92. Zero tolerance: Can suspension and expulsion keep schools safe?* (pp. 17–43). San Francisco: Jossey-Bass.

Slee, P. T., & Rigby, K. (1992). Australian school children's self appraisal of interpersonal relations: The bullying experience. *Child Psychiatry and Human Development, 23,* 273–282.

Smith, P. K., & Brain, P. (2000). Bullying in schools: Lessons from two decades of research. *Aggressive Behavior, 26,* 1–9.

Sourander, A., Helstela, L., Helenius, H., & Piha, J. (2000). Persistence of bullying from childhood to adolescence: A longitudinal 8-year follow-up study. *Child Abuse and Neglect, 24,* 873–881.

Tebo, M. G. (2000, April). Zero tolerance, zero sense. *American Bar Association Journal.* Retrieved May 1, 2002, from www.abanet.org/journal/apr00/04FZERO.html

Unnever, J., & Cornell, D. G. (2003). The culture of bullying in middle school. *Journal of School Violence, 2,* 5–27.

Unnever, J., & Cornell, D. (in press). Middle school victims of bullying: Who reports being bullied? *Aggressive Behavior.*

U.S. Department of Education, Office of Elementary and Secondary Education, Safe and Drug-Free Schools and Communities Program. (2002). Report on state/territory implementation of the Gun-Free Schools Act for school year 1999–2000. Washington, DC: U.S. Department of Education. Retrieved August 12, 2004, from http://www.ed.gov/about/reports/annual/gfsa/index.html

U.S. Surgeon General. (2001). *Youth violence: A report of the Surgeon General.* Rockville, MD: U.S. Department of Health and Human Services.

Virginia Department of Education. (2003). Annual report for the school year 2001–02: Incidents of crime, violence and substance abuse in Virginia's public schools. Richmond: Virginia Department of Education.

Vossekuil, B., Fein, R. A., Reddy, M., Borum, R., & Modzeleski, W. (2002). *The final report and findings of the* Safe School Initiative: *Implications for the prevention of school attacks in the United States*. Washington, DC: U.S. Secret Service and U.S. Department of Education.

Whitehead, J. W. (2001). Zero common sense school discipline rules cheapen students' humanity. Charlottesville, VA: The Rutherford Institute. Retrieved August 12, 2004, from http://www.rutherford.org/articles_db/commentary.asp?record_id=99

Williams, S. S., Mulhall, P. F., Reis, J. S., & DeVille, J. O. (2002). Adolescents carrying handguns and taking them to school: Psychosocial correlates among public school students in Illinois. *Journal of Adolescence, 25,* 551–567.

Wilson, D. B., Gottfredson, D. C., & Najaka, S. S. (2001). School-based prevention of problem behaviors: A meta-analysis. *Journal of Quantitative Criminology, 17,* 247–272.

Wilson, S. J., Lipsey, M. W., & Derzon, J. H. (2003). The effects of school-based intervention programs on aggressive behavior: A meta-analysis. *Journal of Consulting and Clinical Psychology, 71,* 136–149.

4

BARRY KRISBERG AND ANGELA M. WOLF

Juvenile Offending

Few social issues are more subject to false perceptions than juvenile offending. Fueled by inflated media accounts that overemphasize the extent of juvenile participation in violent crime, the general public holds the view that juveniles account for the vast majority of violent crime. In several presentations before citizen audiences, we have used a brief quiz to test the knowledge of the audience about youthful offending. Despite years of declining juvenile arrests, most audiences believe that youth crime is increasing at an alarming rate. They also believe that teenagers account for over two thirds of all arrests for murder, forcible rape, robbery, and aggravated assault. In fact, minors comprise less that 15% of those arrested for the most serious crimes. Our audiences are usually shocked to find out that more children are killed by their parents or guardians than by other youngsters. Virtually no one guesses that teenagers are more often the victims of crime than any other population age group.

Getting the facts straight about juvenile offending is a crucial precursor to formulating intelligent and effective strategies to prevent juvenile crime and to construct appropriate control and treatment agendas. In this chapter we attempt to summarize some of those key facts. Current trends in juvenile crime are reviewed. The relative strengths and weaknesses of research based on official arrest statistics and on youth self-report data are assessed. Research on the etiology of delinquent behavior is summarized, along with empirical insights into why some youth desist from offending behavior.

Other important topics examined include the very small core of offenders who account for the majority of juvenile offenses, sometimes called serious, violent, and chronic offenders; the special role of juvenile gangs in propelling youth further into lives of serious and chronic offending; and the "cycle of violence"—young people as victims of crime, rather than as offenders, and the role of victimization in future offending. Finally, data are reviewed on the vastly disproportionate representation of youth of color in the juvenile justice system. The social policy implications of this disproportionality are briefly examined.

Current Trends in Juvenile Offending

The best available data for assessing trends in juvenile offending come from police departments that report juvenile arrests to the Federal Bureau of Investigation (FBI; Snyder, 2002). An analysis of recent trends in juvenile offending that is based on this data source follows a discussion of its relative strengths and weaknesses. However, it is important to note that arrest statistics have significant limitations that may bias conclusions that are based on these data. These limitations are discussed below.

FBI arrest data over the last two decades have revealed major changes in juvenile offending behavior (Snyder, 2002). For example, if we look at the Violent Crime Index (consisting of arrests for murder, forcible rape, robbery, and aggravated assault), the number of arrests per 100,000 juveniles ages 10–17 was fairly stable through most of the 1980s. Beginning in 1988 the juvenile violent arrest rate increased dramatically and peaked in 1994. Arrests of juveniles for weapons law violations were similar to the trends in the Violent Crime Index. This sudden rise, not seen since the early 1970s, led to a nationwide focus on juvenile violence. Some speculated that a new wave of juvenile "superpredators" was storming the gates. But the rise in juvenile violence was quickly reversed, and juvenile arrests for violent crimes have declined every year between 1994 and 2000. Preliminary FBI data suggest that this decline in juvenile arrests for violent offenses is continuing in the early years of the new millennium. Considering the period from 1991 to 2000, arrests in the Violent Crime Index declined by 17%. The largest drop was in arrests for homicide, which fell by 65% during this time. Between 1991 and 2000 juvenile arrests for forcible rape and robbery also decreased by 26 and 2%, respectively. Juvenile arrests for aggravated assault declined by 7%.

While no one can say for sure, the general decline in juvenile crime did correspond with a significant improvement in the economy and a decline in teenage unemployment. Unlike the case of other violent offenses, the number of juveniles who were arrested for minor assaults did not decrease during the latter part of the 1990s, a period in which the youth population increased. Other potential explanations for the decline in juvenile violence include speculation that (a) trafficking in "crack" cocaine that was associated with high levels of gang violence declined in the late 1990s, (b) improved enforcement of gun laws kept weapons out of the hands of juveniles, (c) tougher juvenile sentencing policies exerted a deterrent effect, or (d) expanded violence prevention programs reduced youthful violence. There is scant evidence supporting or refuting any of these claims.

Interestingly, violent arrests for adults also decreased during the 1991–2000 period—a drop of 10%. The decline in adults arrested for homicide was 37%; declines in adult arrests for forcible rape and robbery were 30 and 32%, respectively. The number of adult arrests for aggravated assault was also down, though only slightly (1%).

The rate of juvenile arrests for serious property offenses was relatively stable in the 1980s and early 1990s, but then declined by 37% between 1994 and 2000. By the end of the 1990s, juvenile arrests for serious property crime reached levels lower than those at any time since the 1960s. The drop in arrests was especially noteworthy for burglary. Between 1991 and 2000 arrests for burglary for both juveniles and adults decreased by about one third. Juvenile motor vehicle arrests peaked in 1990, but dropped by 54% by 2000. There was a smaller decline in adult arrests for car theft during this same period (23%). Arrests of juveniles for arson and larceny were more stable over the decade of the 1990s, although some decreases were observed in the latter part of the decade. Trying to account for the drop in property crimes committed by juveniles is nearly impossible. There were many factors that might be possible explanations for the decline in juvenile property crimes, such as reduced teenage unemployment, expanded home-owner efforts to "burglarproof" their homes, or greater law enforcement attention to arresting juveniles for violent crimes versus property offenses. There is even speculation that juveniles found drug trafficking more lucrative than burglaries and auto thefts during this time frame. Since drug crimes are less likely to result in arrests than other offenses, a shift in offending behavior might appear as a crime drop if the more popular crimes are less subject to police apprehension.

A great deal of public attention and funding has been directed at reducing drug abuse among young people as part of the much touted "War on Drugs." Juvenile arrests for drug crimes were stable from 1980 through 1993. But between 1993 and 2000, this rate grew by 78%, peaking in 1997. During the entire decade of the 1990s, arrests of adults for drug crimes grew by 42% compared to a 145% increase in juvenile drug-related arrests during the same period.

Female Offenders

Another important trend that can be seen in the arrest data is the growing number of young women who were arrested, even though they comprise a much smaller proportion of those arrested than do their male counterparts. Between 1980 and 2000, juvenile arrests increased proportionately more for girls than for boys. During this period, overall arrests for young females rose by 35% compared to 11% for young males. This difference was especially pronounced for certain violent crimes. The increase in girls arrested for aggravated assault was 121% compared to 28% for boys; for weapons offenses there was a 70% increase in arrests of girls compared to a 20% increase for boys. Young males, however, bore the largest share of the increase in juvenile drug arrests, with a 70% increase for boys versus a 47% increase for girls.

No simple answer exists for the trends in arrests by young women. Again, a wide range of speculation exists, running the gamut from the adverse impact of the women's liberation movement to tougher juvenile justice policies aimed at female offenders. There are just insufficient data to honestly interpret these trends.

Juvenile Crime Data Collection and Research Methods

Typically, crime is measured through three methods. These methods include self-report from the perpetrator, official arrest data, and self-report of victimization. Self-report surveys collect the type, frequency, and severity level of delinquent acts from individual respondents and often collect a variety of descriptive and contextual information, such as the relationship between the victim and offender, the nature of the crime, and the location of the crime. Official measures include data collected through official sources, such as arrest and incarceration records. Official measures capture only data that come to the attention of authorities and are often confined to characteristics of the offense. Self-report victimization surveys access the level of victimization in a population and thus measure crime regardless of whether the crime has been reported to authorities. Like self-report delinquency scales, self-report victimization data allow for more details about crimes, such as their context, the relationship between offender and victim, and the like.

Data collected from each of these sources are an essential component of criminal justice research. Measures of delinquency and criminal activity are used to describe community crime levels, to assess the ramifications of policy change, and to evaluate criminal justice programs and practices. At its best, juvenile justice research affects corrections and public policy, the development of prevention and intervention services for at-risk and delinquent youth, and public perception of social problems. Given the potential impact of delinquency research on the lives of young people, appropriate measurement of offense variables is crucial. Each method of measurement has utility but has different meanings and distinct shortcomings. The following section discusses each approach.

Self-Report Measures

Thornberry and Krohn (2000) described the development and use of self-report measures as one of the most important contributions to criminal justice research in the 20th century. Self-report data attempt to measure all delinquent behaviors, not only those behaviors that come to the attention of police or court officials. For measurement of undetected delinquent behavior, self-report measures are reasonably accurate and valid. Although respondents may not have been able or willing to disclose the exact number of crimes committed, respondents usually distinguished reliably between low and high frequency (Kelly, Huizinga, Thornberry, & Loeber, 1997).

One of the significant advantages of self-report measures is their measurement of all offending rather than only behavior detected by officials (Kelly et al., 1997). This is particularly important because the majority of delinquent behavior does not result in an official record (Thornberry & Krohn, 2000). Also, it captures the low-level and infrequent offending that is more likely to escape police intervention (Elliott & Ageton, 1980).

However, self-report measures also suffer from shortcomings. Self-report measures may underreport crime, as these measures rely on the memory of the offender and the willingness to disclose unlawful behaviors. Possible reasons for this underreporting include an intentional positive response bias—respondents may be reluctant to paint themselves in a negative light (Elliott & Ageton, 1980). Additionally, self-report measures are vulnerable to problems with recall (Blumstein, Cohen, Roth, & Visher, 1986) and may be particularly suspect when used with youth with low cognitive abilities.

Official Delinquency Data

Official measures of delinquency are composed of police and court records, such as arrest data. Data can be gathered to measure delinquency for a specific population, such as participants in an intervention, or they can be collected across a community or even nationwide. One commonly cited source is the Uniform Crime Reports (UCR). The UCR have been collected from local police departments and compiled by the Federal Bureau of Investigation since 1929. The UCR include data on known offenses and arrests. Official measures of delinquency such as the UCR have certain advantages over self-report data. They are not subject to the response bias of the offender and, for some research, it is desirable to measure only those behaviors that receive official intervention and system response; an example is a study measuring the effects of official intervention.

Official measures of delinquent and criminal behavior suffer from a number of limitations. Arrests represent only a fraction of the actual number of offenses that occur. National data suggest that victims report about one third of the most serious offenses to the police (Krisberg, in press). For some offenses, such as drug crimes, gun sales, or minor assaults, the level of underreporting is much higher. The police actually make arrests in a small fraction of cases (about 50% of reported violent crimes and about 20% of property offenses; Krisberg, in press), so arrest statistics are missing a large, submerged segment of the crime problem. It is not clear what portion of this uncounted criminal behavior is attributable to juveniles. Further, changes in law enforcement practices, such as crackdowns on specific types of crimes, can lead to a significant increase in arrests even if the underlying behavior among youth has not changed. This is a very serious problem in interpreting juvenile crime trends because there are often periodic law enforcement campaigns against such delinquent behavior as underage drinking, adolescent drug use, truancy, curfew violations, and juvenile gangs. The recent popularity among adults of "zero tolerance" policies at schools has led to many minor offenses previously resolved on campuses being referred to police agencies for formal action. The arrest trends will vary with policy shifts, but it is unclear whether the behavior of youth is changing.

Although arrest statistics may underestimate the amount of crime committed by juveniles due to unsolved crimes, underreporting, or variable enforcement patterns, these statistics may also exaggerate the amount of juvenile offending. FBI arrest data typically count the number of persons taken into custody for a given offense. Thus, if seven juveniles in a car are arrested for robbing a convenience store, the number of robbery arrests is counted as seven—even if only one of the juveniles actually committed the offense. It has been well documented that juveniles tend to commit crimes in groups (Zimring, 1981), and this fact inflates the actual participation of juveniles in crime statistics. For example, if the police arrest five youth in a stolen car, this event will be recorded as if there were five separate auto thefts. In fact, only one of the juveniles might actually be adjudicated for the offense. Further, arrests do not automatically result in youngsters being adjudicated or convicted of that crime. Most arrests are not prosecuted. Less than half of juvenile arrests go to court, and about half of these court referrals result in dismissals (Krisberg, in press). This illustrates that arrest is a very imperfect measure of juvenile crime trends. However, many researchers argue that the proximity of the arrest decision to the actual criminal event makes these data a bit more reliable than numbers generated from later points in the juvenile justice process (e.g., juvenile court statistics or correctional data).

Official statistics are incident-based as opposed to person-based. They provide data only on particular incidents and not about contextual factors, such as length of time the offender has been committing crimes or frequency of an individual's criminal behavior (Hawkins, Laub, Lauritsen, & Cothern, 2000).

Self-Report Measures of Victimization

Self-report measures of victimization such as the National Crime Victimization Survey (NCVS) conducted by the U.S. Department of Justice's Bureau of Justice Statistics are also used in criminal justice research. These measures assess crime from the victim's point of view and often include crimes that escape the attention of authorities. Like the UCR, the NCVS is an important social indicator, as it captures our national level of victimization.

Characterizing Young Offenders

Using any measure of delinquency, it appears that delinquent behaviors are common during adolescence. Most people limit their offending behaviors to adolescence, move through this period of offending with few if any lasting ramifications, and go on to lead productive and essentially crime-free lives in adulthood (Moffitt, 1993; Moffitt & Caspi, 2001). However, there is a small group of offenders that continues to commit crimes through their youth and into adulthood. This group is sometimes referred to as "life-course-persistent offenders."

Persisters Versus Desisters

The majority of youthful offenders can be categorized as those who limit their offending behaviors to adolescence. For young people, participation in some delinquent behaviors is developmentally normal, common, and temporary (Arnett, 1992; Moffitt & Caspi, 2001) and will likely cease over time. In contrast, for a small group of offenders, the trajectory toward unlawful behavior begins young and continues throughout their lifetime. These life-course-persistent offenders begin to demonstrate antisocial behavior during early childhood, and this behavior escalates over time (Moffitt, Caspi, Harrington, & Milne, 2002).

Moffitt and colleagues have explored these offender typologies at length and postulated that the majority of youthful offenders desist their unlawful behaviors as they mature. They theorized that delinquent behavior often begins during puberty, a time when young people experience tension between their childhood and their new roles, privileges, and responsibilities as adolescents. This period is termed the "maturity gap." It is during this maturity gap that young people explore autonomy from parents and seek approval from peer groups. While this exploration often translates into involvement in delinquent or antisocial behaviors, the majority of young people move through this stage and assume the appropriate roles and responsibilities of young adulthood (Moffitt, 1993; Moffitt & Caspi, 2001). Specifically, if a youth's childhood is characterized by adequate protective factors and limited risk factors, even an offending young person is likely to desist from criminal behavior and move into a healthy adult role. However, even for desisters, if this normal delinquent behavior causes lasting negative outcomes, such as a criminal record, substance dependence, or injury, the transition toward the desistance of unlawful behaviors may be delayed (Moffitt et al., 2002).

In contrast, for a small group of offenders, antisocial behaviors persist. Moffitt and colleagues argued that, for this group, antisocial behavior begins early in life and is exacerbated by high-risk home and social environments. These risk factors may include poor parenting, lack of parental affection and bonds, and poverty. As the young person develops, he or she is likely to be negatively affected by further risk factors, such as delinquent peer groups and community crime and violence (Moffitt et al., 2002). Risk factors and protective factors are discussed more extensively later in this chapter.

Compared to desisters, life-course-persistent offenders typically begin offending at a younger age, commit more offenses, more severe offenses, and more frequent offenses, and their offending persists for a longer period (Blumstein et al., 1986). Life-course-persistent offenders also are at a greater risk for a variety of other problems, including substance abuse, school failure, employment problems, mental health problems, and adult criminal careers (Elliott, Huizinga, & Menard, 1989).

This persister versus desister typology is a useful way to distinguish offenders who are displaying normal developmental patterns from those offenders who are at risk for continued criminal activity. Another typology used to describe youth at high risk for lifelong criminal activities is that of the serious, violent, and chronic offender.

Serious, Violent, and Chronic Offenders

These offenders receive a disproportionate amount of attention from researchers, corrections officials, and policy-makers. One reason for this is that such youth represent a small proportion of juvenile offenders but account for the majority of juvenile offenses (Howell, Krisberg, & Jones, 1995; Loeber, Farrington, & Waschbusch, 1998). They also are involved in the crimes most likely to receive media coverage. It is important to note that the definition of serious, violent, and chronic offender varies across studies. Both local laws and the opinions of experts affect these definitions. With this is mind, common definitions and descriptions are explored below.

Serious offenders are usually defined as individuals who commit offenses such as burglary, auto theft, drug trafficking, or possession of a weapon (Loeber et al., 1998). Minor offenses, such as status offenses, vandalism, disorderly conduct, and motor vehicle violations are usually excluded from the category of serious offenses. *Violent offenders* are a category of serious offenders who commit acts of violence, including homicide, aggravated assault, kidnapping, and rape. Although there is some debate over the definition of a violent offense, minor acts of aggression such as simple assault are typically excluded (Loeber et al., 1998). It is generally agreed that *chronic offenders* are repeat offenders of relatively serious crimes (Loeber et al., 1998).

Although these three categories of offenders are sometimes used separately, it is important to note that there is substantial overlap between them (Farrington, 1991; Snyder, 1998). In a review of official court records, Snyder (1998) found that fewer than 30% of juveniles were serious, nonviolent offenders, 15% were identified as chronic offenders, and 8% were violent offenders; most of the sample (64%) were arrested for only nonserious offenses. In this study, Snyder found that approximately 30% of chronic offenders were also violent offenders; more than half of violent offenders were also chronic offenders; and 35% of serious offenders were also chronic offenders. In a subsequent review of crimes committed by chronic offenders, Loeber and colleagues (1998) found that chronic offenders comprised between 7 and 25% of delinquent youth.

Given that such a large proportion of offenses during the peak years of offending are committed by a relatively small number of offenders (Howell et al., 1995), it is important to examine the differences between these serious and chronic offenders and youth who do not engage in serious delinquent activities. Serious, violent, and chronic offenders are plagued with a number of serious problems, including truancy, substance use, and mental health problems (Loeber & Farrington, 2000), and they are disproportionately victims of violence (Loeber, Kalb, & Huizinga, 2001). These youth tend to begin their offending careers younger than other delinquents (Ge, Donnellan, & Wenk, 2001; Loeber & Farrington, 2000) and these careers tend to persist over time (Moffitt et al., 2002). In the following sections, we examine the developmental pathways and risk factors affecting the development of serious and lasting delinquent careers. These factors have important prevention and intervention implications (Lipsey & Derzon, 1998).

Pathways to Criminal Behavior

For many troubled youth, the pathway toward a career of serious or chronic juvenile offending begins early in life. Child delinquents (offenders under 12 years of age) are at significantly increased risk of developing serious criminal behaviors and engaging in these unlawful behaviors for a longer time. Recently, predictive trajectories for the development of serious delinquent careers have been developed through the important work of Loeber and colleagues. They have used factor and cluster analyses of delinquent behavior to identify three primary pathways to more serious delinquent careers (Loeber & Farrington, 2000; Loeber, Wei, Stouthamer-Loeber, Huizinga, & Thornberry, 1999).

The first is defined as an overt pathway. This pathway, typified by physical aggression, begins with minor acts of aggression and escalates to physical fighting and then more serious violent behavior. The second is defined as a covert pathway. This pathway begins with minor mischief, such as shoplifting or frequent lying, and escalates to acts such as property damage and then to increasingly serious acts of delinquent behavior. The third pathway is defined as the authority conflict pathway, which begins with stubborn behavior and moves toward disobedience and avoidance of authority (Loeber & Farrington, 2000; Loeber et al., 1999; Tolan & Gorman-Smith, 1998).

Loeber and colleagues postulated that along any of these pathways, two qualitative changes occur when youth escalate to increasingly serious acts of delinquency. First, delinquent and disruptive behaviors start at home and then progress outside of the home to the youth's school and/or broader community. Second, youth begin with antisocial behavior toward those close to them, such as relatives and peers; then, over time, they harm strangers in the neighborhood and, then, strangers increasingly far from home (Loeber & Farrington, 2000).

Understanding these pathways is important for targeting resources toward reversing this destructive path. However, further exploration of how children begin to progress down these trajectories is critical. In the following sections, the major risk factors contributing to the development of serious and lifelong careers are explored.

Risk Factors for Criminal Behavior

Several thorough reviews of risk and protective factors that affect the development of delinquency have recently been published (see Hawkins et al., 1998; Lipsey & Derzon, 1998; Stouthamer-Loeber, Loeber, Wei, Farrington, & Wikstrom, 2002). Across numerous studies, certain individual, family, and neighborhood/community characteristics have been identified as risk factors.

INDIVIDUAL RISK FACTORS

CHILDHOOD ANTISOCIAL BEHAVIORS. One of the mostly commonly discussed risk factors for serious offending is childhood delinquency and behavior problems, including antisocial behavior (Elliott et al., 1989; Farrington, 1989; Lipsey & Derzon, 1998; Patterson, Forgatch, Yoerger, & Stoolmiller, 1998; Sampson & Laub, 1993; Snyder & Sickmund, 1999). Sampson and Laub (1993) reported that the perpetration of childhood delinquency is significantly related to adolescent and adult criminal behavior. Specifically, youth who engaged in childhood delinquency were 3 to 4 times more likely to commit crimes during adulthood. Childhood offenders also commit more serious offenses during adolescence. Snyder and Sickmund (1999) found that childhood offenders are responsible for the majority of serious juvenile offenses. Other studies have found that the number of early onset antisocial behaviors, regardless of severity, is related to subsequent delinquent involvement (Farrington, 1989).

COGNITIVE ABILITIES. Several studies have indicated that poor cognitive development and neurocognitive problems are related to serious and persisting delinquency (Farrington & Hawkins, 1991; Farrington, Jolliffe, Loeber, Stouthamer-Loeber, & Kalb, 2001; Moffitt & Caspi, 2001; Moffitt, Lynam, & Silva, 1994). Measures of cognitive ability, such as IQ measurements taken during childhood, are a significant predictor of later delinquency (Farrington, 1995; Ge et al., 2001; Moffitt et al., 1994; Sigurdsson, Gudjonsson, & Peersen, 2001).

SUBSTANCE USE. Substance use has long been associated with delinquent and criminal behaviors. Substance abusing behaviors, including both alcohol and illicit drug use, significantly predict delinquency (Hirschi, 1969; Lipsey & Derzon, 1998). In fact, through a meta-analysis, Lipsey and Derzon (1998) found that substance use was one of the strongest predictors of serious and persistent delinquency.

SCHOOL FAILURE. Academic failure, including poor school performance and dropping out of school, is significantly related to serious delinquency (Farrington, 1989; Hawkins et al., 1998; Lipsey & Derzon, 1998; Thornberry, Moore, & Christenson, 1985). For example, Farrington's (1989) research indicated that high truancy rates and discipline problems were associated with the perpetration of violent offenses.

DELINQUENT PEERS. Association with delinquent peers, including siblings, is related to serious offenses during adolescence (Farrington, 1989; Hawkins et al., 1998; Maguin & Loeber, 1996). Further, the lack of appropriate strong social ties with peers and adults is a significant predictor of serious delinquent offenses (Lipsey & Derzon, 1998).

FAMILY RISK FACTORS

FAMILY STRUCTURE AND SIZE. A study assessing risk and protective factors in childhood delinquency revealed that single-parent homes, families with a large number of children, and divorced parents are all risk factors for child delinquency (Wasserman et al., 2003). A combination of more siblings, less parental influence, and greater antisocial peer associations have been attributed with increased delinquency (Fleener, 1999).

PARENTING PRACTICES. Sampson and Laub (1993) identified four parenting factors that predicted youth offending. These included erratic and harsh discipline practices, lack of parental supervision, parental rejection, and weak bonds between parent and child. In another study, three specific family practices were found to be particularly associated with conduct problems. These included high levels of parent-child conflict, poor monitoring of children, and low levels of positive parental involvement (Wasserman et al., 2003).

Other studies have found similar evidence that some parenting practices are a risk factor for delinquency (Wolfgang, Figlio, & Sellin, 1972), including inadequate parenting and family management skills (Hawkins et al., 1998; Moffitt & Caspi, 2001; Patterson, Crosby, & Vuchinich, 1992), an adverse family environment (Ge et al., 2001), lack of parental supervision (Farrington, 1995; McCord, 1996; Sampson & Laub, 1993), and lack of parental affection (McCord, 1996).

A study by Baker, Tabacoff, and Tornusciolo (2003) demonstrated that family systems that encourage secrecy and deception can contribute to the development of particular types of delinquency. For example, they found that adjudicated sexual offenders were more likely to have been told lies by their families, to have had their families exhibit taboo behaviors, and to have many family myths than a group of young people with conduct disorders (Baker et al., 2003).

Research has documented that there is a path from child abuse to juvenile offending. Specifically, physical abuse and neglect of children are significant predictive factors of later juvenile offense (Stewart, Dennison, & Waterson, 2002). Child abuse in unhealthful family environments is associated with more juvenile and adult arrests.

ANTISOCIAL PARENTS. Youth who have parents who model antisocial behaviors are at risk for delinquency and antisocial behaviors. Several studies have found that having an antisocial parent or a parent with a criminal history was related to youth who commit violent offenses or are seriously delinquent (Farrington et al., 2001; Hawkins et al., 1998; Lipsey & Derzon, 1998). Furthermore, antisocial adults tend to choose other antisocial adults as their partners and thus create family environments that are increasingly conflictive (Wasserman et al., 2003).

SOCIOECONOMICS. Family poverty is also a predictor of delinquency outcomes (Hawkins et al., 1998; Lipsey & Derzon, 1998; Stouthamer-Loeber et al., 2002). Derzon's meta-analysis (1997) demonstrated that socioeconomic status is a predictor of violent behavior in youth between the ages of 6 and 12 as well as of those between 12 and 15. Socioeconomic status was a better single predictor of violent behavior than other family characteristics, IQ of the youth, and broken home factors in both age groups (Derzon, 1997).

NEIGHBORHOOD OR COMMUNITY FACTORS

NEIGHBORHOOD POVERTY AND SOCIAL DISORGANIZATION. Being raised in an impoverished neighborhood has been associated with involvement in crime and violence (Farrington, 1989; Stouthamer-Loeber et al., 2002). Living in a neighborhood that is characterized by availability of drugs and firearms, adult joblessness, and adult criminal behavior can also contribute to rates of delinquency and violence (Thornberry, Huizinga, & Loeber, 1995). Impoverished neighborhoods are generally more likely to suffer from neighborhood disorganization. Neighborhood disorganization is generally characterized by weak social control networks that are unable to cope with criminal activity (Wasserman et al., 2003). Another study on community social organization found that juveniles who were raised in communities with high levels of sense of community were more likely to participate in prosocial behavior (Cantillon, Davidson, & Schweitzer, 2003).

VICTIMIZATION. Another important risk factor for delinquency is childhood and adolescent victimization. Research investigating the cyclical nature of violence suggested that victimization is linked to subsequent delinquency (Woodward & Fergusson, 2000). Children who have experienced family violence in their homes are twice as likely to engage in violent, criminal behaviors, thus creating a "cycle of violence" (Widom, 1989). Although young offenders are often portrayed as violent criminals and "juvenile predators," young people are actually disproportionately *victims* of violent crimes (Wordes & Nunez, 2002). In fact, teenagers are twice as likely as other age groups to be victims of violent crimes (Bureau of Justice Statistics, 2001). One survey conducted in 1995 indicated that up to 20% of adolescents were victims of violent crimes in the past year (Sieving et al., 2000). Therefore, an important step in preventing the development of violent delinquent careers may be the prevention of childhood and adolescent victimization. Some of the national dialogue on youthful offenders should be redirected toward victimization against our nation's young people.

Gangs

Interest in juvenile gangs has been longstanding. A recent Academy Award–nominated movie, *Gangs of New York*, is based on a classic study of juvenile gangs by Herbert Asbury that was first published in 1927. Gangs galvanize popular interest via the entertainment and news media, and they often have been the focus of public policy discussions about youthful offending. Social scientists have described different aspects of gang behavior and attempted to understand the etiology of these groups. At one time, many believed that gangs were largely a phenomenon specific to a few urban centers and largely confined to those areas of cities that had large concentrations of minority youth and new immigrants. Gangs were predominately male social groupings and were focused principally on protection of neighborhood "turfs." More recent surveys (see Howell in Howell et al., 1995) suggest that gangs are located more often in suburban areas and rural towns, female gangs are becoming more prevalent, and gangs are increasingly involved in drug trafficking activities. Over the last several years there has been a sense that the gang problem is increasing and that gangs are moving into smaller communities. Whether this perception is accurate or an artifact of greater law enforcement attention to gangs is a difficult issue to resolve.

Gangs remain an elusive phenomenon because teenagers frequently congregate, and some of their group behaviors involve illegal activities. Thus, entities as diverse as neo-Nazis, high school fraternities, radical political movements, street corner groups, and adolescent sports teams might, under some definitions, be considered "gangs." There is no universally accepted definition of what constitutes a gang, and the boundaries between juvenile gangs and other group-oriented criminal behaviors are "fuzzy" (Klein, 1995). Critics of law enforcement antigang campaigns have argued that these efforts are directed primarily at minority and immigrant youngsters because the police choose to define the gang-like behavior of White middle-class youth as more benign "clubs" or cliques. However, some of the school shootings that have involved mostly White youth from more prosperous communities suggest the existence of gangs in these communities.

Should we worry about gangs? Definitely. Research in Rochester, New York, and Denver, Colorado (Esbensen & Huizinga, 1993; Thornberry, Krohn, Lizotte, & Chard-Wierschem, 1993), indicates that participation in gangs adds additional risk factors to otherwise delinquency-prone youth. Further, these studies indicate that gang involvement is associated with more frequent illegal acts and more violent behavior among teenagers.

Can we worry too much about gangs? Probably. There has been a pernicious tendency to suggest that youth gangs are becoming national and even international criminal syndicates. It has been suggested that juvenile street gangs dominate the drug trade and that gangs account for almost all the murders in most communities. Few of these allegations have withstood empirical investigation (Klein, 1995). Law enforcement agencies have developed elaborate fictions about massive gang conspiracies that resonate with their own organizational agendas for greater levels of staffing and funding. Some of these gang stories are derived from police listening to adolescents with rich imaginations who are more than willing to tell, and embellish, stories about the fantastic exploits of their peers to law enforcement officials.

Young people tend to be joiners. Gangs provide a way for youth who are not fitting into socially acceptable groups to band together to shore up fragile adolescent self-images. Gangs also can provide a sense of protection from school and playgroup bullies. During most of the time these youth spend with their gangs, they are engaging in noncriminal behavior. Gangs are a vehicle to gain access to commodities, though illegal, and to earn money, though outside the legitimate labor market. But gangs can also facilitate crime by introducing novices to more criminally sophisticated young adults or by creating a climate in which social inhibitions are lessened. Periodically we have witnessed examples of group-incited adolescent violence, such as group rapes, riots at high school sporting events, or mass looting or vandalism that begins during celebrations.

While there is a rich literature about gangs, we are a long way from understanding the pushes and pulls into and out of gang behavior. More needs to be known about the different levels of youthful gang involvement. Although there is usually a very small core of regular gang members, most youth belong to gangs in an occasional and episodic manner. The relationship between juvenile gangs and adult criminal groups is another important topic for further study. In some locales, it appears that gangs that form in prisons and youth correctional facilities later spill out into communities. Last, there is very little consensus about what social interventions are effective in reducing the negative aspects of gang behavior.

Overrepresentation of Minority Youth

Disproportionate minority representation is one of the largest problems plaguing the juvenile justice system. In response to growing concern with this issue, the federal Juvenile Justice Act was amended in 1992 to require states seeking funding from the Office of Juvenile Justice and Delinquency Prevention to examine disproportionate minority confinement in their juvenile justice systems. Participating states were also encouraged to make efforts to ameliorate the problem. Disproportionate representation exists, not only in confinement, but at every stage of the juvenile justice system, beginning with arrest rates. In a national review of dozens of state-specific studies, Hamparian and Leiber (1997) found that the overrepresentation of minority youth increased progressively from the arrest stage through adjudication. The largest gap between White youth and children of color occurs at early stages of the justice process, at the point of arrest, court intake, and detention (Poe-Yamagata & Jones, 2000). However, these initial disparities are exacerbated at later stages of the process, adding to the disadvantage experienced by minority youth in the juvenile justice system.

Racial disparities cannot be explained by higher levels of offending by minority groups (Huizinga & Elliott, 1987). Although African American youth self-reported modestly higher frequencies of offending than White youth, the differences were not statistically significant, and they could not explain the discrepancy between groups in arrest rates or at other stages of juvenile processing.

If not driven by an offense pattern, why are minorities disproportionately represented at every stage of juvenile processing? The answer is complex and likely includes subjective decision making (by police, intake workers, prosecutors, and judges), intentional or unintentional profiling, biased policies, economic disadvantage, and inadequate community resources. More research needs to be conducted to increase understanding of this issue, but what is needed even more than that is research pointing to solutions. There are few issues more salient in the need to reform juvenile justice practices than disproportionate minority representation.

Conclusion

In this chapter we have reviewed some key empirical data on juvenile offending. The field of juvenile crime is often dominated by media portrayals and public policy discussions that are not grounded in solid research. For example, recent trends in juvenile arrest data show a steady decline in youth participation in the most serious crimes since the mid-1990s. Yet the popular myth is that rates of juvenile delinquency are rising out of control. We have also noted that young people are more likely to be victims than perpetrators of violent crime. Nevertheless, many in the general public see teenagers as fearsome "superpredators."

During the past decade there has emerged a significant body of longitudinal studies that reveal a great deal about pathways into and out of serious and chronic juvenile offending. Although episodic involvement in delinquency is pervasive among many adolescents, only a small fraction of these young people persist in serious and chronic law breaking. The emerging research gives us new clues to accurately gauging the risk and protective factors for chronic offending. Specifically, we have seen how issues such as negative peer influences, exposure to family violence, and early problem behavior can exacerbate delinquent careers. Gang involvement also has been identified as a crucial causal factor.

These data and recent research provide a solid foundation for programs to prevent serious juvenile offending and to treat juvenile law violators. Current early intervention and juvenile justice strategies need to be reexamined in light of the evolving scientific data. Finally, there are remaining measurement issues about official data and self-report surveys that must be confronted before a more robust empirical picture of juvenile offending can emerge.

References

Arnett, J. (1992). Reckless behavior in adolescence: A developmental perspective. *Developmental Review, 12,* 339–373.

Baker, A. J. I., Tabacoff, R., & Tornusciolo, G. (2003). Family secrecy: A comparative study of juvenile sex offenders and youth. *Family Process, 42,* 105–116.

Blumstein, A., Cohen, J., Roth, J. A., & Visher, C. A. (1986). *Criminal careers and "career criminals."* Washington, DC: National Academy Press.

Bureau of Justice Statistics. (2001). *Criminal victimization in the United States, 1999 statistics tables: National Crime Victimization Survey.* Washington, DC: U.S. Department of Justice, Office of Justice Programs.

Cantillon, D., Davidson, W. S., & Schweitzer, J. H. (2003). Measuring community social organization: Sense of community as a mediator in social disorganization theory. *Journal of Criminal Justice, 31,* 321–339.

Derzon, J. H. (1997). *The developmental trajectory for violence: Predictive relationships across two life stages.* Nashville, TN: Vanderbilt Institute for Public Policy Studies.

Elliott, D., & Ageton, S. (1980). Reconciling race and class differences in self-reported and official estimate of delinquency. *American Sociological Review, 45,* 95–110.

Elliott, D. S., Huizinga, D., & Menard, S. (1989). *Multiple problem youth: Delinquency, substance use, and mental health problem.* New York: Springer-Verlag.

Esbensen, F. A., & Huizinga, D. (1993). Gangs, drugs, and delinquency in a survey of urban youth. *Criminology, 31,* 565–589.

Farrington, D. P. (1989). Early predictors of adolescent aggression and adult violence. *Violence and Victims, 4,* 79–100.

Farrington, D. P. (1991). Childhood aggression and adult violence. Early precursors and later-life outcomes. In D. J. Pepler & K. H. Rubin (Eds.), *The development and treatment of childhood aggression* (pp. 5–29). Hillsdale, NJ: Erlbaum.

Farrington, D. P. (1995). The development of offending and antisocial behavior from childhood: Key findings from the Cambridge Study in Delinquent Development. *Journal of Child Psychology and Psychiatry, 360,* 929–964.

Farrington, D. P., & Hawkins, J. D. (1991). Predicting participation, early onset and later persistence in officially recorded offending. *Criminal Behavior and Mental Health,* 1, 1–33.

Farrington, D. P., Jolliffe, D., Loeber, R., Stouthamer-Loeber, M., & Kalb, L. M. (2001). The concentration of offenders in families, and family criminality in the prediction of boys' delinquency. *Journal of Adolescence,* 24, 579–596.

Fleener, F. T (1999). Family as a factor in delinquency. *Psychological Reports,* 85, 80–81.

Ge, X., Donnellan, M. B., & Wenk, E. (2001). The development of persistent criminal offending in males. *Criminal Justice and Behavior,* 28, 731–755.

Hamparian, D., & Leiber, M. (1997). *Disproportionate confinement of minority juveniles in secure facilities: 1996 national report.* Champaign, IL: Community Research Associates.

Hawkins, D. F., Laub, J. H., Lauritsen, J. L., & Cothern, L. (2000). *Race, ethnicity, and serious and violent juvenile offending.* Washington, DC: U.S. Department of Justice, Office of Justice Programs, Office of Juvenile Justice and Delinquency Prevention.

Hawkins, J. D., Terrenkohl, T., Farrington, D. P., Brewer, D., Catalano, R. F., & Harachi, T. W. (1998). A review of predictors of youth violence. In R. Loeber & D. P Farrington (Eds.), *Serious and violent juvenile offenders. Risk factors and successful interventions* (pp. 313–345). Thousand Oaks, CA: Sage.

Hirschi, T. (1969). *Causes of delinquency.* Berkeley: University of California Press.

Howell, J. C., Krisberg, B., & Jones, M. (1995). Trends in juvenile crime and youth violence. In J. C. Howell, B. Krisberg, J. D. Hawkins, & J. J. Wilson (Eds.), *Sourcebook on serious, violent, and chronic juvenile offenders* (pp. 1–35). Thousand Oaks, CA: Sage.

Huizinga, D., & Elliott, D. S. (1987). Juvenile offenders: prevalence, offender incidence, and arrest rates by race. *Crime and Delinquency,* 33, 206–223.

Kelly, B. T., Huizinga, D., Thornberry, T. P., & Loeber, R. (1997). *Epidemiology of serious violence.* Washington, DC: U.S. Department of Justice, Office of Justice Programs, Office of Juvenile Justice and Delinquency Prevention.

Klein, M. W. (1995). *The American street gang: Its nature, prevalence, and control.* New York: Oxford University Press.

Krisberg, B. (in press). *Redeeming our children.* Woodland Hills, CA: Sage.

Lipsey, M. W., & Derzon, J. H. (1998). Predictors of violent or serious delinquency in adolescents and early adulthood: A synthesis of longitudinal research. In R. Loeber & D. P. Farrington (Eds.), *Serious and violent juvenile offenders. Risk factors and successful interventions.* Thousand Oaks, CA: Sage.

Loeber, R., & Farrington, D. P. (2000). Young children who commit crime: Epidemiology, developmental origins, risk factors, early interventions, and policy implications. *Development and Psychopathology,* 12, 737–762.

Loeber, R., Farrington, D. P., & Waschbusch, D. A. (1998). Serious and violent juvenile offenders. In R. Loeber & D. P. Farrington (Eds.), *Serious and violent juvenile offenders. Risk factors and successful interventions.* Thousand Oaks, CA: Sage.

Loeber, R., Kalb, L., & Huizinga, D. (2001). *Juvenile delinquency and serious injury victimization.* Washington, DC: U.S. Department of Justice, Office of Justice Programs, Office of Juvenile Justice and Delinquency Prevention.

Loeber, R., Wei, E., Stouthamer-Loeber, M., Huizinga, D., & Thornberry, T. (1999). Behavioral antecedents to serious and violent juvenile offending: Joint analyses from the Denver Youth Survey, Pittsburgh Youth Study, and the Rochester Development Study. *Studies in Crime Prevention,* 8, 245–263.

Maguin, E., & Loeber, R. (1996). Academic performance and delinquency. In M. Tonry (Ed.), *Crime and justice: A review of research* (Vol. 20, pp. 145–264). Chicago: University of Chicago Press.

McCord, J. (1996). Family relationship, juvenile delinquency, and adult criminality. *Criminology, 29,* 397–417.

Moffitt, T. E. (1993). "Life-course-persistent" and "adolescence-limited" antisocial behavior: A developmental taxonomy. *Psychological Review, 100,* 674–701.

Moffitt, T. E., & Caspi, A. (2001). Childhood predictors differentiate life-course persistent and adolescence-limited antisocial pathways among males and females. *Development and Psychopathology, 13,* 355–375.

Moffitt, T. E., Caspi, A., Harrington, H., & Milne, B. J. (2002). Males on the life-course-persistent and adolescent-limited antisocial pathways: Follow-up at age 26. *Development and Psychopathology, 14,* 179–207.

Moffitt, T. E., Lynam, D., & Silva, P. A. (1994). Neuropsychological tests predicting persistent male delinquency. *Criminology, 32,* 277–300.

Patterson, G. R., Crosby, L., & Vuchinich, S. (1992). Parenting, peers, and the stability of antisocial behavior in preadolescent males. *Developmental Psychology, 28,* 510–521.

Patterson, G. R., Forgatch, M. S., Yoerger, K. L., & Stoolmiller, M. (1998). Variables that initiate and maintain an early-onset trajectory for juvenile offending. *Development and Psycholopathology, 10,* 531–547.

Poe-Yamagata, E., & Jones, M. (2000). *And justice for some.* San Francisco: National Council on Crime and Delinquency.

Sampson, R., & Laub, J. (1993). *Crime in the making: Pathways and turning points through life.* Cambridge, MA: Harvard University Press.

Sieving, R. E., Beuhring, T., Resnick, M. D., Bearinger, L. H., Shew, M., Ireland, M., et al. (2000). Development of adolescent self-report measures from the National Longitudinal Study of Adolescent Health. *Journal of Adolescent Health, 28,* 73–81.

Sigurdsson, J. F., Gudjonsson, G. H., & Peersen, M. (2001). Differences in the cognitive ability and personality of desisters and re-offenders: A prospective study among young offenders. *Psychology, Crime & Law, 7,* 33–43.

Snyder, H. N. (1998). Serious, violent, and chronic juvenile offenders: An assessment of extent of and trends in officially recognized serious criminal behavior in a delinquent population. In R. Loeber & D. P. Farrington (Eds.), *Serious and violent juvenile offenders. Risk factors and successful interventions* (pp. 68–85). Thousand Oaks, CA: Sage.

Snyder, H. N. (2002). *Juvenile arrests 2000.* Washington, DC: U.S. Department of Justice, Office of Justice Programs, Office of Juvenile Justice and Delinquency Prevention.

Snyder, H. N., & Sickmund, N. (1999). *Juvenile offenders and victims: 1999 national report.* Washington, DC: U.S. Department of Justice, Office of Justice Programs, Office of Juvenile Justice and Delinquency Prevention.

Stewart, A., Dennison, S., & Waterson, E. (2002). Pathways from child maltreatment to juvenile offending. *Trends and issues in crime and criminal justice.* Canberra, Australia: Australian Institute of Criminology.

Stouthamer-Loeber, M., Loeber, R., Wei, E., Farrington, D. P., & Wikstrom, P. H. (2002). Risk and promotive effects in the explanation of persistent serious delinquency in boys. *Journal of Consulting and Clinical Psychology, 70,* 111–123.

Thornberry, T. P., Huizinga, D., & Loeber, R. (1995). The prevention of serious delinquency and violence: Implications from the Program of Research on the Causes and Correlates of Delinquency. In J. C. Howell, B. Krisberg, J. D. Hawkins, & J. J. Wilson (Eds.), *Sourcebook on serious, violent, and chronic juvenile offenders* (pp. 213–237). Thousand Oaks, CA: Sage.

Thornberry, T. P., & Krohn, M. D. (2000). The self-report method for measuring delinquency and crime. *Measurement and Analysis of Crime and Justice, 4,* 33–83.

Thornberry, T. P., Krohn, M. D., Lizotte, A. J., & Chard-Wierschem, D. (1993). The role of juvenile gangs in facilitating delinquent behavior. *Journal of Research in Crime and Delinquency, 30,* 55–87.

Thornberry, T. P., Moore, M., & Christenson, R. L. (1985). The effect of dropping out of high school on subsequent criminal behavior. *Criminology, 23,* 3–18.

Tolan, P. H., & Gorman-Smith, D. (1998). Development of serious and violent offending careers. In R. Loeber & D. P. Farrington (Eds.), *Serious and violent juvenile offenders. Risk factors and successful interventions* (pp. 68–85). Thousand Oaks, CA: Sage.

Wasserman, G. A., Keenan, K., Tremblay, R. E., Coie, J. D., Herrenkohl, R. L., & Petechuk, D. (2003). Risk and protective factors of child delinquency. *Child delinquency.* Bulletin. Washington, DC:, U.S. Department of Justice, Office of Juvenile Justice and Delinquency Prevention.

Widom, C. S. (1989). The cycle of violence. *Science, 244,* 160–166.

Wolfgang, M. E., Figlio, R., & Sellin, T. (1972). *Delinquency in a birth cohort.* Chicago: University of Chicago Press.

Woodward, L. J., & Fergusson, D. (2000). Childhood peer relationship problems and later risks of educational under-achievement and unemployment. *Journal of Child Psychology and Psychiatry, 41,* 191–201.

Wordes, M., & Nunez, M. (2002). *Our vulnerable teenagers: Their victimization, its consequences, and directions for prevention and intervention.* Oakland, CA: National Council on Crime and Delinquency.

Zimring, F. (1981). Kids, groups, and crime: Some implications of a well-known secret. *Journal of Criminal Law and Criminology, 72,* 867.

5

Naomi E. Sevin Goldstein, Oluseyi Olubadewo,
Richard E. Redding, and Frances J. Lexcen

Mental Health Disorders
The Neglected Risk Factor in Juvenile Delinquency

Once a neglected area of study, the relationship between mental health and delinquency has recently become a major focus in juvenile justice jurisprudence. Lawyers, judges, and policy-makers have expressed concern about the unmet mental health needs of juvenile delinquents. Juvenile justice research has repeatedly suggested that inadequate attention to mental health problems may lead to recidivism and future adult offending (Lexcen & Redding, 2000; Wierson, Forehand, & Frame, 1992). For example, a comparison between male juvenile delinquents receiving adequate mental health care and those receiving insufficient care revealed that the latter group committed twice as many adult offenses and twice as many violent crimes (Lewis, Yeager, Lovely, Stein, & Cobham-Portorreal, 1994).

Attention to the mental health of juvenile delinquents is particularly important because rates of mental illness in this population are substantially higher than those found in the general adolescent population. The rate of mental illness in the general adolescent population is approximately 20% (U.S. Department of Health and Human Services, 2001), and although estimates in the juvenile offender population vary greatly, rates are at least twice those associated with nonoffending youth (Cocozza & Skowyra, 2000).

This chapter reports the prevalence and characteristics of common mental health disorders in this population and describes the most promising mental health treatment options for juvenile delinquents. Further, risk factors that predispose juveniles to delinquent behavior and mental health problems are reviewed. Finally, the higher rates of mental health-related problems among female juvenile offenders are addressed.

Mental Disorder Prevalence Rates Among Juvenile Offenders

Research has shown prevalence rates of "mental illness" among juvenile offenders ranging from 20% (Cocozza & Skowyra, 2000) to 100% (McManus, Alessi,

Grapentine, & Brickman, 1984). This wide variability in rates is largely attributed to the inconsistent samples and methods used across studies (Goldstein et al., 2003a). The most common disorders among youthful offenders are conduct, mood, substance use, and attention-deficit hyperactivity disorders (Lexcen & Redding, 2000; Teplin, Abram, McClelland, Dulcan, & Mericle, 2002; Ulzen & Hamilton, 1998; Wasserman, McReynolds, Lucas, Fisher, & Santos, 2002), with conduct disorder being the most frequent. Symptoms of conduct disorder, such as stealing and destroying property, may often be the actions that result in arrests (Wierson et al., 1992). Because the symptoms of conduct disorder may directly result in arrest and because delinquent behaviors are symptoms of conduct disorder, the high prevalence of this disorder is expected, with rates ranging from 87 to 91% in the chronic juvenile offender population (Lexcen & Redding, 2000). Other disruptive behavior disorders diagnosed among juvenile offenders are oppositional defiant disorder (14.5% for boys, 17.5% for girls) (Teplin et al., 2002) and mania (2.2% for boys, 1.8% for girls) (Teplin et al., 2002), associated with bipolar disorder (Lexcen & Redding, 2000). Despite the overlap between conduct disorder and juvenile delinquency, conduct disorder is not necessarily the primary diagnosis of youth in this population. Mood disorders, such as major depressive disorder and dysthymia, have been identified in some studies (e.g., McManus et al., 1984) as more common primary diagnoses than conduct disorder. This is especially true among girls in the juvenile justice system (Lexcen & Redding, 2000).

Stable prevalence rates are difficult to obtain for this population because research results vary widely. Several factors contribute to the range of rates (Cocozza, 1992; Teplin et al., 2002). First, the timing of studies varies widely. Whether youth were tested within 12 hours of entering a facility or 12 months after admittance may have affected the appearance of symptoms, their intensities, and the lengths of time those symptoms had been experienced, as stress levels can vary with different phases of the juvenile process, and mental health symptoms can be exacerbated by stress (Deardorff, Gonzales, & Sandler, 2003).

Second, the gender, ethnicity, and ages of subjects vary widely across studies. Prevalence rates can be dramatically affected by gender. Compared to boys, 2 to 3 times as many female juvenile offenders are diagnosable with a mental illness (i.e., exceed clinical cutoff scores on standardized diagnostic instruments) (Timmons-Mitchell et al., 1997), and female juvenile offenders are typically diagnosed with more comorbid mental health problems (Grisso, 1999; Lexcen & Redding, 2000). Likewise, diagnoses and mental health-related problems can vary by race and ethnicity (Teplin et al., 2002). For instance, smaller proportions of African American incarcerated adolescents met criteria for anxiety disorders and for some types of substance abuse than did other incarcerated youth (Domalanta, Risser, Roberts, & Risser, 2003), and White male offenders were 3 times more likely to attempt suicide than were African American male offenders (Kempton & Forehand, 1992). Additionally, age may affect prevalence rates of disorders, as some disorders have later ages of onset than others. Thus, prevalence rates may vary according to the demographic characteristics of juvenile offender samples.

Third, prevalence rates may also be influenced by the settings in which studies are conducted. Community-based detention centers, state-run detention centers, outpatient court clinics, foster care or halfway housing, and state-sponsored disciplinary schooling offer various levels of confinement. Restriction of freedom may affect the intensity of juvenile offenders' symptoms or, alternatively, judges may adjudicate youth to specific programs based, in part, on whether they present with or have a history of mental health symptoms.

Fourth, the method of sampling employed (i.e., random sampling vs. convenient sampling) may affect obtained prevalence rates, as different methods may affect sample size and, consequently, the representativeness of the sample. Additionally, different assessment procedures were used to obtain diagnoses across studies, such as record reviews, clinical interviews, self-reports, observational ratings, or a combination of methods (Teplin et al., 2002). The reliability, validity, and sensitivity of these methods vary considerably, further contributing to the inconsistency of findings across studies.

Despite such variability, it is clear that compared to adolescents in the general population, at least twice as many juvenile delinquents are diagnosable with mental health disorders (Cocozza, 1992). Furthermore, of youth diagnosed with mental health disorders, the number of diagnoses for juvenile offenders far exceeds the number for adolescents in the general population (Wierson et al., 1992).

Substance Abuse

Many high school students report the occasional use of substances (e.g., alcohol, marijuana, cocaine) (National Clearinghouse for Alcohol and Drug Information [NCADI], 1999). Juvenile offenders, however, report significantly higher rates of substance dependence and abuse than do their peers (Ulzen & Hamilton, 1998). Substance abusing juvenile offenders often experience recurrent legal problems resulting from their use of substances (American Psychiatric Association, 1994). In addition to arrests for possession or use of alcohol or illicit drugs, juvenile offenders may be high or intoxicated during the commission of the crimes for which they are arrested (National Institute of Justice, 2003).

Substance abuse and dependence account for a substantial portion of the clinical diagnoses among juvenile offenders. Teplin and colleagues (2002) found similar rates of substance abuse disorder for both boys (50.7%) and girls (46.8%) in this population. Another study of seriously delinquent juveniles found that 63% concurrently abused more than one drug (McManus et al., 1984). A third study found that 40% of incarcerated adolescents met criteria for alcohol dependence (Ulzen & Hamilton, 1998). The majority of youth in this third sample also reported using both marijuana and street drugs, such as cocaine, crack, and speed. This finding of multiple drug use among adolescent offenders appears consistent across studies (e.g., Brunelle, Brochu, & Cousineau, 2000; McManus et al., 1984; Neighbors, Kempton, & Forehand, 1992).

The direction of causality between substance abuse and delinquency is un-

clear. Many researchers assert that, based on empirical evidence, juvenile delinquency is a strong predictor of future substance abuse (Wierson et al., 1992),
whereas other researchers hold the view that drug addiction precedes delinquent
behaviors (Brunelle et al., 2000). Substance intoxication reduces inhibition,
impairs judgment (Wierson et al., 1992), and may increase a youth's willingness
to commit crimes, particularly violent crimes (Lexcen & Redding, 2000). In
addition, continued drug use requires substantial amounts of money; therefore,
youth may need to commit crimes, such as theft, drug dealing, or prostitution, to
maintain drug habits.

Regardless of the direction of causality, researchers generally agree that substance use and delinquency are interdependent (Wierson et al., 1992). More
serious delinquency is associated with more serious drug use (Johnson, Wish,
Schmeidler, & Huizinga, 1991), and use of specific types of drugs is associated
with particular types of crime (Smart, Mann, & Tyson, 1997). A greater number
of offenses and more violent crimes tend to occur with the use of prescription
pills, cocaine, or amphetamines, whereas minor offenses and nonviolent crimes
tend to occur with the use of alcohol or when no substances have been con-
sumed (Brunelle et al., 2000; Dawkins, 1997; Johnson et al., 1991).

Substance abuse frequently co-occurs with other disorders in adolescent offenders. For instance, use of multiple drugs is related to the number of depressive symptoms reported by incarcerated adolescents. Juvenile offenders using
either alcohol or marijuana reported fewer depressive symptoms than did offenders using more than one drug (other than alcohol or marijuana) concurrently
(Neighbors et al., 1992). Substances may be used to cope with depression (Green
& Ritter, 2000; Pollock, Maisto, Cornelius, & Martin, 2000), and three quarters
of offenders in one sample reported using drugs to alleviate feelings of sadness
and depression (Farrow & French, 1986). However, other studies also have
demonstrated that substance use can trigger episodes of depression (Miller, 2001;
Rodell, Benda, & Rodell, 2001; Silberg, Rutter, D'Onforio, & Eaves, 2003).
Thus, it is possible that depression and substance use feed off one another bidi-
rectionally, with each problem exacerbated by the other. Substance abuse also
appears as a symptom of conduct disorder (Lexcen & Redding, 2000), and adolescents diagnosed with both substance abuse and conduct disorder are much
more likely to become involved with the juvenile justice system than are youth
suffering solely from either substance abuse or conduct disorder (Grilo, Fehon,
Walker, & Martino, 1996; Lexcen & Redding, 2000).

Common substance abuse programs for juvenile offenders include inpatient and outpatient treatment, behavioral family therapy, multisystemic therapy,
and drug courts. Inpatient treatment may initially seem desirable for young
offenders because so many exhibit low motivation to change and poor social
functioning and come from distressed homes. However, inpatient treatment has
been found no more effective than outpatient treatment (Jainchill, 2000;
Williams & Chang, 2000), and, in fact, it may interfere with the youth's access to
natural environments to practice coping and other therapeutic skills.

Behavioral family therapy involves teaching family members to alter contingency patterns in response to a youth's desirable and undesirable behaviors in

order to maximize cooperation and reduce social noncompliance, delinquency, and drug use. The basis for this treatment is that drug-abusing adolescents typically receive more attention from parents when they are embroiled in substance abuse crises than when they are functioning well. This approach to treatment teaches parents to assign responsibilities for behavior with contingent privileges, including bonuses for superior performance and punishment for inferior performance. Families work together to identify the behaviors parents desire and rewards youth would like to receive. Negotiation skills are taught as part of the process, as are record-keeping skills to monitor the completion of the behavioral contract (Rueger & Liberman, 1984). Behavioral family therapy has been found to be an effective treatment for psychological disorders (Smith, Sayger, & Szykula, 1999). In children ages 5 to 14, Smith and colleagues (1999) found significant differences between pre- and posttreatment levels of internalizing behaviors (i.e., depression and anxiety) and externalizing behaviors (i.e., aggressiveness and delinquency). However, they did not find differences in levels of substance abuse, and behavioral family therapy was not significantly more effective than were other methods of family therapy.

Multisystemic therapy (MST) for substance abusing delinquents may provide the most reliable and valid data on treatment effectiveness for substance abusing juvenile offenders; MST has been studied with large numbers of adolescents in multiple geographic locations. MST conceptualizes the adolescent as a product of a set of nested systems, including home, school, peers, neighborhood, and the larger community (Henggeler et al., 1991), with treatment addressing the dysfunctional transactions across these systems. Intervention requires engaging family members, teachers, social service agencies, and others who have significant contact with the adolescent (Henggeler et al., 1991). Research results suggest MST is an effective and promising treatment (Henggeler, Clingempeel, Brondino, & Pickrel, 2002), and detailed findings are available in chapter 11 in this volume.

Another intervention option is the use of juvenile drug courts to handle juvenile delinquents with substance abuse problems. This treatment's popularity grew out of the success of adult drug courts and is patterned closely after the adult system's structure (Cooper & Bartlett, 1998). Requirements for completion often involve approximately 1 year of consistent compliance. Generally, the juvenile must maintain a set period of sobriety, establish a stable living situation, and obtain a high school diploma or GED certificate in order to graduate from drug court and have their charges dropped. Some programs also require successful completion of community service hours, completion of alcohol and drug treatment, and workforce preparation (Cooper & Bartlett, 1998). Involuntary termination usually occurs after repeated failures to adhere to the program requirements (Cooper & Bartlett, 1998). See Tate and Redding (ch. 7 in this volume) for a more detailed review of diversionary strategies, such as drug courts.

Treatment dropout for families of substance-dependent or abusing juvenile offenders is a persistent problem (Pompi, 1994). Strategies for improving completion rates include acceptance into treatment programs earlier in the course of the disorder, higher levels of parental involvement with treatment providers, and concrete program planning (Stark, 1992; Szapocznik et al., 1988). Incorporating MST or facets of this treatment (e.g. family-directed goal planning, continuous access to service providers) has been found effective in terms of both outcome and cost when compared with traditional community services (Henggeler, Pickrel, Brondino, & Crouch, 1996). Henggeler and colleagues (1996) noted that successful implementation of this program requires a high level of commitment by service providers, as demonstrated by increased family engagement and time involvement.

Treatment programs should incorporate relapse prevention techniques in order to prevent loss of effective treatment gains. Such techniques include participation in therapeutic booster sessions, learning how to recognize and avoid triggers of drug use, and participation in community-based programs to maintain access to drug-free experiences (Goldstein et al., 2003b). One study demonstrated the effectiveness of booster sessions for relapse prevention, finding that after a brief period of relapse after 6 months of initial treatment, subjects receiving booster sessions had lower rates of substance use and academic problems (Bry & Krinsley, 1992).

Depression and Suicidal Behavior

Depression is the most common mood disorder among juvenile delinquents. Depression in adolescents is characterized by depressed mood, changes in sleep and appetite, impaired cognitive processes, and suicidal ideation (Weiss & Garber, 2003). Depressed adolescents' thought processes are often marked by hopelessness, fatalistic or catastrophic thinking, and negative automatic thoughts (Belsher, Wilkes, & Rush, 1995; Curry & Craighead, 1990; Garber, Weiss, & Shanley, 1993; Pinto & Francis, 1993). Depression is also frequently comorbid with other disorders, such as conduct disorder, alcohol and substance abuse, and attention-deficit/hyperactivity disorder, or ADHD (Biederman, Faraone, Mick, Moore, & Lelon, 1996; King et al., 1996; Patterson, Crosby, & Vuchinich, 1992). Depressed delinquent males are more likely to have comorbid diagnoses of substance dependence, ADHD, posttraumatic stress disorder (PTSD), and other anxiety disorders than nondepressed boys (Kashani et al., 1980). The onset of the comorbid disorder(s) frequently predates the depressive disorder (Biederman et al., 1996).

Self-ratings of depression in juvenile offenders correlate highly with clinician diagnoses ($r = .73$) (McManus et al., 1984), suggesting that adolescents' complaints of despondent mood, suicidal ideation, or changes in sleep, appetite, or energy should be taken seriously as indicators of potential depression. It has been reported that studies using clinical interviews with delinquent subjects found much higher prevalence rates of affective disorder diagnoses (32 to 78%) than those employing record data without client interviews (2 to 12%) (Otto, Greenstein, Johnson, & Friedmen, 1992). Although depression is of concern for male juvenile offenders, it is found much more frequently among girls in this population (Lexcen & Redding, 2000). Prevalence rates of depression in female juvenile delinquents range from 21.6% (Teplin et al., 2002) to 67% (Myers, Burket, Lyles, Stone, & Kemph, 1990), with most studies' estimates falling on the higher end (Goldstein et al., 2003a).

Delinquency and childhood depression are associated (Loeber & Keenan, 1994; Ryan & Redding, 2003; Wierson et al., 1992). Depressed children are more likely to engage in delinquent acts, such as physical aggression and stealing, than are nondepressed children (Loeber & Keenan, 1994; Wierson et al., 1992). Depressed children also exhibit greater rates of conduct problems, impulsivity, and hyperactivity (Wierson et al., 1992). With respect to the relationship between depression and antisocial behavior, it has been suggested that disruptive behavior is a symptom of childhood depression (Takeda, 2000; Tisher, 1995), particularly in boys, and that depression can contribute to or exacerbate delinquent behavior (Ryan & Redding, in press). However, others have found that conduct disorder often predates depression (Loeber & Keenan, 1994). Symptoms of conduct disorder emerge earlier in depressed boys, even when accounting for a period of withdrawal and abstinence from substances (Riggs, Baker, Mikulich, Young, & Crowley, 1995).

Suicidal ideation and behaviors are frequently associated with depression (Lexcen & Redding, 2000; Kempton & Forehand, 1992; Wierson et al., 1992). Depression is significantly associated with suicide among White male juvenile offenders (Kempton & Forehand, 1992) and also significantly associated with suicidal ideation among female juvenile offenders (Goldstein et al., 2003a). Both male and female suicide attempters are often diagnosed with depression, often with accompanying substance abuse, conduct disorder, and feelings of hopelessness (Kempton & Forehand, 1992; Rohde, Mace, & Seeley, 1997). In addition, the environmental stressors commonly experienced by juvenile delinquents, such as limited social support and histories of physical and sexual abuse, may predispose these youth to view suicide as a viable solution to their problems (Rohde et al., 1997).

The strongest predictor of future suicide attempts is a history of past attempts and other suicidal behavior (Rohde et al., 1997). Rates of suicidal ideation and behavior among juvenile delinquents range from 17 to 61% (Kempton & Forehand, 1992; Rohde et al., 1997), far exceeding the 2.6 to 19% rate for the general adolescent population (Gould, Greenberg, Velting, & Shaffer, 2003). In a study in which 36.7% of a juvenile delinquent sample had attempted suicide, 75% of the attempters reported that they had believed their efforts would not be fatal (Memory, 1989). The high rate of nonlethal attempts does not, however, negate the seriousness of the behavior, as self-injurious behaviors may unintentionally become lethal. The prevalence rate of completed suicides among juvenile offenders is 4.6 times greater than the rate among adolescents in the general population (Memory, 1989; see also Penn, Esposito, Schaeffer, Fritz, & Spirito, 2003). One explanation for the elevated rates of self-injurious and suicidal behavior among juvenile offenders is that this population's high rates of mental health disorders and environmental stressors predispose them to attempt suicide (Rohde et al., 1997).

Empirically supported treatments for unipolar depression include cognitive-behavioral therapy and/or medication (Kaslow, McClure, & Connell, 2002).

Cognitive-behavioral therapy addresses the distorted thought processes that maintain the depression and attempts to increase the frequency of pleasant activities (Kaslow et al., 2002). In addition to improving mood, medication can alleviate physical symptoms, such as insomnia, psychomotor retardation, and loss of appetite (Ryan & Redding, in press).

Depression in adolescents can range from an uncomplicated diagnosis with good response to comorbid diagnoses with psychotic symptoms and high-risk treatment needs. For instance, the initial presentation of depression may represent a depressive episode of bipolar disorder, and, if misdiagnosed, treatment with antidepressants can aggravate the condition and its prognosis (Cusack, 2002; Kusumakar, 2002).

Externalizing Problems: Conduct Disorder and ADHD

Conduct disorder, characterized by persistent violation of age-appropriate societal rules or a disregard for others' rights, is common among juvenile offenders. Adolescents with conduct disorder differ from typical adolescents in their perceptions, cognitions, and social relationships. Neuropsychological deficits associated with frontal cortex impairment and a lack of problem-solving flexibility are commonly found in conduct-disordered youth (Caspi, Lynam, Moffitt, & Silva, 1993; Kandel & Freed, 1989; Lueger & Gill, 1990; Moffitt, 1993). This impairment is associated with several perceptual and behavioral disruptions, including difficulties generating alternative solutions to problems and adapting behavior to changing environmental contingencies (Lueger & Gill, 1990).

ADHD is characterized by symptoms of inattention, hyperactivity, and/or impulsivity (American Psychiatric Association, 1994). Adolescents with ADHD typically have impaired school performance, reduced participation in extracurricular activities, and disrupted social relationships (Barkley, 2002; Barkley, Fischer, Edelbrock, & Smallish, 1990; Fischer, Barkley, Edelbrock, & Smallish, 1990). Children and young adults (up to 22 years of age) with ADHD perform more poorly on tests of problem-solving abilities and attentional capacities, skills associated with frontal and prefrontal cortex areas, even when controlling for comorbid diagnoses (Seidman, Biederman, Faraone, Weber, & Ouellette, 1997; Shue & Douglas, 1992). The long-term prognosis for ADHD is poor; behaviors can be managed but cannot be cured, and behavioral management does not generalize across situations (Barkley et al., 1990). ADHD in adults is associated with psychiatric illness, impaired social skills, job failures, and marital problems (Barkley, 2002).

The occurrence among juvenile delinquents of each externalizing disorder is more frequent than that in the general juvenile population. Prevalence estimates of conduct disorder in males range from 6 to 16%, and in females from 2 to 9% (American Psychiatric Association, 1994). Among school children, 3 to 5% are diagnosable with ADHD (American Psychiatric Association, 1994), and the majority of such children (70 to 80%) meet diagnostic criteria in adolescence as well as adulthood (Ingram, Hechtman, & Morgenstern, 1999). In contrast to these rates in the general population, conduct disorder was diagnosed in approximately 90% of one juvenile offender sample (Eppright, Kashani, Robinson, & Reid, 1993) and 55% of another sample of juvenile offenders (Zagar, Arbit, Hughes, Busell, & Busch, 1989). On the lower side, although still much higher than rates obtained from the general population of adolescents, Teplin and colleagues (2002) found that 37.8% of male juvenile offenders and 40.6% of female juvenile offenders in their large sample met diagnostic criteria for conduct disorder; 16.6% of male juvenile offenders and 21.4% of female juvenile offenders met criteria for ADHD.

ADHD and conduct disorder are often comorbid; 30 to 35% of adolescents diagnosed with ADHD also receive a diagnosis of conduct disorder (Biederman, Newcorn, & Sprich, 1991; O'Shaughnessy, 1992), and approximately 19% of incarcerated juveniles with conduct disorder are also diagnosed with ADHD (Hollander & Turner, 1986). ADHD and conduct disorder can be distinguished from one another, and from a comorbid diagnosis of the two, by conducting structured mental health assessments, examining longitudinal outcomes, and reviewing a statistical summary of symptoms (Abikoff & Klein, 1992). Careful diagnostic assessment is essential to planning special education services and treatment of behavior disorders.

Although the presenting symptoms of ADHD and conduct disorder may appear similar, ADHD predicts more cognitive functioning problems, whether diagnosed alone or comorbidly with conduct disorder. For instance, Aronowitz and colleagues (1994) found more neuropsychological impairment and neurological soft signs (i.e., slight abnormalities in behavior, such as speech disturbances, awkward gait, hyperactivity, poor balance, lack of coordination, low muscle tone) (SSM Rehabilitative Institute, 2003) in children with both conduct disorder and ADHD than in children with conduct disorder alone. Furthermore, children with comorbid conduct disorder and ADHD had lower intellectual and academic skills and entered the juvenile justice system earlier than did those youth having only conduct disorder (Aronowitz et al., 1994). These patterns suggest that, although conduct disorder may account for behavioral problems that result in involvement with the justice system, ADHD can contribute to the poor intellectual functioning that may exacerbate behavioral disorders (Forehand, Wierson, Frame, Kempton, & Armisted, 1991). A diagnosis of ADHD alone suggests impairments in cognitive abilities that affect academic and, possibly, social performance. A diagnosis of conduct disorder alone may indicate antisocial and developmental behavioral problems. But a comorbid diagnosis of these two externalizing disorders may yield cognitive impairment, impulsivity, and hyperactivity in youth with antisocial predispositions and aggressive tendencies (Foley, Carlton, & Howell, 1996; Forehand et al., 1991; Klein & Mannuzza, 1991).

Given the frequent comorbidity of these two disorders and the prevalence of these diagnoses among youthful offenders, it is crucial to examine prognoses for this population. A diagnosis of conduct disorder appears to predict more criminal outcomes for juveniles than does one of ADHD (Foley et al., 1996). In a review of literature on ADHD, conduct disorder, and juvenile delinquency,

Foley and colleagues (1996) concluded that, when controlling for the comorbidity between these two disorders, ADHD is not as strong a predictor of offending behavior as is conduct disorder. Distinguishing these two diagnoses is essential, as accurate diagnosis is a prerequisite to effective treatment, although there is some overlap among the effective treatments for ADHD and conduct disorder.

Several medications are effective in treating adolescents with ADHD, including antidepressants; neuroleptics; stimulants, such as dextroamphetamine, methylphenidate, and pemoline; and adrenergic agonists, such as clonidine and guanfacine (Brown & La Rosa, 2002; Conners, 2002; Greenhill, 1992; Jacobvitz, Sroufe, Stewart, & Leffert, 1990; Steingard, Biederman, Spencer, Wilens, & Gonzolez, 1993). These medications have not traditionally been prescribed for conduct disorder, but when compared to a placebo, methylphenidate effectively reduced most conduct disorder symptoms, regardless of the severity of comorbid ADHD symptoms (Klein et al., 1997).

Other treatments for ADHD include psychosocial interventions, such as classroom-based behavior modification, social skills training, cognitive skills training, and parent training/home-based interventions (Wierson et al, 1992). Multimodal treatment has produced superior results compared to medication alone (Hinshaw, Klein, & Abikoff, 2002).

Traditional treatment for conduct disorder has been limited to nonpharmacological interventions (Klein et al., 1997). In a review of research on psychosocial treatments, Kazdin (1997) noted that the dysfunctions associated with conduct are often due, in part, to living conditions, such as poor housing and education. These economic and environmental difficulties cause stress in both parents and children, putting strain on their relationships and fostering and maintaining antisocial behavior in children. Parent training-based, cognitive-behavioral treatments can help by teaching parents practical skills to navigate conflicts through improved communication, administration of contingent responses to desirable and undesirable behaviors, and appropriate interpersonal responses (Barkley, Edwards, & Robin, 1999). Reviews of outcome studies revealed significant reductions in antisocial and aggressive behaviors following participation in such cognitive-behavioral treatment interventions (Baer & Nietzel, 1991; Durlak, Furhman, & Lampman, 1991).

Youth-based interventions for conduct disorder are frequently conducted in a group format. However, peer-group therapy has been shown to have iatrogenic effects with juvenile offenders because it exposes them to more deviant peers and negative peer influences (Dishion, McCord, & Poulin, 1999). Should group therapy occur, a maximum of 10 members is the recommended size for psychotherapy groups of adolescents in the general population (Carlin, 1996). However, given the high prevalence of conduct disorder in the juvenile delinquent population and the limited numbers of personnel and resources in justice facilities, groups often have more than 10 members (Carlin, 1996).

Therapists may encounter difficulty controlling such groups because of their size and the volatility of the population, and these youth will often exhibit difficulty paying attention and remembering rules. Therefore, at every meeting, rules should be read, and immediate consequences for infringement administered (Carlin, 1996). Goldstein and colleagues (2003b) also recommended dispensing immediate tangible rewards for compliance with group rules. Another characteristic of juvenile delinquent groups for youth with conduct disorder is low educational achievement (Lexcen & Redding, 2000). Such low achievement is associated with youths' limited abilities to use and understand sophisticated vocabulary words and abstract verbal concepts (Snowling, Adams, Bowyer-Crane, & Tobin, 2000). Rather than relying on written materials, Goldstein and colleagues (2003b) recommended reliance on role-playing scenarios and visual stimuli, such as pictures and videotaped vignettes, to convey information and practice skills.

Finally, leaders should be prepared to deal with these youths' verbally and physically aggressive coping styles, attributable, in part, to environmental influences and cognitive deficits and dysfunctions (Carlin, 1996). For instance, in a prospective study, cognitive deficits were observed in infants who later became aggressive children and adolescents (Lyons-Ruth, 1992). Additionally, in a study of aggressive boys, a bias to perceive hostile intent in ambiguous interpersonal situations was attributed to two cognitive errors: selective recall of hostile social cues and impulsive decision making (Dodge & Newman, 1981). In such situations, these youth may respond with unanticipated aggression to nonprovocative behaviors, perhaps because they are familiar with fewer behavioral options (Dodge, Price, Bachorowski, & Newman, 1990). Among male adolescents in maximum security facilities, these cognitive biases were specifically associated with undersocialized aggressive conduct disorder (a psychiatric diagnosis of childhood antisocial personality disorder characterized by fighting, hitting, assaultive behavior, temper tantrums, and destructiveness; Quay, 1999) and violent interpersonal criminal acts, but not with nonviolent crimes and socialized conduct disorder (characterized primarily by negative peer associations, truancy, gang membership, curfew violations, and lying and cheating; Quay, 1999) (Dodge et al., 1990). Thus, conduct disorder appears to be associated with cognitive deficits related to misperceptions of social situations and poorly planned responses to interpersonal interactions.

Other well-recognized treatments for conduct disorder include parent management training (PMT), functional family therapy (FFT), and MST. PMT involves teaching parents to respond consistently to children and interrupting maladaptive interactional habits that maintain aggressive or antisocial behaviors (Kazdin, 1997). PMT, which is effective for younger children, has shown short-term effectiveness for promoting prosocial behaviors in children and using discipline to minimize maladaptive behaviors (Froehlich, Doepfner, & Lehmkuhl, 2002; Kazdin, 1997). FFT expands the premises of PMT to include family therapy. MST extends even further to include school and community settings as elements of the adolescent's environment (Kazdin, 1997). See Redding and Mrozoski (ch. 11 in this volume) for a detailed explanation of these treatments and associated research.

Female Juvenile Offenders

In 2000, girls constituted 28% of the 2.4 million juvenile arrests (Office of Juvenile Justice and Delinquency Prevention [OJJDP], 2002a). Recent statistics indicate that adolescent girls represent a rapidly growing population in the justice system (Teplin et al., 2002). The 2000 Violent Crime Index (offenses of murder and nonnegligent manslaughter, forcible rape, robbery, and aggravated assault) arrest rate for female youth was 66% above its 1980 level, whereas the rate for male youth was 16% below its 1980 level (OJJDP, 2002b). The arrest rates for property crimes (offenses of burglary, larceny-theft, motor vehicle theft, and arson) increased 3% from 1980 to 2000 for female youth, while it decreased 46% for males (OJJDP, 2002c). Between 1992 and 2001, there was an 18.8% increase in the number of female delinquents arrested (compared with a 9.2% decrease for males) (Federal Bureau of Investigation, 2001). In addition, between 1985 and 1994, the number of cases in which courts ordered delinquent female offenders to be placed in residential facilities increased 47%, and the number of probation cases increased 67% (U.S. Justice Department, 1998).

The rate of mental health problems among female offenders is 2 to 3 times that of male offenders (Timmons-Mitchell et al., 1997). This increased rate may be due to the unique characteristics of girls in this population. Such gender-specific characteristics include greater prevalence of physical, emotional, and sexual abuse histories; pregnancy and sexually transmitted diseases, sometimes attributable to the abuse; and issues of self-esteem and body image (Ackerman, Newton, McPherson, Jones, & Dyckman, 1998; Acoca, 1998). The mental health problems most common among female juvenile offenders are depression, anxiety, substance use, difficulties associated with sexual and physical abuse histories, suicidal ideation and self-mutilation, and conduct disorder/oppositional defiant disorder (Goldstein et al., 2003b). Rates of self-mutilation and suicide attempts are high among female juvenile offenders. One study found that over half the girls in justice facilities attempted suicide at least once, with half of those attempting multiple times (Myers et al., 1990).

Depression is the most frequent psychiatric diagnosis among female juvenile offenders, with other mood disorders, adjustment disorders, and anxiety disorders following close behind (Myers et al., 1990; Timmons-Mitchell et al., 1997). Additionally, the prevalence of substance abuse among female juvenile offenders ranges from 47% (Teplin et al., 2002) to 87% (Myers et al., 1990); more than 50% of female offenders in one sample reported using drugs during the crimes that led to their incarcerations (Fejes-Mendoza, Miller, & Eppler, 1995). Alcohol also poses a problem for this population, as one study found that female juvenile offenders met criteria for alcohol dependence (63.6%) at more than twice the rate of male juvenile offenders (31.6%) (Ulzen & Hamilton, 1998), and other studies have found similar proportions (Kakar, Friedemann, & Peck, 2002; Prinz & Kerns, 2003; Teplin et al., 2002).

In addition, more than half the girls in juvenile facilities studied by the

American Correctional Association (1986) reported histories of physical or sexual abuse, primarily by family members (see also Acoca, 1998; Teplin et al., 2002). Victimization of female adolescents frequently is a significant factor in their entry into the juvenile justice system. For example, 92% of female juvenile offenders interviewed in a 1998 study reported that they had been subjected to some form of emotional, physical, and/or sexual abuse (Acoca & Dedel, 1998). There is a strong relationship between physical, sexual, and emotional victimization and specific high-risk behaviors, such as drug use, school failure, and gang membership (Acoca, 1998). In fact, the age that female adolescent offenders begin using drugs coincides with the age at which they are most likely to be abused (Acoca & Dedel, 1998). Acoca and Dedel (1998) found that girls were most likely to be beaten stabbed, shot, or raped at ages 13 and 14, and 75% of women offenders interviewed reported that regular use of drugs and alcohol began at approximately age 14. These women reported frequent attempts to self-medicate and alleviate the pain resulting from victimization and abuse.

Abusive experiences and drug use correlate highly with multiple risky be-haviors, including truancy, unsafe sexual activity, and gang involvement. For abused girls, joining gangs may fill a social function, allowing young women to feel accepted and protected (Acoca, 1998), but it also typically results in acts of crime and violence (Acoca & Dedel, 1998). These behaviors and, in particular, status offenses (i.e., behaviors deemed illegal solely based on the young age of the offender) often lead to the detainment and arrest of female adolescents (American Bar Association and National Bar Association, 2001).

In an effort to address the unique needs of the increasing female adolescent offender population, the 1992 amendment to the Juvenile Justice and Delin-quency Prevention Act of 1974 was passed. In this amendment, Congress re-quired states to include in their analysis of juvenile crime problems "(i) an analy-sis of gender-specific services for the prevention and treatment of juvenile delinquency, including the types of such services available and the need for such services for females; and (ii) a plan for providing needed gender-specific services for the prevention and treatment of juvenile delinquency" (OJJDP, 1998, 1992 Reauthorization of the JJDP Act section, para. 1). This amendment led to new efforts to better serve this population.

Despite such efforts, treatment services for female juvenile offenders are limited, particularly in residential placements. States generally have several fa-cilities available for boys but often only have one facility available for girls (Gold-stein et al., 2003a). In 1997, 15% of juvenile residential facilities housed only females, while 52% of the facilities housed only males (Scahill, 2000). The limited number of facilities available for girls may restrict the variety of treat-ment options that can be made available to this population. In addition, little mental health intervention research has been conducted with female juvenile offenders (Goldstein et al., 2003a), presenting a significant challenge for states and programs wishing to identify effective gender-specific treatments for this population.

Risk and Protective Factors for Delinquency and Mental Health Problems

Developmental risk factors for delinquency, such as habitual lying, low academic achievement, and aggression, have been identified to predict delinquency in children as young as elementary school age (Bartol, 2001; Moeller, 2001). Youth who commit delinquent behaviors were often aggressive and hostile as children (Bartol, 2001). Because of such aggressiveness, they were largely unpopular in school and tended to alienate their peers (Benda, 2003). Such alienation removed opportunities for prosocial engagement, and the child instead engaged in deviant behaviors, such as truancy, lying, and stealing (Bartol, 2001). These deviant behaviors in young children are strongly associated with future juvenile delinquency (Benda, 2003; Huesmann, Eron, & Dubow, 2003).

Socioeconomic status also sometimes is used to explain how predictors of delinquency are fostered in young, underprivileged children. The Interactional Theory of Delinquency holds that children from underprivileged backgrounds are born into social structures lacking necessary family, social, and educational characteristics (Thornberry & Krohn, 2001). To further compound this situation, children do not experience one or two such deficits but, rather, an array of simultaneously interacting deficits. For example, inadequate social support, financial instability, and the absence of consistent parental figures may all lead to weak familial and social bonds. Unlike more privileged children, these children do not have many protective factors to shield them from the effects of their difficult environments (Thornberry & Krohn, 2001).

Related to risk factors for mental health problems among juvenile offenders, and consistent with the Interactional Theory of Delinquency, juvenile delinquents tend to experience a great deal of family dysfunction, such as parental conflict, physical and sexual abuse, parental arrest and incarceration, inconsistent living situations, and ineffective parental supervision and discipline (Moeller, 2001; Redding, 2003). In a survey of serious juvenile delinquents, 72% of youth lost a parent through death, separation, or divorce. Furthermore, almost half reported experiencing some form of physical abuse, neglect, or abandonment. Female delinquents were significantly more likely to experience physical abuse or neglect and subsequent removal from their homes before the age of 10 (McManus et al., 1984).

Parental and sibling substance use also serves as a risk factor for juvenile offenders' substance use disorders. Substance use by parents of juvenile offenders is greatly elevated compared to use by parents of adolescents in the general population (Ulzen & Hamilton, 1998). Excessive drinking was reported by adolescents for 22% of parents of incarcerated youth, compared to 2% of parents of the general population of youth (Ulzen & Hamilton, 1998). Likewise, approximately 15% of parents of juvenile offenders reported using drugs, compared to 4% of parents of the general adolescent population (Ulzen & Hamilton, 1998). In another study, having 2 generations (parents and grandparents) with histories of alcohol abuse and dependence was predictive of greater delinquency in offspring, earlier onset of alcohol and marijuana use, and greater frequency of cocaine and marijuana use by age 18 (Windle, 1996).

Exposure to family violence, as well as to community violence, is very common among juvenile offenders. This risk factor is significantly related to PTSD symptoms in juvenile delinquents (Wood, Foy, Layne, Pynoos, & James, 2002). The majority of youth in one study qualified for partial PTSD (multiple symptoms of PTSD, yet not enough to qualify for a clinical diagnosis), with 24% qualifying for full PTSD (Burton, Foy, Bwanausi, Johnson, & Moore, 1994). Almost three quarters of the sample reported having been victims of violent acts by gangs or the perpetrators of violence (more than 80% of the sample belonged to gangs). Other major sources of exposure to violence included physical abuse, being a victim of weapons violence, and witnessing the death of a bystander, enemy, or friend. Many youth experienced more than one form of violence. The more violence to which a youth was exposed, the greater the likelihood that he or she would qualify for a diagnosis of full PTSD (Burton et al., 1994). Additionally, inadequate social support was significantly related to higher levels of PTSD. Those with full PTSD were more likely to have high levels of family conflict, while those delinquents without PTSD symptoms had the highest levels of family solidarity (Burton et al., 1994).

Risk factors for depression in adolescents include low self-esteem, low parental support, poor relationships with parents and peers, and a history of trauma or abuse (Ryan & Redding, in press). Additionally, depression has been associated with genetic factors, parental conflict, and general family discord (Faraone & Biederman, 1997). Although little research has been conducted on risk factors of depression in incarcerated youth, gang membership and offense history (i.e., higher levels of recidivism) were most strongly associated with depression in one study (Fernandez, 2001).

Parental depression is a significant risk factor for conduct disorder in adolescents (Fendrich, Warner, & Weissman, 1990). Developmental studies have shown that conduct disorder in children was predicted by difficult temperament at 2 years of age, poverty, child–parent separation, and level of maternal stress (Bagley & Mallick, 1997). Other developmental risk factors include maternal substance abuse during pregnancy, child maltreatment, and large family size coupled with poverty (Olds et al., 1998). Although research exists on predictors of persistent offending and aggression among juvenile offenders (e.g., Broidy et al., 2003; Stouthamer-Loeber & Loeber, 2002), to our knowledge, there are no published studies identifying predictors of conduct disorder in juvenile offenders. However, much of the research on risk factors for delinquency would be relevant.

For instance, special education needs have been associated with juvenile delinquency. Up to 35% of incarcerated juveniles require special education services for learning disabilities (Dunivant, 1982). Meltzer, Levine, Karniski, Palfrey, and Clark (1984) found that juvenile delinquents had documented academic difficulties beginning in elementary school, demonstrating that these needs are often long-standing. Subjects had problems with reading (45%) and spelling (38%) by the second grade, problems with truancy (19%) by the fifth grade, and overall academic delays (50%) by junior high school (Meltzer et al. 1984). Additionally, math deficits have been found to be associated with recidivism in females (Archwamety & Katisiyannis, 1998).

On measures of intelligence, juvenile delinquents scored significantly lower (about one-half standard deviation) than nondelinquents (Moffitt, 1993; Redding & Arrigo, in press). Violent juvenile offenders obtained even lower IQ scores— about 17 points lower than nondelinquent adolescents (Moffitt, 1993). Low intelligence alone does not predict delinquency, but the relationship remains robust even when ethnicity and socioeconomic status are accounted for (Lynam, Moffitt, & Stouthamer-Loeber, 1993). Conversely, IQ can act as a mediating factor for older adolescents who are at risk of becoming delinquent, with higher IQ serving as a protective factor (Rohde, Noell, & Ochs, 1999). Compared to nondelinquent youth, delinquent youth scored significantly lower on measures of language skills, verbal abilities, and visual–spatial and visual–motor integration skills; they also appeared to be relatively poor in attending to or ignoring competing tasks in receptive and expressive domains (Davis, Sanger, & Morris-Friehe, 1991; Hurt & Naglieri, 1992; Moffitt & Silva, 1988). Slow language acquisition as an infant and reading disabilities also have been found to be predictors of juvenile delinquency (Cornwall & Bawden, 1992; McGee, Share, Moffitt, Williams, & Silva, 1988; Stattin & Klackenberg-Larsson, 1993).

Attentional disorders are primarily predicted by heredity, genetic factors, and neurobiological abnormalities in the brain (Biederman & Faraone, 2002; Faraone & Biederman, 1997; Spencer, Biederman, Wilens, & Faraone, 2002). Additional risk factors of ADHD include maternal depression, parental conflict, family dysfunction, and low income (Faraone & Biederman, 1997). Although there are no published studies on risk factors for ADHD in juvenile offenders specifically, ADHD in this population has been associated with physical aggression and conduct problems (Loeber, Farrington, Stouthamer-Loeber, & Van Kammen, 1998).

Conclusion

Only during the past few years has the mental health of juvenile delinquents become a priority of policy-makers and the justice system. With the juvenile justice system's shift away from rehabilitation and toward retribution, more juveniles are processed in the adult criminal system (Grisso, 1999). In many states, a juvenile's mental health status is a key component in whether the case is heard in juvenile or criminal court, and it impacts many other decisions related to juvenile cases (Grisso, 1999). Juveniles transferred to adult court are now facing legal questions formerly associated primarily with adult defendants, such as competence to stand trial and the insanity defense.

Given these changes, legislatures have taken greater notice of the mental health needs of juvenile delinquents, both pre- and postadjudication. Congress conducted "a series of investigations that documented the consistent inadequacy of mental health care and services in juvenile correctional facilities in a number of states" (Cocozza & Skowyra, 2000, p. 3). Additionally, Congress examined juvenile justice facilities nationwide in an attempt to ascertain the mental health services available to juvenile delinquents at the time. In addition, Congress reviewed several bills concerning the implementation of nationwide mental health and substance abuse assessment and treatment services in juvenile justice facilities (Cocozza & Skowyra, 2000).

Although mental health needs of juvenile delinquents were historically overlooked, the detrimental effects of untreated mental health problems in young offenders have become more obvious to researchers, policy-makers, and juvenile justice administrators. Mental health problems are often associated with and exacerbated by the difficult lives of these youth. Juvenile offenders must often deal with family conflict, abuse, and exposure to community violence. Their failure and disinterest in school contribute to truancy and conduct-disordered behaviors. Juvenile girls face further obstacles, as their heightened vulnerability to victimization may be related to their greater rates of mental health problems. Identifying and understanding the mental health needs of juvenile offenders should assist mental health and criminal justice professionals, as well as policy-makers, develop and implement effective assessment and treatment approaches for juvenile offenders that will reduce offending and recidivism in this population.

References

Abikoff, H., & Klein, R. G. (1992). Attention-deficit hyperactivity and conduct disorder: Comorbidity and implications for treatment. *Journal of Consulting and Clinical Psychology, 60*(6), 881–892.

Ackerman, P. T., Newton, J. E., McPherson, W. B., Jones, J. G., & Dyckman, R. A. (1998). Prevalence of post traumatic stress disorder and other psychiatric diagnoses in three groups of abused children (sexual, physical, and both). *Child Abuse and Neglect, 22*(8), 759–774.

Acoca, L. (1998). Outside/inside: The violation of American girls at home, on the streets and in the juvenile justice system. *Crime and Delinquency, 44*(4), 561–589.

Acoca, L., & Dedel, K. (1998). *No place to hide: Understanding and meeting the needs of girls in the California Juvenile Justice System.* San Francisco: National Council of Crime and Delinquency.

American Bar Association and the National Bar Association. (2001). *Justice by gender: The lack of appropriate prevention, diversion, and treatment alternatives for girls in the justice system.* Washington, DC: Author.

American Correctional Association. (1986). *Public policy for corrections: A handbook for decision makers.* Laurel, MD: Author.

American Psychiatric Association. (1994). *Diagnostic and statistical manual of mental disorders* (4th ed.). Washington, DC: Author.

Archwamety, T., & Katsiyannis, A. (1998). Factors related to recidivism among delinquent females at a state correctional facility. *Journal of Child and Family Studies, 7*(1), 59–67.

Aronowitz, B., Liebowitz, M. R., Hollander, E., Fazzini, E., Durlach-Misteli, C., Frenkel, M., et al. (1994). Neuropsychiatric and neuropsychological findings in conduct disorder and attention-deficit hyperactivity disorder. *Journal of Neuropsychiatry & Clinical Neurosciences, 6*(3), 245–249.

Baer, R. A., & Nietzel, M. T. (1991). Cognitive and behavioural treatment of impulsivity in children: A meta analytic review of the outcome literature. *Journal of Clinical Child Psychology, 20,* 400–412.

Bagley, C., & Mallick, K. (1997). Temperament, CNS problems and maternal stressors: Interactive predictors of conduct disorder in 9-yr.-olds. *Perceptual and Motor Skills, 84*(2), 617–618.

Barkley, R. A. (2002). Major life activity and health outcomes associated with attention-deficit/hyperactivity disorder. *Journal of Clinical Psychiatry, 63*(112), 10–15.

Barkley, R. A., Edwards, G. H., & Robin, A. L. (1999). *Defiant teens: A clinician's manual for assessment and family intervention.* New York: Guilford Press.

Barkley, R. A., Fischer, M., Edelbrock, C. S., & Smallish, L. (1990). The adolescent outcome of hyperactive children diagnosed by research criteria: An eight year prospective follow-up study. *Journal of the American Academy of Childhood and Adolescent Psychiatry, 29,* 546–557.

Bartol, C. R. (2001). *Criminal behaviour: A psychosocial approach.* Upper Saddle River, NJ: Prentice Hall.

Belsher, G., Wilkes, T. C. R., & Rush, A. J. (1995). An open, multisite pilot study of cognitive therapy for depressed adolescents. *Journal of Psychotherapy Practice and Research, 4*(1), 52–66.

Benda, B. B. (2003). A test of three competing theoretical models of delinquency using structural equation modelling. *Journal of Social Service Research, 29*(2), 55–91.

Biederman, J., Faraone, S., Mick, E., Moore, P., & Lelon, E. (1996). Child Behaviour Checklist findings further support comorbidity between ADHD and major depression in a referred sample. *Journal of the American Academy of Child and Adolescent Psychiatry, 35*(6), 734–742.

Biederman, J., & Faraone, S. V. (2002). Current concepts on the neurobiology of ADHD. *Journal of Attention Disorders, 6*(Suppl. 1), 7–16.

Biederman, J., Newcorn, J., & Sprich, S. (1991). Comorbidity of attention deficit hyperactivity disorder with conduct, depressive, anxiety, and other disorders. *American Journal of Psychiatry, 148,* 564–577.

Broidy, L. M., Nagin, D. S., Tremblay, R. E., Bates, J. E., Brame, B., Dodge, K. A., et al. (2003). Developmental trajectories of childhood disruptive behaviors and adolescent delinquency: A six-site, cross-national study. *Developmental Psychology, 39*(2), 222–245.

Brown, R. T., & La Rosa, A. (2002). Recent developments in the pharmacotherapy of attention-deficit/hyperactivity disorder (ADHD). *Professional Psychology—Research and Practice, 33*(6), 591–595.

Brunelle, N., Brochu, S., & Cousineau, M. (2000) Drug-crime relations among drug-consuming juvenile delinquents: A tripartite model and more. *Contemporary Drug Problems, 27*(4), 835–867.

Bry, B. H., & Krinsley, K. E. (1992). Booster sessions and long-term effects of behavioural family therapy on adolescent substance use and school performance. *Journal of Behaviour Therapy and Experimental Psychiatry, 23*(3), 183–189.

Burton, D., Foy, D. W., Bwanausi, C., Johnson, J., & Moore, S. (1994). The relationship between traumatic exposure, family dysfunction, and post-traumatic stress symptoms in male juvenile offenders. *Journal of Traumatic Stress, 7*(1), 83–93.

Carlin, M. E. (1996). Large group treatment of severely disturbed/conduct-disordered adolescents. *International Journal of Group Psychotherapy, 46*(3), 379–397.

Caspi, A., Lynam, D., Moffitt, T., & Silva, P. (1993). Unravelling girls' delinquency: Biological, dispositional, and contextual contributions to adolescent misbehaviour. *Developmental Psychology, 29,* 19–30.

Cocozza, J. J. (1992). *Responding to the mental health needs of youth in the juvenile justice system.* Seattle, WA: The National Coalition for the Mentally Ill in the Criminal Justice System.

Cocozza, J. J., & Skowyra, K. R. (2000). Youth with mental health disorders: Issues and emerging responses. *Juvenile Justice, 7*(1), 3–13.

Conners, C. K. (2002). Forty years of methylphenidate treatment in attention-deficit/hyperactivity disorder. *Journal of Attention Disorders, 6*(Suppl. 1), S-17–S-30.

Cooper, C. S., & Bartlett, S. (1998). *Juvenile and family drug courts: profile of program characteristics and implementation issues.* Washington, DC: Office of Justice Programs Drug Court Clearinghouse and Technical Assistance Project.

Cornwall, A., & Bawden, H. N. (1992). Reading disabilities and aggression: A critical review. *Journal of Learning Disabilities, 25*(5), 281–288.

Curry, J. F., & Craighead, W. E. (1990). Attributional style in clinically depressed and conduct disordered adolescents. *Journal of Consulting and Clinical Psychology, 58*(1), 109–115.

Cusack, J. (2002). Challenges in the diagnosis and treatment of bipolar disorder. *Drug Benefit Trends, 14*(10), 34–38.

Davis, A. D., Sanger, D. D., & Morris-Friehe, M. (1991). Language skills of delinquent and non-delinquent adolescent males. *Journal of Communication Disorders, 24*(4), 251–266.

Dawkins, M. P. (1997). Drug use and violent crime among adolescents. *Adolescence, 32*(126), 395–405.

Deardorff, J., Gonzales, N. A., & Sandler, I. W. (2003). Control beliefs as a mediator of the relation between stress and depressive symptoms among inner-city adolescents. *Journal of Abnormal Child Psychology, 31*(2), 205–217.

Dishion, T. J., McCord, J., & Poulin, F. (1999). When interventions harm: Peer groups and problem behavior. *American Psychologist, 54,* 755–764.

Dodge, K. A., Price, J. M., Bachorowski, J., & Newman, J. P. (1990). Hostile attributional biases in severely aggressive adolescents. *Journal of Abnormal Psychology, 99*(4), 385–392.

Dodge, R., & Newman, J. P. (1981). Biased decision-making processes in aggressive boys. *Journal of Abnormal Psychology, 90*(4), 375–379.

Domalanta, D. D., Risser, W. L., Roberts, R. E., & Risser, J. M. H. (2003). Prevalence of depression and other psychiatric disorders among incarcerated youths. *Journal of the American Academy of Child and Adolescent Psychiatry, 42,* 477–484.

Dunivant, N. (1982). *The relationship between learning disabilities and juvenile delinquency.* Williamsburg, VA: National Center for State Courts.

Durlak, J. A., Furhman, T., & Lampman, C. (1991). Effectiveness of cognitive behavioural therapy for maladapting children: A meta-analysis. *Psychological Bulletin, 110,* 204–214.

Eppright, T. D., Kashani, J. H., Robinson, B. D., & Reid, J. C. (1993). Comorbidity of conduct disorder and personality disorders in incarcerated juvenile populations. *American Journal of Psychiatry, 150*(8), 1233–1236.

Faraone, S. V., & Biederman, J. (1997). Do attention deficit hyperactivity disorder and major depression share familial risk factors? *Journal of Nervous and Mental Disease, 185*(9), 533–541.

Farrow, J., & French, J. (1986). The drug abuse-delinquency connection revisited. *Adolescence, 21*(84), 951–960.

Federal Bureau of Investigation. (2001). *Crime in the United States.* Washington, DC: U.S. Government Printing Office.

Fejes-Mendoza, K., Miller, D., & Eppler, R. (1995). Portraits of dysfunction: Criminal educational, and family profiles of juvenile female offenders. *Education and Treatment of Children, 18*(3), 309–321.

Fendrich, M., Warner, V., & Weissman, M. M. (1990). Family risk factors, parental depression, and psychopathology in offspring. *Developmental Psychology, 26*(1), 40–50.

Fernandez, P. J. (2001). Incarcerated adolescents and young adults: Examining gang membership status, type of crime committed, offense history, and length of incarceration as predictors of depression. *Dissertation Abstracts International, 61*(8-B), 4401.

Fischer, M., Barkley, R. A., Edelbrock, C. S., & Smallish, L. (1990). The adolescent outcome of hyperactive children diagnosed by research criteria: II. Academic, attentional, and neuropsychological status. *Journal of Consulting and Clinical Psychology, 58,* 580–588.

Foley, B. A., Carlton, C. O., & Howell, R. J. (1996). The relationship of attention deficit hyperactivity disorder and conduct disorder to juvenile delinquency: Legal implications. *Bulletin of the American Academy of Psychiatry and Law, 24*(3), 333–345.

Forehand, R., Wierson, M., Frame, C., Kempton, T., & Armisted, L. (1991). Juvenile delinquency entry and persistence: Do attention problems contribute to conduct problems? *Journal of Behavioural Therapy and Experimental Psychiatry, 22,* 261–264.

Froehlich, J., Doepfner, M., & Lehmkuhl, G. (2002). Effects of combined cognitive behavioural treatment with parent management training in ADHD. *Behavioural and Cognitive Psychotherapy, 30*(1), 111–115.

Garber, J., Weiss, B., & Shanley, N. (1993). Cognitions, depressive symptoms and development in adolescents. *Journal of Abnormal Psychology, 102*(1), 47–57.

Goldstein, N. E., Arnold, D. H., Weil, J., Mesiarik, C., Peuschold, D., Grisso, T., et al. (2003a). Comorbid symptom patterns in female juvenile offenders. *International Journal of Law and Psychiatry, 26,* 565–582.

Goldstein, N. E. S., Thomson, M., Appleton, C., Weil, J., Osman, D., Strachan, M., et al. (2003b). The delinquency intervention and assessment (DIA) program for girls: An empirically-based, court-mandated, gender-specific treatment for female juvenile offenders. Manuscript submitted for publication.

Gould, M. S., Greenberg, T., Velting, D. M., & Shaffer, D. (2003). Youth suicide risk and preventive interventions: A review of the past 10 years. *American Academy of Child and Adolescent Psychiatry, 42*(4), 386–405.

Green, B., & Ritter, C. (2000). Marijuana use and depression. *Journal of Health and Social Behavior, 41*(1), 40–49.

Greenhill, L. L. (1992). Pharmacotherapy: Stimulants. *Child and Adolescent Psychiatric Clinics of North America, 1,* 411–448.

Grilo, C. M., Fehon, D. C., Walker, M., & Martino, S. (1996). A comparison of adolescent inpatients with and without substance abuse using the Millon Adolescent Clinical Inventory. *Journal of Youth & Adolescence, 25*(3), 379–388.

Grisso, T. (1999). Juvenile offenders and mental illness. *Psychiatry, Psychology and Law, 6*(2), 143–151.

Henggeler, S. W., Borduin, C. M., Melton, G. B., Mann, B. J., Smith, L. A., Hall, J. A., et al. (1991). Effects of multisystemic therapy on drug use and abuse in serious juvenile offenders: A progress report from two outcome studies. *Family Dynamics of Addiction, 1*(3), 40–51.

Henggeler, S. W., Clingempeel, W. G., Brondino, M. J., & Pickrel, S. G. (2002). Four-year follow-up of multisystemic therapy with substance-abusing and substance-dependent juvenile offenders. *Journal of American Academy of Child Psychiatry*, 41(7), 868–874.

Henggeler, S. W., Pickrel, S. G., Brondino, M. J., & Crouch, J. L. (1996). Eliminating (almost) treatment dropout of substance abusing or depending delinquents through home-based multisystemic therapy. *American Journal of Psychiatry*, 153(3), 427–428.

Hinshaw, S. P., Klein, R. G., & Abikoff, H. B. (2002). Childhood attention-deficit hyperactivity disorder: Nonpharmacological treatments and their combination with medication. In P. E. Nathan & J. M. Gorman (Eds.), *A guide to treatments that work*. London: Oxford University Press.

Hollander, H. E., & Turner, F. D. (1986). Characteristics of incarcerated delinquents: Relationship between development disorders, environmental and family factors, and patterns of offense and recidivism. *Journal of American Academy of Child Psychiatry*, 24(2), 222–226.

Huesmann, L., Eron, L. D., & Dubow, E. F. (2003). Childhood predictors of adult criminality: Are all risk factors reflected in childhood aggressiveness. *Criminal Behavior and Mental Health*, 12(3), 185–208.

Hurt, J., & Naglieri, J. A. (1992). Performance of delinquent and nondelinquent males on planning, attention, simultaneous, and successive cognitive processing tasks. *Journal of Clinical Psychology*, 48(1), 120–128.

Ingram, S., Hechtman, L., & Morgenstern, G. (1999). Outcome issues in ADHD: Adolescent and adult long-term outcome. *Mental Retardation and Developmental Disabilities Research Reviews*, 5(3), 243–250.

Jacobvitz, D., Sroufe, L. A., Stewart, M., & Leffert, N. (1990). Treatment of attentional and hyperactivity problems in children with sympthomimetic drugs: A comprehensive review. *Journal of the American Academy of Child and Adolescent Psychiatry*, 29, 677–688.

Jainchill, N. (2000). Substance dependency treatment for adolescents: Practice and research. *Substance Use and Misuse*, 35(12–14), 2031–2060.

Johnson, B. D., Wish, E. D., Schmeidler, J., & Huizinga, D. (1991). Concentration of delinquent offending: Serious drug involvement and high delinquency rates. *Journal of Drug Issues*, 21(2), 205–229.

Kakar, S., Friedemann, M., & Peck, L. (2002). Girls in detention: The results of focus group discussion interviews and official records review. *Journal of Contemporary Criminal Justice*, 18(1), 57–73.

Kandel, E., & Freed, D. (1989). Frontal-lobe dysfunction and antisocial behaviour: A review. *Journal of Clinical Psychology*, 45(3), 404–413.

Kashani, J. H., Manning, G. W., McKnew, D. H., Cytryn, L., Simons, J. F., & Wooderson, P. C. (1980). Depression among incarcerated delinquents. *Psychiatry Resident*, 3, 185–190.

Kaslow, N. J., McClure, E. B., & Connell, A. M. (2002). Treatment of depression in children and adolescents. In I. H. Gotlib & C. L. Hammen (Eds.), *Handbook of depression*. New York: Guilford Press.

Kazdin, A. E. (1997). Practitioner review: Psychosocial treatment for conduct disordered children. *Journal of Child Psychology and Psychiatry*, 38(2), 161–178.

Kempton, T., & Forehand, R. L. (1992). Suicide attempts among juvenile delinquents: The contribution of mental health factors. *Behavior Research and Therapy*, 30(5), 537–541.

King, C. A., Ghazuiddin, N., McGovern, L., Brand, E., Hill, E., & Naylor, M. (1996). Predictors of comorbid alcohol and substance abuse in depressed adolescents. *Journal of the American Academy of Child and Adolescent Psychiatry*, 35(6), 743–751.

Klein, R. G., Abikoff, H., Klass, E., Ganeles, D., Seese, L. M., & Pollack, S. (1997). Clinical efficacy of methylphenidate in conduct disorder with and without attention deficit hyperactivity disorder. *Archives of General Psychiatry, 54*, 1073–1080.

Klein, R. G., & Mannuzza, S. (1991). Long-term outcome of hyperactive children. A review. *Journal of the American Academy of Child and Adolescent Psychiatry, 30*(3), 383–387.

Kusumakar, V. (2002). Antidepressants and antipsychotics in the long-term treatment of bipolar disorder. *Journal of Clinical Psychiatry, 63*(Suppl. 10), 23–28.

Lewis, D. O., Yeager, C. A., Lovely, R., Stein, A., & Cobham-Portorreal, C. S. (1994). A clinical follow-up of delinquent males: Ignored vulnerabilities, unmet needs and the perpetuation of violence. *Journal of the American Academy of Child and Adolescent Psychiatry, 33*, 518–528.

Lexcen, F., & Redding, R. E. (2000). Mental health needs of juvenile offenders. *Juvenile Correctional Mental Health Report, 3*(1), 1, 2, 8–16.

Loeber, R., Farrington, D. P., Stouthamer-Loeber, M., & Van Kammen, W. B. (1998). Multiple risk factors for multiproblem boys: Co-occurrence of delinquency, substance use, attention deficit, conduct problems, physical aggression, covert behavior, depressed mood, and shy/withdrawn behavior. In R. Jessor (Ed.), *New perspectives on adolescent risk behavior* (pp. 90–149). New York: Cambridge University Press.

Loeber, R., & Keenan, K. (1994). Interaction between conduct disorder and its comorbid conditions: Effects of age and gender. *Clinical Psychology Review, 14*(6), 497–523.

Lueger, R. J., & Gill, K. J. (1990). Frontal-lobe cognitive dysfunction in conduct disorder adolescents. *Journal of Clinical Psychology, 46*(6), 696–706.

Lynam, D., Moffitt, T., & Stouthamer-Loeber, M. (1993). Explaining the relation between IQ and delinquency: Class, race, test motivation, school failure or self-control? *Journal of Abnormal Psychology, 102*(2), 187–196.

Lyons-Ruth, K. (1992). Maternal depressive symptoms, disorganized infant-mother attachment relationships and hostile-aggressive behavior in the preschool classroom: A prospective longitudinal view from infancy to age five. In D. Cicchetti & S. L. Toth (Eds.), *Developmental perspectives on depression. Rochester symposium on developmental psychopathology* (pp. 131–171). Rochester, NY: University of Rochester Press.

McGee, R., Share, D., Moffitt, T. E., Williams, S., & Silva, P. A. (1988). Reading disability, behaviour problems and juvenile delinquency. In D. H. Saklofske & S. B. G. Eysenck, (Eds.), *Individual differences in children and adolescents*. New Brunswick, NJ: Transaction.

McManus, M., Alessi, N. E., Grapentine, W. L., & Brickman, A. (1984). Psychiatric disturbances in serious delinquents. *Journal of the American Academy of Child and Adolescent Psychiatry, 23*, 602–615.

Meltzer, L. J., Levine, M. D., Karniski, W., Palfrey, J. S., & Clark, S. (1984). An analysis of the learning styles of adolescent delinquents. *Journal of Learning Disabilities, 17*(10), 600–608.

Memory, J. (1989). Juvenile suicides in secure detention facilities: Correction of published rates. *Death Studies, 13*, 455–463.

Miller, C. (2001). Toxicant-induced loss of tolerance. *Addiction, 96*(1), 115–139.

Moeller, T. G. (2001). *Youth aggression and violence: A psychological approach.* Mahwah, NJ: Erlbaum.

Moffitt, T. E. (1993). Adolescence-limited and life-course-persistent antisocial behaviour: A developmental taxonomy. *Psychological Review, 4*, 674–701.

Moffitt, T. E., & Silva, P. A. (1988). Neuropsychological deficit and self-reported delinquency in an unselected birth cohort. *Journal of the American Academy of Child and Adolescent Psychiatry, 27*(2), 233–240.

Myers, W. C., Burket, R. C., Lyles, B., Stone, L., & Kemph, J. P. (1990). *DSM-III* diagnoses and offences in committed female juvenile delinquents. *Bulletin of the American Academy of Psychiatry and Law, 18,* 47–54.

National Clearinghouse for Alcohol and Drug Information. (1999). *Youth Risk Behaviour Surveillance, United States, 1995.* Retrieved January 20, 2002, from http://www.health.org/pubs/yrbbs7index.htm

National Institute of Justice. (2003). 2000 Arrestee drug abuse monitoring: Annual report. Retrieved October 17, 2003, from http://www.ncjrs.org/pdffiles1/nij/193013.pdf

Neighbors, B., Kempton, T., & Forehand, R. (1992). Co-occurrence of substance abuse with conduct, anxiety, and depression disorders in juvenile delinquents. *Addictive Behaviours, 17,* 379–386.

Office of Juvenile Justice and Delinquency Prevention. (1998, October). *National efforts to address the needs of the adolescent female offender.* Retrieved March 15, 2002, from http://ojjdp.ncjrs.org/pubs/gender/oview-3.html

Office of Juvenile Justice and Delinquency Prevention. (2002a). *Statistical briefing book.* Retrieved January 20, 2002, from http://ojjdp.ncjrs.org/ojstatbb/html/qa250.html

Office of Juvenile Justice and Delinquency Prevention. (2002b). *Statistical briefing book.* Retrieved March 15, 2002, from http://ojjdp.ncjrs.org/ojstatbb/asp/JAR_Display.asp?ID=qa2301031502

Office of Juvenile Justice and Delinquency Prevention. (2002c). *Statistical briefing book.* Retrieved March 15, 2002, from http://ojjdp.ncjrs.org/ojstatbb/asp/JAR_Display.asp?ID=qa2306031502

Olds, D., Pettitt, L. M., Robinson, J., Henderson, C., Eckenrode, J., Kitzman, H., et al. (1998). Reducing risks for antisocial behavior with a program of prenatal and early childhood home visitation. *Journal of Community Psychology, 26*(1), 65–83.

O'Shaughnessy, R. J. (1992). Clinical aspects of forensic assessment of juvenile offenders. *Psychiatric Clinics of North America, 15,* 721–735.

Otto, R. K., Greenstein, J. J., Johnson, M. K., & Friedmen, R. M. (1992). Prevalence of mental disorders in the juvenile justice system. In J. J. Cocozza (Ed.), *Responding to the mental health needs of youth in the juvenile justice system.* Seattle, WA: The National Coalition for the Mentally Ill in the Criminal Justice System.

Patterson, G. R., Crosby, L., and Vuchinich, S. (1992). Parenting, peers, and the stability of antisocial behavior in preadolescent males. *Developmental Psychology, 28,* 510–521.

Penn, J., Esposito, C. L., Schaeffer, L. E., Fritz, G. K., & Spirito, A. (2003). Suicide attempts and self-mutilative behavior in a juvenile correctional facility. *Journal of the American Academy of Child and Adolescent Psychiatry, 42*(7), 762–769.

Pinto, A., & Francis, G. (1993). Cognitive correlates of depressive symptoms in hospitalised adolescents. *Adolescence, 28*(111), 661–672.

Pollock, N. K., Maisto, S. A., Cornelius, J. R., & Martin, C. S. (2000). Predictors of different definitions of alcohol relapse in adolescents. *Alcoholism: Clinical and Experimental Research, 24,* 80A.

Pompi, K. F. (1994). Adolescents in therapeutic communities: Retention and posttreatment outcomes. *NIDA Research Monograph, 144,* 128–161.

Prinz, R. J., & Kerns, S. E. U. (2003). Early substance abuse by juvenile offenders. *Child Psychiatry and Human Development, 33*(4), 263–267.

Quay, H. C. (1999). Classification of disruptive behaviour disorders. In H. Quay & A. Hogan (Eds.), *Handbook of disruptive behaviour disorders* (pp. 3–21). Coral Gables, FL: University of Miami.

Redding, R. E. (2003). Youth violence through the lens of normal and pathological development. *Contemporary Psychology, 47,* 286–289.

Redding, R. E., & Arrigo, B. (in press). Multicultural perspectives on delinquency: Etiology and intervention. In C. Frisby and C. Reynolds (Eds.), *Handbook of multicultural school psychology.* New York: Wiley.

Riggs, P. D., Baker, S., Mikulich, S. K., Young, S. E., & Crowley, T. J. (1995). Depression in substance-dependent delinquents. *Journal of the American Academy of Child and Adolescent Psychiatry, 34*(6), 764–771.

Rodell, D., Benda, B., & Rodell, L. (2001). Effects of alcohol problems on depression among homeless veterans. *Alcoholism Treatment Quarterly, 19*(3), 65–81.

Rohde, P., Mace, D. E., & Seeley, J. R. (1997). The association of psychiatric disorders with suicide attempts in a juvenile delinquent sample. *Criminal Behaviour and Mental Health, 7,* 187–200.

Rohde, P., Noell, J., & Ochs, L. (1999). IQ scores among homeless older adolescents: Characteristics of intellectual performance and associations with psychosocial functioning. *Journal of Adolescence, 22*(3), 319–328.

Rueger, D. B., & Liberman, R. P. (1984). Behavioural family therapy for delinquent and substance-abusing adolescents. *Journal of Drug Issues, 2,* 403-418.

Ryan, E. P., & Redding, R. E. (in press). Mood disorders in juvenile offenders. *Psychiatric Services.*

Scahill, M. C. (2000). Female delinquency cases, 1997. OJJDP Fact Sheet 16. Retrieved March 15, 2003, from http://www.ncjrs.org/pdffiles1/ojjdp/fs200016.pdf

Seidman, L. J., Biederman, J., Faraone, S. V., Weber, W., & Ouellette, C. (1997). Toward defining a neuropsychology of attention deficit hyperactivity disorder: Performance of children and adolescents in a large clinically referred sample. *Journal of Consulting and Clinical Psychology, 65*(1), 150–160.

Shue, K. L., & Douglas, V. I. (1992). Attention deficit hyperactivity disorder and frontal lobe function. *Brain and Cognition, 20,* 104–124.

Silberg, J., Rutter, M., D'Onofrio, B., & Eaves, L. (2003). Genetic and environmental risk factors in adolescent substance use. *Journal of Child Psychology and Psychiatry and Allied Disciplines, 49*(5), 664–676.

Smart, R. G., Mann, R. E., & Tyson, L. A. (1997). Drugs and violence among Ontario students. *Journal of Psychoactive Drugs, 29*(4), 369–373.

Smith, W. J., Sayger, T. V., & Szykula, S. A. (1999). Child-focused family therapy: Behavioral family therapy versus brief family therapy. *Australian and New Zealand Journal of Family Therapy, 20*(2), 83–87.

Snowling, M., Adams, J., Bowyer-Crane, C., & Tobin, V. (2000). Levels of literacy among juvenile offenders: The incidence of specific reading difficulties. *Criminal Behaviour and Mental Health, 10*(4), 229–241.

Spencer, T. J., Biederman, J., Wilens, T. E., & Faraone, S. V. (2002). Overview and neurobiology of ADHD. *Journal of Clinical Psychiatry, 63*(Suppl. 112), 3–9.

SSM Rehabilitative Institute. (2003). *Index of medical terms.* Retrieved August 18, 2003, from http://www.ssmrehab.com/internet/home/ssmrehab.nsf/0/9333EF005B436DCA6256C93005F2813?OpenDocument

Stark, M. J. (1992). Dropping out of substance abuse treatment: A clinically oriented view. *Clinical Psychology Review 12*(1), 93–116.

Stattin, H., & Klackenberg-Larsson, I. (1993). Early language and intelligence development and their relationship to future criminal behaviour. *Journal of Abnormal Psychology, 102*(3), 369–378.

Steingard, R., Biederman, J., Spencer, T., Wilens, T., & Gonzalez, A. (1993). Comparison of clonidine response in the treatment of attention deficit hyperactivity disorder with and without comorbid tic disorders. *Journal of the American Academy of Child and Adolescent Psychiatry, 32*, 350–353.

Stouthamer-Loeber, M., & Loeber, R. (2002). Lost opportunities for intervention: Undetected markers for the development of serious juvenile delinquency. *Criminal Behaviour and Mental Health, 12*(1), 69–82.

Szapocznik, J., Perez-Vidal, A., Brickman, A. L., Foote, F. H., Santisteban, D., Hervis, O., et al. (1988). Engaging adolescent drug abusers and their families in treatment: A strategic structural systems approach. *Journal of Consulting and Clinical Psychology, 56*, 552–557.

Takeda, Y. (2000). Aggression in relation to childhood depression: A study of Japanese 3rd-6th graders. *Japanese Journal of Developmental Psychology, 11*(1), 1–11.

Teplin, L. A., Abram, K. M., McClelland, G. M., Dulcan, M. K., & Mericle, A. A. (2002). Psychiatric disorders in youth in juvenile detention. *Archives of General Psychiatry, 59*, 1133–1143.

Thornberry, T. P., & Krohn, M. D. (2001). The development of delinquency: An interactional perspective. In S. White (Ed.), *Handbook of youth and justice* (pp. 289–305). New York: Kluwer Academic/Plenum.

Timmons-Mitchell, J., Brown, C., Schulz, C., Webster, S. E., Underwood, L. A., & Semple, W. E. (1997). Comparing the mental health needs of female and male incarcerated juvenile delinquents. *Behavioural Sciences and the Law, 15*(2), 195–202.

Tisher, M. (1995). Teacher's assessments of prepubertal childhood depression. *Australian Journal of Psychology, 47*(2), 93–96.

U.S. Department of Health and Human Services. (2001). *Mental health: A report of the Surgeon General*. Rockville, MD: Author.

U.S. Justice Department. (1998). *Women in the criminal justice system: A twenty year update: A special report*. Rockville, MD: National Criminal Justice Reference Service.

Ulzen, T. P. M., & Hamilton, H. (1998). The nature and characteristics of psychiatric .comorbidity in incarcerated adolescents. *Canadian Journal of Research, 43*, 57–63.

Wasserman, G. A, McReynolds, L. S, Lucas, C. P, Fisher, P., & Santos, L. (2002). The voice DISC-IV with incarcerated male youths: Prevalence of disorder. *Journal of the American Academy of Child and Adolescent Psychiatry, 41*, 314–321.

Weiss, B., & Garber, J. (2003). Developmental differences in the phenomenology of depression. *Development and Psychopathology, 15*(2), 403–430.

Wierson, M., Forehand, R. L., & Frame, C. L. (1992). Epidemiology and treatment of mental health problems in juvenile delinquents. *Advanced Behavioural Research and Therapy, 14*, 93–120.

Williams, R., & Chang, S. (2000). A comprehensive and comparative review of adolescent substance abuse treatment outcome. *Clinical Psychology: Science and Practice, 7*(2), 138–166.

Windle, M. (1996). On the discriminative validity of a family history of problem drinking with index with a national sample of young adults. *Journal of Studies on Alcohol, 57*(4), 378–386.

Wood, J., Foy, D. W., Layne, C., Pynoos, R., & James, C. B. (2002). An examination of the relationships between violence exposure, posttraumatic stress symptomatology, and delinquent activity: An "ecopathological" model of delinquent behavior among incarcerated adolescents. *Journal of Aggression, Maltreatment and Trauma, 6*(1), 127–147.

Zagar, R., Arbit, J., Hughes, J. R., Busell, R. E., & Busch, K. (1989). Developmental and disruptive behaviour disorders among delinquents. *Journal of the American Academy of Child and Adolescent Psychiatry, 28,* 437–440.

6

KIRK HEILBRUN, RIA LEE, AND CINDY C. COTTLE

Risk Factors and Intervention Outcomes

Meta-Analyses of Juvenile Offending

Research on juvenile offending has been conducted in two broad areas that are particularly important in this book: prediction and risk reduction. Studies in the former area seek to identify risk factors and protective factors for juveniles and link them empirically with outcomes as specific as juvenile offending and as broad as antisocial behavior. In the latter area, research has focused on interventions delivered to juvenile offenders that are designed to reduce the risk of such offending and behavior. The use of large-scale reviews of empirical research in both areas is particularly important for several goals of this book: identifying future research directions, distilling implications for policy, and addressing "best practices" for assessment, intervention, and decision making with juveniles that are informed by empirical research.

In this chapter, we identify research in the targeted areas of prediction and intervention. We also specify subpopulations within adolescent offenders and seek to identify studies describing outcomes as narrow as offending and as broad as antisocial behavior. We use these distinctions to create a matrix that describes various areas of research on juvenile delinquency. Using this matrix, we then apply the tool of meta-analysis to describe cumulative trends of empirical research within these areas, populations, and outcomes.

Nature and Value of Meta-Analysis

Meta-analysis is a form of statistical analysis that estimates the strength of relationships among predictive or outcome variables across a number of studies. By combining the results of a number of primary studies, meta-analysis can be used to summarize research findings in a way that is more powerful than that in any single study. However, the value of meta-analysis is determined by the number and quality of existing primary studies. When such studies are numerous, well designed, and effectively implemented, then meta-analysis can be a particularly powerful tool for identifying findings that transcend the idiosyncrasies of any single study. By contrast, however, when there are relatively few available primary studies, or the studies are methodologically flawed, then the value of a meta-analysis is reduced accordingly.

There are several considerations in conducting a meta-analysis. First, researchers must take active steps to avoid bias in selecting studies; this can be accomplished by using multiple data bases for computer searches, cross-referencing studies, contacting authors and experts, and searching for unpublished studies (Rosenthal, 1991). By including a wide range of studies and by contacting researchers whose reports include only a partial listing of findings, researchers can minimize the likelihood of bias in favor of studies reporting statistically significant relationships.

A second consideration concerns the reliability and validity of the meta-analytic findings. This involves examining the comparability of the studies, using inclusion criteria that are clearly defined, and evaluating the reliability of these criteria across studies (Stock, 1994). Important criteria in any meta-analysis include the time period covered in the review, the quality and design of the study, and a list of included variables and their operational definitions. In the area of juvenile recidivism, researchers conducting meta-analyses should pay particular attention to the definition of juvenile ($\leq$18 years old vs. $\leq$21 years old), recidivism (e.g., rearrest vs. reconviction), and the length of time participants are at risk for reoffending.

Second, researchers must decide how the studies should be analyzed and the effect size that will be used in reporting the results. In the simplest terms, studies can be summarized and an overall mean effect size representing the association between two variables or groups of variables can be reported. However, as meta-analytic methods and primary study methodologies become more sophisticated, researchers can conduct more complex analyses. For example, researchers can include analyses of moderators, such as gender or treatment type, and can also estimate true mean effect sizes after correcting or controlling for measurement or sampling error, methodological differences across studies, and between-studies differences in study design (e.g., the duration of treatment).

There are at least six important areas to which meta-analysis can be applied in the investigation of juvenile offending. These areas include (a) predictors of general recidivism, (b) predictors of sexual recidivism, (c) predictors of violent recidivism, (d) effects of interventions on general recidivism, (e) effects of interventions on sexual recidivism, and (f) effects of interventions on violent recidivism (see Table 6.1). The following sections provide a review of the findings of meta-analyses that have been conducted in these areas.

Meta-Analyses on Predictors of Juvenile Recidivism

Predictors of General Recidivism

The relationship between various predictors and general reoffending (for any offense) in juveniles has been considered in a recent meta-analysis (Cottle, Lee,

TABLE 6.1 Meta-Analytic Research on Juvenile Recidivism: Prediction Versus Intervention Impact and Different Outcomes

Recidivism	Study
Predictors of	
General	Cottle et al. (2001)
Sexual	Present chapter
Violent	Present chapter
Effects of intervention on	
General	Lipsey (1992)
Sexual	Not yet possible[a]
Violent	Lipsey & Wilson (1998)

[a]A review of the literature yielded an insufficient number of empirical treatment outcome studies to conduct a meta-analysis. Only three such studies were located (see Borduin, Henggeler, Blasker, & Stein, 1990; Kahn & Chambers, 1991; Worling & Curwen, 2000).

& Heilbrun, 2001). A total of 23 published studies met inclusion criteria by considering juveniles ranging in age from 12 to 21 with a prior arrest history and providing data on reoffense. Since one team of researchers published two studies using data collected from the same sample (Dembo et al., 1998; Dembo, Williams, Schmeidler, Getreu, & Berry, 1991), we decided to include only the study with the longer outcome period (Dembo et al., 1998) to avoid double counting the sample data. For the remaining 22 studies (marked with one asterisk in the References section), data about reoffense were considered if they resulted in reincarceration, rearrest, or probation or parole violations, as obtained from official records or self-report. The length of the outcome periods ranged considerably across studies (1–192 months), with a mean follow-up of approximately 45 months. There was also a wide range in the number of participants in each study (45–9,176), with a mean sample size of approximately 688 participants. The total number of participants was 15,265, the majority of whom (93%) were male. Participants' ages ranged from 6 to 21 years, with a mean age of 14.7 years, and the racial breakdown of the sample was 46% White, 37% African American, and 18% who were classified as "other." Seventeen studies included in the meta-analysis reported comparable recidivism rates, which ranged from 22 to 75%, with an overall mean recidivism rate of 48%.

The Cottle et al. (2001) review identified a total of 30 predictor variables, which were categorized into the following domains: *demographic information* (including gender, race, and socioeconomic status), *offense history* (age at first contact with the law, age at first commitment, number of prior arrests, number of prior commitments, type of crime committed, and length of first incarceration), *family and social factors* (having been a victim of physical or sexual abuse, living with a single parent, parental pathology, number of out-of-home placements, family problems such as impaired intrafamilial relationships, effective use of leisure time, and having delinquent peers), *educational factors* (history of special education, school attendance, and school achievement as determined by teachers' reports, grade point average, and grade placement), *standardized test scores* (achievement scores and verbal, performance, and full scale IQ scores), *substance abuse history* (substance use and abuse), and *clinical factors* (severe pathology such as psychosis and suicidality, nonsevere pathology such as stress and anxiety, conduct problems, and treatment history). We found only a small number of studies that examined formal measures of risk assessment. As a result, the composite variable "formal risk assessment" was created to represent research that investigated relevant variables as predictors of recidivism.

This meta-analysis identified strong relationships between a number of predictor variables and general reoffending behavior in juveniles. In particular, the study found that all of the variables in the first domain, demographic information, were significantly associated with recidivism. Specifically, male gender ($Z_r = .11$, $p < .001$) and membership in a minority race ($Z_r = .07$, $p < .001$) were positively related to recidivism. Similarly, a low socioeconomic background also increased the reoffense risk among juveniles ($Z_r = -.07$, $p < .001$). In order to determine whether race would continue to be significant when controlling for socioeconomic status (SES), a hierarchical regression analysis was conducted, and both gender and SES were entered in the equation before race. This analysis revealed that after controlling for the effect of SES, race did not retain a significant association with recidivism (F change $= 1.80$, $p = .25$).

The meta-analysis further showed a significant association between recidivism and each of the offense history variables. Juveniles who were younger when they experienced their first contact with the law ($Z_r = -.34$, $p < .001$) and younger at the time of their first commitment ($Z_r = -.35$, $p < .001$) were at an increased risk of recidivism. Those with more prior arrests ($Z_r = .06$, $p < .001$), more previous commitments ($Z_r = .17$, $p < .001$), and longer incarcerations ($Z_r = .19$, $p < .001$), as well as those who committed more serious crimes ($Z_r = .16$, $p < .001$), also showed an increased recidivism risk.

The majority of the family and social variables were also found to be significant predictors of recidivism. Specifically, juveniles with a history of being victims of physical or sexual abuse ($Z_r = .11$, $p < .001$) and those raised in a single-parent home ($Z_r = .07$, $p < .001$), having more out-of-home placements ($Z_r = .18$, $p < .001$), or having significant family problems ($Z_r = .23$, $p < .001$) were at increased risk of recidivism. Furthermore, juveniles who failed to effectively use their leisure time ($Z_r = .23$, $p < .001$) and those with delinquent peers ($Z_r = .20$, $p < .001$) were also at increased risk. The presence of parental pathology ($Z_r = .05$, $p = $ ns) was the only variable that was not a significant predictor of recidivism in this domain.

A history of special education ($Z_r = .13$, $p < .01$) was the only variable significantly related to recidivism among the educational factors. School attendance ($Z_r = -.05$, $p = $ ns) and school reports of academic achievement ($Z_r = -.03$, $p = $ ns) were not found to be significant predictors. With respect to standardized test scores, three of the four variables were significantly associated with recidivism. In particular, juveniles with lower standardized achievement test scores ($Z_r = -.11$, $p < .001$), lower full scale IQ scores ($Z_r = -.14$, $p < .001$), and lower verbal IQ scores ($Z_r = -.11$, $p < .01$) were at greater risk of recidivism. However, performance IQ scores ($Z_r = -.03$, $p = $ ns) were not significantly associated with recidivism.

Within the substance use domain, substance *abuse* was significantly related to recidivism ($Z_r = .15$, $p < .001$). However, substance *use* was not found to increase recidivism risk significantly ($Z_r = .01$, $p = $ ns). Among the clinical factors, two variables were significantly associated with recidivism risk. Specifically, a history of conduct problems ($Z_r = .26$, $p < .001$) and nonsevere pathology ($Z_r = .31$, $p < .001$) increased the risk of reoffending. Having a history of severe pathology ($Z_r = .07$, $p = $ ns) or a history of psychiatric treatment ($Z_r = .02$, $p = $ ns), however, was not significantly related to recidivism. Finally, the composite variable representing any type of formal risk assessment was a significant predictor of recidivism ($Z_r = .12$, $p < .001$).

One important goal of the Cottle et al. (2001) meta-analysis was to identify risk factors with the strongest association with general recidivism risk among juvenile offenders. We addressed this by rank ordering the factors according to Z-score magnitude and determining the number of additional participants with null results that would be needed to change the significance of the results. The findings indicate that a younger age at first commitment was the strongest predictor variable, followed by age at first contact with the law and history of nonsevere pathology. Overall, the results showed that variables within the history and the family and social-factors domains were most consistently predictive of juvenile general recidivism (see Table 6.2).

Furthermore, we determined that the minimum number of participants in an unretrieved study with a Z value of zero needed to nullify the significance ranged from 473 to 81,345. This substantial range is a reflection of the variability in the power of the studies included in the meta-analysis.

All of the participants in this meta-analysis were juveniles who had previously been adjudicated delinquent. As a result, the overall sample was substantially more homogenous than might by typical in a study of first-time juvenile offenders. These particular sample characteristics may be responsible for the somewhat unexpected findings that variables such as substance use, school attendance and achievement, and treatment history showed only weak associations with juvenile recidivism; the discriminative power of these predictors was probably decreased as a result of sample homogeneity.

Predictors of Sexual Recidivism

A second meta-analysis, conducted for this chapter, considered predictors of recidivism among juvenile sexual offenders. The studies incorporated into two categories: those describing juvenile sexual offenders and those considering juvenile violent (but nonsexual) offenders. Meta-analysis on the latter group of studies is discussed later in this chapter. Next, we created outcome-specific categories for (a) violent, nonsexual reoffending and (b) nonviolent, sexual reoffend-

TABLE 6.2 Predictors of Recidivism in Juveniles (N = 15,265) by Effect Size Strength

Variable	Zr	N	κ	Studies
Age at first commitment	−.346***	720	3	Archwamety & Katsiyannis (1998); Katsiyannis & Archwamety (1997); Towberman (1994)
Age at first contact with the law	−.341***	1225	8	Archwamety & Katsiyannis (1998); Duncan, Kennedy, & Patrick (1995); Hanson, Henggeler, Haefele, & Rodick (1984); Katsiyannis & Archwamety (1997); Minor, Hartmann, & Terry (1997); Myner, Santman, Cappelletty, & Perlmutter (1998); Niarhos & Routh (1992)
Nonsevere pathology	.305***	953	7	Bleker (1983); Duncan et al. (1995); Hanson et al. (1984); Jung & Rawana (1999); Niarhos & Routh (1992); Steiner et al. (1999); Wierson & Forehand (1995)
Family problems	.277***	1054	5	Hanson et al. (1984); Hoge et al. (1996); Jung & Rawana (1999); Niarhos & Routh (1992); Towberman (1994)
Conduct problems	.255***	1667	7	Duncan et al. (1995); Myner et al. (1998); Niarhos & Routh (1992); Stattin & Magnusson (1989); Towberman (1994); Repo & Virkkunen (1997); Wierson & Forehand (1995)
Effective use of leisure time	−.233***	588	2	Hoge, Andrews, & Leschied (1996); Jung & Rawana (1999)
Delinquent peers	.204***	1525	7	Archwamety & Katsiyannis (1998); Hoge, Andrews, & Leschied (1996); Jung & Rawana (1990); Katsiyannis & Archwamety (1997); Myner et al. (1998); Niarhos & Routh (1992); Towberman (1994)
Length of first incarceration	.187***	641	3	Archwamety & Katsiyannis (1996); Katsiyannis & Archwamety (1997); Myner et al. (1998)
Number of out-of-home placements	.184***	424	2	Myner et al. (1998); Towberman (1994)
Number of prior commitments	.174***	585	3	Archwamety & Katsiyannis (1998); Duncan et al. (1995); Katsiyannis & Archwamety (1997)
Type of crime	.159***	10,267	7	Archwamety & Katsiyannis (1998); Dembo et al. (1998); Katsiyannis & Archwamety (1997); Minor et al. (1997); Myner et al. (1998); Niarhos & Routh (1992); Wierson & Forehand (1995)

TABLE 6.2 *(continued)*

Variable	Zr	N	κ	Studies
Standardized achievement score	−.153***	506	3	Archwamety & Katsiyannis (1998); Duncan et al. (1995); Katsiyannis & Archwamety (1997)
Substance abuse	.149***	1111	6	Archwamety & Katsiyannis (1998); Duncan et al. (1995); Katsiyannis & Archwamety (1997); Myner et al. (1998); Niarhos & Routh (1992); Wierson & Forehand (1995)
Full scale IQ score	−.142***	1756	5	Archwamety & Katsiyannis (1998); Duncan et al. (1995); Katsiyannis & Archwamety (1997); Niarhos & Routh (1992); Stattin & Magnusson (1989)
History of special education	.130**	432	2	Archwamety & Katsiyannis (1998); Katsiyannis & Archwamety (1997)
Risk assessment instruments	.118***	10,353	6	Archwamety & Katsiyannis (1998); Ashford & LeCroy (1988); Dembo et al. (1998); Dembo, Williams, Fagan, & Schmeidler (1994); Jung & Rawana (1999); Katsiyannis & Archwamety (1997)
History of abuse	.112***	9949	5	Archwamety & Katsiyannis (1998); Dembo et al. (1998); Katsiyannis & Archwamety (1997); Myner et al. (1998); Towberman (1994)
Gender (male)	.111***	9671	3	Dembo et al. (1998); Hoge et al. (1996); Minor et al. (1997)
Verbal IQ score	−.111**	716	4	Archwamety & Katsiyannis (1998); Bleker (1983); Hanson et al. (1984); Katsiyannis & Archwamety (1997)
Single parent	.070***	10,501	5	Dembo et al. (1998); Minor et al. (1997); Myner et al. (1998); Niarhos & Routh (1992); Putnins (1984)
Severe pathology	.069	346	2	Archwamety & Katsiyannis (1998); Niarhos & Routh (1992)
Race (minority	.067***	10,121	6	Archwamety & Katsiyannis (1998); Dembo et al. (1998); Katsiyannis & Archwamety (1997); Minor et al. (1997); Myner et al. (1998); Niarhos & Routh (1992)
SES	.065***	10,363	3	Dembo et al. (1998); Myner et al. (1998); Stattin & Magnusson (1989)
Number of prior arrests	.058***	10,155	7	Archwamety & Katsiyannis (1998); Dembo et al. (1998); Duncan et al. (1995); Jung & Rawana (1999); Katsiyannis & Archwamety (1997); Niarhos & Routh (1992); Wierson & Forehand (1995)

TABLE 6.2 (continued)

Variable	Zr	N	κ	Studies
School attendance	−.048	299	2	Myner et al. (1998); Towberman (1994)
Parent pathology	.047	529	3	Hoge et al. (1996); Myner et al. (1998); Niarhos & Routh (1992)
Performance IQ score	−.031	491	2	Archwamety & Katsiyannis (1998); Katsiyannis & Archwamety (1997)
School report of achievement	−.028	10,025	6	Myner et al. (1998); Dembo et al. (1998); Duncan et al. (1995); Jung & Rawana (1999); Niarhos & Routh (1992); Hoge et al. (1996)
History of treatment	.019	9366	2	Dembo et al. (1998); Towberman (1994)
Substance use	.014	9366	2	Dembo et al. (1998); Towberman (1994)

Note. Zr = weighted mean effect size; κ = number of unique samples. *Source*: From "The Prediction of Criminal Recidivism in Juveniles: A Meta-Analysis," by C. Cottle, R. Lee, and K. Heilbrun, 2001, *Criminal Justice and Behavior, 28*. Copyright 2001 by Sage. Reprinted with permission.

$**p < .01. ***p < .001.$

ing to allow identification of predictors that could distinguish between violent and sexual offending. Sexual reoffending tends to be categorized as either violent ("hands-on") or nonviolent ("hands-off"), so violent sexual reoffending constitutes an area of overlap between the two categories.

We located nine studies on juvenile sexual recidivism that met our inclusion criteria for the meta-analysis. These studies are marked with two asterisks in the References section. Inclusion criteria were as follows: (a) incorporating adolescents aged 7–21 with one or more prior arrests for sexual offending, (b) defining reoffense as any new offense that resulted in reincarceration, rearrest, or parole violation, and (c) providing reoffense data from official records, self-report, or both.

The sample sizes of the included studies ranged from 16 to 221 participants, with a mean of 128.9. The follow-up periods varied in length from 24 to 228 months, with a mean outcome period of 54.2 months. The total number of participants was 1,160, approximately 97% of whom were male. The participants ranged in age from 7 to 20 years, with a mean age of 14.6 years. Several studies failed to report demographic data such as age, gender, and racial background. Among the studies that provided this information, the racial breakdown of the sample included 73.4% White, 12.3% African American, and 14.3% who were categorized as "other."

Overall mean recidivism rates were reported for sexual reoffending (14.3%), nonsexual reoffending (41.0%), and any reoffending (48.7%). The total reoffense rate does not equal the sum of all sexual and nonsexual reoffending rates, as some studies did not report recidivism rates for nonsexual reoffending, and other studies did not report recidivism rates for any reoffending.

The variables in this meta-analysis were categorized into several domains, as we did previously in the meta-analysis on general recidivism in juveniles (Cottle et al., 2001). A total of nine predictor variables were identified in the following broad domains: offense history, family and social factors, and intervention. The offense history domain included five variables: age at first sexual offense, type of initial sexual offense (contact vs. noncontact), age of youngest victim, relationship to victim (acquaintance or stranger), and number of prior nonsexual arrests. The family and social factors domain included three factors: social problems, having been the victim of physical abuse, and having been the victim of sexual abuse. In this context, the variable "social problems" was measured as functional deficits (e.g., lack of social skills and inadequate sexual knowledge; Kahn & Chambers, 1991), social maladjustment (e.g., level of peer support and partici-pation in community-based treatment group activities; Smith & Monastersky, 1986), or according to scores on a self-report measure of social competencies and problem behaviors (Achenbach Youth Self-Report, social problems subscale; Worling & Curwen, 2000). Relatively few studies were located that investigated comparable interventions for juvenile sexual offenders. As a result, this domain could not be divided into distinct factors reflecting specific types of interventions such as multisystemic, individual, or group treatments. The predictor "interven-tion" was therefore created as a composite variable, incorporating studies that considered any form of treatment focused on decreasing rates of sexual recidi-vism among juvenile offenders.

The results of the meta-analysis indicated that three of the five predictors in the offense history domain were significantly associated with recidivism in juve-nile sexual offenders. Specifically, the age of the offender ($Z_r = -.069$, $p < .05$) was negatively related to reoffending, as younger adolescents were at higher risk for recidivism. A positive association was determined between the type of the ini-tial sexual offense ($Z_r = .126$, $p < .01$) and recidivism, in that juveniles who com-mitted less serious sexual offenses (e.g., indecent liberties or noncontact of-fenses) were more likely to reoffend both sexually and nonsexually than juveniles who committed more serious offenses, such as rape. The results also showed that the relationship between the juvenile offenders and their victims ($Z_r = .184$, $p < .001$) was significantly associated with reoffending; those who com-mitted offenses against acquaintances were more likely to reoffend than juve-niles who committed offenses against either relatives or strangers. The only non-significant factors in this domain were the age of the victim ($Z_r = -.077$, $p = $ ns) and the juvenile's offense history ($Z_r = .083$, $p = $ ns).

None of the predictors in the family and social factors domain was signifi-cantly associated with recidivism: social problems ($Z_r = .024$, $p = $ ns), history of sexual abuse ($Z_r = .063$, $p = $ ns), and history of physical abuse ($Z_r = .016$, $p = $ ns). However, the composite intervention variable ($Z_r = -.158$, $p < .001$) was signifi-cantly negatively related to recidivism, suggesting that interventions were effec-tive in decreasing the risk of reoffending among juvenile sexual offenders.

The predictor variables were also considered individually and rank ordered according to their Z-score magnitudes. The relationship between offender and victim was the strongest predictor of recidivism among juvenile sexual offenders. Specifically, those who victimized acquaintances were at higher risk of reoffending than juveniles who offended against strangers. The intervention variable was the second strongest predictor of recidivism (those receiving intervention were at lower risk), followed by type of initial sex offense and criminal history.

One conclusion drawn from this meta-analysis was that several limitations continue to impede meta-analytic reviews of juvenile sexual offenders. For instance, many studies do not provide basic descriptive data, and much of the published research lacks consistency in defining and measuring outcome variables; both preclude meaningful comparisons. In a similar vein, predictors vary considerably across studies, limiting consistency and thus impeding meta-analytic comparisons. The findings of the Lee, Cottle, and Heilbrun (2001) meta-analysis must be considered with these limitations in mind, as well as with the limits on its generalizability resulting from the small overall sample size.

Predictors of Violent Recidivism Among Violent Offenders

The third area of juvenile recidivism, violent reoffending, was also considered for the purposes of this chapter. As with general and sexual recidivism, we used meta-analysis to identify the strongest predictors of juvenile violent reoffending. To distinguish studies investigating violent juvenile reoffending from those that examined sexual reoffending, we conducted the violent reoffending meta-analysis using only studies investigating violent, nonsexual reoffending.

We located only four published studies (marked with three asterisks in the References section) examining nonsexual, violent juvenile reoffending. Inclusion criteria for a potential study to be included in this meta-analysis were as follows: (a) considering juveniles aged 7–21 with at least one prior arrest for a violent offense and (b) providing data on subsequent offending that resulted in rearrest, reincarceration, or revocation of parole (c) as obtained from official records or self-reports. The majority of the studies included in the meta-analysis used official records to obtain data on reoffending.

Only one of these four studies used violent reoffending as the outcome; the other three used *any* reoffending. Among the studies investigating juvenile violent reoffending, only one predictor could be used for meaningful meta-analysis for predicting this outcome ("any recidivism"). We created this variable ("intervention") as a composite to encompass any intervention delivered to reduce recidivism risk among violent adolescent offenders. Such interventions included treatments such as cognitive or family therapy, as well as no-treatment control groups, which were typically described as "usual services" (e.g., probation or incarceration in juvenile correctional facilities).

There was a total of 380 participants across the four studies investigating violent juvenile offenders, with a mean sample size of 95.0 and a range of 60–155. The outcome periods ranged from 14 to 24 months, with a mean of 17.6 months. Only one of the studies included in the meta-analysis reported a recidivism rate for violent reoffending; the others reported recidivism rates for any or general reoffending. The mean recidivism rate for general recidivism among all four studies was 34.9%. A total of 61.5% of the participants were male; participants' mean age was 15.6 years. Only three of the studies reported a racial breakdown of the sample, indicating that 10.2% of the participants were White, 66.6% were African American, and 23.2% were classified as "other."

Within the "intervention" variable, we distinguished between "family and cognitive therapy" services and "usual services" for violent offenders. The distribution of effect sizes was homogeneous ($\chi^2 = 2.51$, $p = .47$). This indicates a good fit for the model, suggesting that there were no significant differences across the studies. The average effect size for the studies included in the meta-analysis was small ($r = .14$, $SD = .08$), and the group mean differences were significantly related to recidivism ($t = 3.49$, $p < .05$). The binomial effect size display (BESD) suggested that family and cognitive therapies (BESD = .57, or 57% success rate) tend to be more successful in reducing recidivism rates among juveniles than usual services (BESD = .43, or 43% success rate).

These results suggest that specific treatment interventions, such as cognitive and family therapies, were more effective in reducing recidivism rates than provision of usual services only. This finding suggests that clinical interventions (e.g., individual or family therapy) provided in addition to usual services (e.g., probation or incarceration) have a greater effect on reducing recidivism rates among violent juvenile offenders, although this finding does not rule out the possibility that more intensive (but not necessarily clinical) intervention is responsible for the bulk of the observed risk reduction. It should be noted, however, that this finding is consistent with the results of ongoing research investigating the effectiveness of specialized clinical interventions, such as multisystemic therapy (e.g., Borduin, 1999; Henggeler, 1999), among juvenile offenders. It should also be observed that we found the number and breadth of existing studies on violent juvenile offenders to be extremely limited, thereby restricting the scope of meta-analytic review. One of these limits concerns the measurement of outcome. Despite the use of violent juvenile offenders as participants in these studies, only one of four investigators used a meaningful specific variable (violent reoffending) that could easily have been recorded specifically, rather than considering outcome very broadly (general reoffending). This failure to distinguish type of reoffending means that no meta-analysis can be conducted on an important question: are violent juvenile offenders more likely to become violent juvenile reoffenders?

Several other limitations constrain the ability to conduct meta-analytic reviews in the areas of sexual and violent juvenile recidivism as well. The failure of investigators to provide basic descriptive data, the selection of risk factors that are limited and not consistent with those used by other investigators, and the inconsistency in operationalizing important variables all limit meaningful meta-analysis. We suggested several remedies for these problems (Lee et al., 2001), including providing relevant descriptive data (e.g., recidivism rates, sample characteristics) and operational definitions (e.g., predictors and their measurement, outcomes and their measurement) and the means by which other investigators can determine effect size (e.g., bivariate correlation coefficients for the relationship between predictor and outcome variables; Z-scores, t scores, F values, or specific p values). We also suggested including the results of variables that are *not* significant; the results of a meta-analysis will be skewed if investigators fail to provide such data.

Meta-Analyses on Interventions to Reduce Risk

Effects of Interventions on General Recidivism

Meta-analyses conducted to assess the effects of interventions on general recidivism among juvenile offenders first appeared in the 1980s, when previous qualitative literature reviews reported that interventions were not effective in reducing recidivism rates among juvenile offenders. It was even suggested that some interventions might be harmful to recipients (for a review see, e.g., Garrett, 1985; Lipsey, 1992). More recent reviews have used improved methodologies and have more clearly communicated results, attempting to answer more specific questions about factors associated with the impact of the interventions being studies. The following summarizes the results of five meta-analyses conducted between 1985 and 2000 investigating the effects of interventions on recidivism among juvenile offenders.

EFFECTS OF RESIDENTIAL TREATMENT ON ADJUDICATED DELINQUENTS: GARRETT (1985)

One of the first large-scale meta-analyses investigating the effects of interventions on general recidivism among juvenile offenders was conducted by Garrett (1985). It included 111 studies between 1960 and 1983 investigating adjudicated delinquents placed in residential facilities, including group homes and halfway houses. To be included in the meta-analysis, a study must have employed a control or comparison group. The final sample of studies included 13,055 participants and a variety of treatment interventions (e.g., individual, group, family, contingency management, cognitive-behavioral, drug/alcohol, vocational, outdoor) and outcome measures (e.g., recidivism, psychological adjustment, institutional adjustment, community adjustment, academic improvement, and vocational adjustment). The majority (81.1%) of the treatments took place in an institutional setting, while the remainder (18.9%) took place in a community residential setting.

Results of the Garrett (1985) meta-analysis indicate that juveniles receiving treatment, regardless of treatment type, setting, offender type, or outcome measure, performed an average of 0.37 SD above the level of untreated juveniles across all outcome measures. When recidivism was used as the specific outcome variable, which occurred in 34 studies, an effect size of 0.13 SD was observed. There was no effect of treatment on vocational adjustment. Other outcome measures produced larger effect sizes: institutional adjustment (.41), psychological adjustment (.52), and community adjustment (.63). However, as the author notes, these effect sizes could be inflated due to reactivity (impact of assessment) of the participants. Other factors, such as the inconsistency of various measures of adjustment across studies, were also described as problematic.

Garrett (1985) also investigated the types of treatments provided, by considering both broad categories of treatments (e.g., psychodynamic, behavioral, life skills, and other, such as music therapy and undifferentiated skills training programs) and specific types of treatments (e.g., individual, group, family, contingency management, outdoor, and milieu). Treatments in the *behavioral* category produced the greatest change among juveniles (effect size = .63), followed by *life skills* interventions (effect size = .31), *other* interventions (effect size = .30), and *psychodynamic* treatments (effect size = .17). Garrett notes, however, that when the rigor of the study is considered, the effectiveness of these categories is changed. For more rigorous studies (i.e., those using randomly assigned participants), the magnitude of effect sizes favors life skills interventions (.32), followed by behavioral (.30), other treatments (.27), and psychodynamic treatments (.17). For less rigorous studies (e.g., those using nonrandom assignment, convenience samples, and the like), other interventions (1.20) appear superior, followed by behavioral (.86), life skills (.31), and psychodynamic (.31). Despite such variation in effect sizes, it seems clear that more behaviorally oriented treatments are useful in reducing recidivism among certain groups of juvenile offenders, and psychodynamic approaches consistently produced more marginal effect sizes. Among the specific types of treatments reported by Garrett (1985), contingency management (.86), family therapy (.81), and cognitive-behavioral therapy (.58) were among the most successful in reducing recidivism among juvenile offenders. Other treatments that appear to have a significant effect on recidivism among juvenile offenders include academic (.39), substance abuse (.28), and outdoor (.38) programs.

JUVENILE CORRECTIONAL TREATMENT: WHITEHEAD AND LAB (1989)

Whitehead and Lab (1989) analyzed 50 delinquency studies published between 1975 and 1984 investigating diversion programs, probation, and residential and community-based treatments. To be included in the analysis, studies had to use a control/comparison group and describe recidivism rates as an outcome measure. The type of treatment was classified as behavioral or nonbehavioral, and the recency and quality of the research design were also considered.

Using the phi coefficient as the measure of effect size, the authors set a coefficient value of .20 or greater as their standard for judging favorable impact of the intervention. Whitehead and Lab reported an average phi coefficient of .12 for studies and concluded that there was not a significant difference between treatment and control groups. Further, they noted that that more rigorous studies showed that treatment effects were even smaller in the more rigorous studies. Finally, the authors indicated that behavioral treatments appear to be no more effective than nonbehavioral approaches in the control of recidivism.

In his review of the Whitehead and Lab meta-analysis, Lipsey (1992) noted that these results do reflect more positive treatment effects when reported in terms more meaningful than phi coefficient effect size estimates. When converted to standard deviation units, a phi coefficient of .12 is equivalent to 0.25 SD units between treatment and control groups, he noted, suggesting that Whitehead and Lab may have been overly conservative in their methodology and, as a consequence, less sanguine about the impact of treatment on recidivism than was warranted.

CORRECTIONAL TREATMENT: ANDREWS ET AL. (1990)

Andrews et al. (1990) reconsidered the Whitehead and Lab (1985) results by observing that "the effectiveness of correctional treatment is dependent upon what is delivered to whom in particular settings" (Andrews et al., 1990, p. 372). After removing overlapping or otherwise methodologically inappropriate samples, Andrews et al. included 45 of the 50 studies used by Whitehead and Lab. Andrews et al. also included an additional 35 studies, to help assess the generalizability of Whitehead and Lab's conclusions. Using the phi coefficient as the effect size estimate, Andrews et al. found that type of treatment contributed significantly to the prediction of effect size (ϕ = .69), even controlling for year of publication, quality of research design, sample of studies used (i.e., Whitehead & Lab original studies vs. the additional 35 studies), treatment setting, justice system (juvenile vs. adult), and behavioral–nonbehavioral intervention (ϕ = .72). The authors also reported that the mean phi coefficient for appropriate correctional service (ϕ = .30, n = 54) was significantly greater than that for criminal sanctions (ϕ = –.07, n = 30), inappropriate service (e.g., those that do not target higher risk populations or that do not focus on criminogenic needs; ϕ = .06, n = 38), and unspecified service (ϕ = .13, n = 32). With respect to type of treatment, Andrews et al. observed that the phi coefficients for behavioral interventions (ϕ = .29, n = 41) were significantly greater than those for nonbehavioral interventions (ϕ = .04, n = 113).

THE VARIABILITY OF EFFECTS: LIPSEY (1992)

Lipsey (1992) conducted an analysis of the effects of interventions on juvenile delinquency and the sources of variability in those effects. This meta-analysis included 443 studies that reported the results of some form of treatment delivered to reduce the risk of delinquency, defined as "behavior chargeable under applicable laws whether or not apprehension occurs or charges are brought," or antisocial behavior, defined as "actions that are threatening, disruptive, or damaging to property, to other persons, or to self" (Lipsey, 1992, p. 88). To be included in the analysis, a study must have included juveniles aged 21 years and younger, employed a control or comparison group, and reported quantitative outcome variables that included at least one delinquency measure.

Lipsey reported that 64.3% of the studies found greater risk reduction for the treatment group, 29.6% of the studies favored the control or comparison group, and the remaining 6.1% of the studies favored neither the treatment nor the control/comparison group. An analysis of the studies (n = 397) allowing for the computation of an effect size estimate yielded an unweighted mean effect size of .172 and an inverse variance weighted mean effect size of .103; both effect sizes were statistically significant. Lipsey observed that although these effect sizes were modest, they were also equivalent to a 10% decrease in delinquency rates for juveniles who receive some form of intervention.

Additional analyses in the Lipsey meta-analysis involved the variability of intervention effects and the sources of that variability. Lipsey analyzed the degree to which reductions in delinquency could be attributed to study characteristics (e.g., publication year, country, author's discipline), methodological variables (e.g., sampling, attrition, outcome measures), or treatment characteristics (e.g., participant characteristics, amount and intensity of treatment, type of treatment conditions, philosophy of the treatment). Using multiple regression, Lipsey found that the cluster of variables related to study characteristics (e.g., publication year, author's discipline, country of origin) were not predictive of treatment effects and that methodological variables accounted for 25% of the variability in effect sizes. The effects of treatment characteristics were added last in the hierarchical multiple regression and accounted for an additional 22% of variability in effect sizes.

Methodological characteristics contributed more strongly when the intervention and comparison groups showed greater differences prior to treatment (R^2 change = .06). Lipsey also found that studies using multiple delinquency outcome measures, longer follow-up periods, and measures with weak reliability and validity were associated with smaller effect sizes (R^2 change = .04). Attrition from either the treatment or comparison group also suppressed effect sizes (R^2 change = .03).

The greatest contribution of treatment characteristics came from treatment modality variables, such as the degree to which the researcher was involved in the treatment setting, which might indicate that highly monitored and better implemented treatments are associated with stronger effect sizes (R^2 change =.11). The role of treatment dosage (e.g., duration, frequency, and amount of treatment) produced a modest effect (R^2 change = .03), indicating that more frequent contact and longer periods of treatment were associated with stronger effect sizes. However, a curvilinear relationship between amount of treatment received and the location of such treatment was observed, such that effect size increased with the amount of treatment up to a level associated with institutional care (continuous and/or frequent contact), but then declined. Lipsey (1992) reported that treatment in an institutional setting was associated with smaller effect sizes than were other categories, such as treatment provider or modality.

With respect to participant characteristics, Lipsey described a slight but nonsignificant tendency for juveniles with higher risk levels to show larger effect sizes.

Considering different types of treatments, Lipsey reported that treatment orientation was only weakly related to effect size (R^2 change = .02). However, more structured and focused treatments and multimodal treatments were more effective than less structured and focused approaches (e.g., counseling), regardless of whether treatment was delivered in a residential facility or in the community.

These forms of treatments resulted in a 20 to 40% decrease in delinquency. Deterrence interventions, such as "shock incarceration" or "scared straight" programs, produced negative treatment effects, however (effect size = −.24).

WILDERNESS CHALLENGE PROGRAMS: WILSON AND LIPSEY (2000)

Wilson and Lipsey analyzed the effects of wilderness challenge programs on recidivism among delinquent youth. Inclusion in the meta-analysis required that the study evaluate a wilderness challenge program geared toward the reduction or prevention of delinquency among juveniles between the ages of 10 and 21. The study also had to use a comparison group, and each wilderness program had to include a physical challenge element and an interpersonal element. A total of 28 studies, including over 3,000 participants, met inclusion criteria for this meta-analysis. The majority of the studies were unpublished (64%) and did not use random assignment (57%). The most frequent duration of treatment was between 3 and 6 weeks (46%); the majority of the programs (64%) did not use a specific form of therapy to enhance the wilderness challenge components; and the most common form of comparison treatment was "institutionalization" (36%), followed by no treatment (29%) and probation (19%).

Among studies using antisocial behavior and delinquency outcomes ($\kappa = 22$), Wilson and Lipsey found a statistically significant, though modest, effect size (.18) in favor of wilderness challenge programs. They described this effect size as equivalent to a recidivism rate of 29% for program participants versus 37% for comparison participants. Using a series of multiple regressions, the authors reported that programs involving more intense physical activities and those incorporating a distinct therapy component (e.g., individual counseling, family therapy) yielded larger reductions in delinquency and antisocial behavior than programs without these components. With the exception of lengthy programs (over 10 weeks), which showed smaller effects, program length was not related to antisocial behavior or delinquency outcomes.

Effects of Interventions on Sexual Recidivism

Despite growing interest in the specialized treatment of juvenile sexual offenders, only a few studies have investigated such interventions. Further, many published "studies" contain only program descriptions or involve uncontrolled evaluations of various treatments. At the time this chapter was written, only three published studies (Borduin et al., 1990; Kahn & Chambers, 1991; Worling & Curwen, 2000) have employed comparison or control groups, probably too few to conduct a meaningful meta-analysis into the efficacy of treatments among juvenile sexual offenders. However, these studies provide the beginning of a foundation for future meta-analysis assessing the impact of interventions with juvenile sexual offenders and are therefore summarized in the remainder of this section.

Borduin et al. (1990) studied 16 male adolescents who had been arrested for a variety of sexual offenses, including exhibitionism, sexual assault, rape, and sodomy. The participants were randomly assigned to receive either multisystemic therapy (MST) or individual therapy. Both forms of therapy addressed a range of issues (e.g., behavioral problems, peer relations, school performance). The primary difference in the treatments was therapy modality, with MST including systemic components such as marital and family therapy and parent training. Participants in the MST condition received an average of 37 hours of treatment, while participants in the individual therapy condition received an average of 45 hours of treatment.

Borduin et al. (1990) reported that 6 of the adolescents (3 in each treatment condition) did not complete treatment; 4 of the 6 adolescents stopped treatment because they were charged with a subsequent offense. The authors indicated that the recidivism rates include data from all 16 adolescents, however, since each participated in treatment for a significant period of time. Evidence for treatment effects was determined by the rate of recidivism, defined as any rearrest, during a mean outcome period of 37 months. Recidivism for the MST group was 12.5% for sexual offenses and 25% for nonsexual offenses; the rates of recidivism for the individual therapy group were 75% for sexual offenses and 50% for nonsexual offenses. The authors suggested that the superior impact of MST might be explained by its focus on changing behavior within the community and on altering the systemic context to support change.

Kahn and Chambers (1991) conducted a retrospective comparison of institution-based versus community-based treatment programs with 221 juvenile sexual offenders. Each of the treatment programs was described as "specialized sexual deviance therapy" (Kahn & Chambers, 1991, p. 336) and included such approaches as confrontation, sex education, anger management, social skills training, development of victim empathy, and behavioral techniques to alter deviant arousal. A total of 44.8% of the juveniles were convicted of a subsequent offense during the follow-up period (mean duration = 28.1 months). Among those who recidivated, 7.5% were convicted of a sexual offense. The authors reported that juveniles who participated in outpatient programs were somewhat less likely than others to be convicted of subsequent sexual offenses; this nonsignificant trend involved juveniles treated in institutional programs being more likely to reoffend than those who were treated in community programs. No significant associations were found between any of the types of disposition (e.g., incarceration, probation, outpatient treatment, restitution) and sexual or total recidivism. However, the authors did observe that all juvenile sexual offenders (number unspecified) diverted from formal adjudication did reoffend.

Worling and Curwen (2000) evaluated the efficacy of a community-based, specialized sexual treatment program that provides individual, group, and family therapy to sexual offenders and victims of sexual abuse. The program, referred to as The Sexual Abuse, Family Education, and Treatment (SAFE-T) Program, uses cognitive-behavioral and relapse prevention strategies and addresses a variety of issues, including denial, deviant sexual arousal, sexual attitudes, victim empathy, social skills, self-esteem, and anger management skills. The authors compared the recidivism rates of those who participated in at least 12 months of the SAFE-T program ($n = 58$) with those who received an assessment only ($n = 46$), refused treatment ($n = 17$), or dropped out before 12 months ($n = 27$). It should be noted, however, that many (67%) of the adolescents in the comparison group reportedly received treatment elsewhere. The follow-up period ranged from 2 to 10 years (mean = 6.23 years). There was a significant difference in the recidivism rates for sexual reoffending between those who participated in the treatment program (5%) and those who dropped out (26%), refused treatment (18%), or received assessment only (13%). There was not a significant difference in the recidivism rates for sexual, violent, or any reoffending among the three comparison groups. Further analyses revealed that juveniles charged with subsequent sexual offenses were more likely to report having (a) been a victim of sexual abuse, (b) more past or present sexual fantasies of children, (c) more child-victim grooming behaviors, and (d) more intrusive sexual assault activities with children. They were also less likely to report recent nonsexual delinquent behavior. These findings may suggest that adolescent sexual offenders include a subgroup of offenders who are more likely to respond favorably to treatment delivered in long-term, specialized treatment programs.

Effects of Interventions on Violent Recidivism

Lipsey and Wilson (1998) and Lipsey (1999) reported the results of the only meta-analysis that has been conducted with violent juvenile offenders. It included studies investigating interventions delivered in both institutional and noninstitutional settings, with juveniles ages 10 to 21.9 years, described as serious (including those with multiple offenses over time, whether violent or not) and/or violent offenders. The number of studies included in the meta-analysis was large ($\kappa = 200$) and somewhat heterogeneous. For example, approximately 20% of the juveniles did not have a history of aggressive behavior and for 16% of juveniles, the aggressive histories were unknown. Thus, the meta-analysis cannot necessarily be interpreted as representing the outcomes of interventions with violent juvenile offenders.

The interventions in this meta-analysis included probation/parole, restitution, deterrence programs (e.g., shock incarceration), counseling, behavioral programs, skills-oriented programs, and multiple services. To be included in the meta-analysis, each study had to include a control or comparison group and use random assignment or report pretreatment group differences. The primary outcome measure for recidivism was police contact, arrest, or a comparable outcome measure, such as contact with a juvenile court.

Results reflect an overall mean recidivism rate for treated juveniles of 44% and a mean recidivism rate of 50% for the control/comparison groups. This represents a statistically significant, although modest, decrease in recidivism among serious juvenile offenders who participated in some form of intervention.

The authors reported that the overall recidivism rates across studies varied substantially as a result of methodological differences, as well as differences in the effectiveness of various interventions. Analyses of the sources of variability in the effects of interventions with serious juvenile offenders indicated that 12% of the variance in effect sizes could be attributed to methodological variables, including the nature of the assignment to experimental groups, attrition, the type of delinquency outcome measure used, sample size, and statistical power. Removing these sources of variance resulted in a larger mean effect size estimate—an 18% decrease in recidivism rates among juveniles receiving some form of intervention.

To assess which variables were associated with reductions in recidivism among serious juvenile offenders, Lipsey and Wilson conducted separate regression analyses investigating interventions with noninstitutionalized juveniles (117 studies) and those with institutionalized juveniles (83 studies). Included variables were offender characteristics (e.g., gender, age, ethnicity, prior offense histories), program characteristics (e.g., age of the program, whether mental health or criminal justice personnel provide treatment), type of treatment employed (e.g., restitution, behavioral programs), and the amount of treatment received (e.g., average number of weeks, frequency of treatment, integrity of treatment implementation).

Among studies investigating interventions with noninstitutionalized juveniles, Lipsey and Wilson reported that variables related to the characteristics of the juveniles who received treatment represented the largest proportion of effect size variance (.40), followed by treatment type (.26), amount of treatment (.20), and program characteristics (.15). Further analyses revealed that treatment effects were larger for juveniles with histories of "mixed" offenses (including more serious crimes) than for those with histories of primarily property offenses. Total duration of treatment was positively associated with treatment effects, but the number of hours of treatment contact per week was negatively associated with treatment effects. Treatments that required more involvement from the research team resulted in larger treatment effect sizes. With respect to the effects of specific types of interventions received among noninstitutionalized juveniles, Lipsey and Wilson noted that consistently positive effects were found for programs involving individual counseling (equated effect size = .46), interpersonal skills training (equated effect size = .44), and behavioral training (equated effect size = .42). Positive but less consistent effects were observed for programs involving multiple services (equated effect size =.29) and restitution and probation/parole (equated effect size = .15). Programs that showed mixed but generally positive effects included those involving employment training/counseling (equated effect size = .22), academic rehabilitation/remediation (equated effect size = .20), advocacy/casework (equated effect size = .19), and family (equated effect size = .19) or group (equated effect size = .10) counseling. Weak or no effects were consistently found for programs that included wilderness/challenge components (equated effect size = .12), early release, probation/parole (equated effect size = .03), deterrence (equated effect size = −.06), and vocational programming (equated effect size = −.18).

Lipsey and Wilson concluded that the most successful interventions for serious, noninstitutional juvenile offenders (individual counseling, interpersonal and behavioral skills training) reduced recidivism rates by approximately 42%. The authors also concluded that interventions that have been reported in the literature to be successful with delinquents of all kinds are also successful with more serious, noninstitutionalized juvenile offenders, with the exception of individual counseling, which does not appear to have a treatment effect for serious, noninstitutional juvenile offenders. Likewise, interventions that have been reported to be unsuccessful with general delinquents of all kinds are also unsuccessful with more serious, noninstitutionalized juvenile offenders.

Different conclusions were drawn for studies investigating interventions with serious juvenile offenders who are institutionalized. First, variables related to juvenile characteristics were not found to contribute significantly to reductions in recidivism rates among institutionalized juveniles. For this group, Lipsey and Wilson reported that variables related to characteristics of the program (.36), the amount of treatment received (.27), and treatment type (.26) accounted for the majority of the effect size variance. Specifically, the authors indicated that more established programs (2 years or older) administered by mental health personnel (as opposed to juvenile justice personnel) with greater treatment integrity, duration of treatment (median of 25 weeks), and continuity of treatment (e.g., weekly contact) were positively associated with larger treatment effects. With respect to types of treatment, the authors observed consistently positive effects for programs involving interpersonal skills training (equated effect size = .42) and participation in a teaching family groups (equated effect size = .26). Positive but less consistent evidence was also reported for behavioral programs (equated effect size = .44), community residential programs (equated effect size = .24), and programs offering multiple services, such as vocational training, skills-oriented education, and work opportunities (equated effect size = .29). Programs that showed mixed but generally positive effects included individual counseling (equated effect size = .19), guided groups (equated effect size = .03), and group counseling (equated effect size = .10). Weak or absent effects were noted for employment-related interventions (equated effect size = .13), drug abstinence (equated effect size = .14), and wilderness/challenge programs (equated effect size = −.01). Milieu therapy consistently showed weak or no effects as well (equated effect size = .13).

For serious, institutionalized juvenile offenders, Lipsey and Wilson reported that the most successful interventions (interpersonal skills training and participation in a teaching family home group) in the meta-analysis reduced recidivism rates by approximately 36%, somewhat lower than the reduction reported for noninstitutionalized offenders (42%). They also observed that institutionalized serious juvenile offenders apparently responded better to treatments that are more skills oriented and systemic, while noninstitutionalized serious juvenile offenders responded more favorably to individual counseling. Interpersonal skills training, often involving a variety of components including modeling, role-playing, social problem solving, and social reinforcement, appeared to be successful for both groups of offenders, reducing recidivism rates by 42% for noninstitutionalized offenders and 38% for institutionalized offenders.

Summary

Results of meta-analyses and other studies described in this chapter suggest that interventions geared toward the reduction of recidivism appear to be successful for a substantial proportion of juvenile offenders. Interventions that are structured and behavioral, and incorporate the juvenile's functioning in his or her immediate environment (e.g., systemic or family treatments) seem particularly promising. In addition, there is evidence to suggest that certain subgroups of offenders, such as sexual and violent offenders, would benefit from specialized treatment programs. However, additional research, particularly that oriented toward a more detailed scrutiny of sexual and violent recidivism studies, is needed to demonstrate such distinct treatment effects with specific populations.

References

Please see text for explanation of asterisks. Not all references are included in text, though all are in the meta-analysis.

Andrews, D., Zinger, I., Hoge, R., Bonta, J., Gendreau, P., & Cullen, F. (1990). Does correctional treatment work? A clinically-relevant and psychologically informed meta-analysis. *Criminology, 28*, 369–404.
*Archwamety, T., & Katsiyannis, A. (1998). Factors related to recidivism among delinquent females at a state correctional facility. *Journal of Child and Family Studies, 7*, 59–67.
*Ashford, J. B., & LeCroy, C. W. (1988). Predicting recidivism: An evaluation of the Wisconsin juvenile probation and aftercare risk instrument. *Criminal Justice and Behavior, 15*, 141–151.
*Ashford, J. B., & LeCroy, C. W. (1990). Juvenile recidivism: A comparison of three prediction instruments. *Adolescence, 25*, 441–450.
*Bleker, E. (1983). Cognitive defense style and WISC-R P>V sign in juvenile recidivists. *Journal of Clinical Psychology, 39*, 1030–1032.
Borduin, C. (1999). Multisystemic treatment of criminality and violence in adolescents. *Journal of the American Academy of Child and Adolescent Psychiatry, 38*, 242–249.
**Borduin, C., Henggeler, S., Blaske, D., & Stein, R. (1990). Multisystemic treatment of adolescent sexual offenders. *International Journal of Offender Therapy and Comparative Criminology, 34*, 105–113.
Cottle, C., Lee, R., & Heilbrun, K. (2001). The prediction of criminal recidivism in juveniles: A meta-analysis. *Criminal Justice and Behavior, 28*, 367–394.
*Dembo, R., Schmeidler, J., Nini-Gough, B., Sue, C. C., Borden, P., & Manning, D. (1998). Predictors of recidivism to a juvenile assessment center: A three year study. *Journal of Child and Adolescent Substance Abuse, 7*, 57–77.
*Dembo, R., Williams, L., Fagan, J., & Schmeidler, J. (1994). Development and assessment of a classification of high risk youths. *Journal of Drug Issues, 24*, 25–54.
Dembo, R., Williams, L., Schmeidler, J., Getreu, A., & Berry, E. (1991). Recidivism among high risk youths: A 2 1/2-year follow-up of a cohort of juvenile detainees. *International Journal of the Addictions, 26*, 1197–1221.
**Dolan, M., Holloway, J., Bailey, S., & Kroll, L. (1996). The psychosocial characteristics of juvenile sexual offenders referred to an adolescent forensic service in the UK. *Medical Sciences and the Law, 36*, 343–352.

*Duncan, R., Kennedy, W., & Patrick, C. (1995). Four-factor model of recidivism in male juvenile offenders. *Journal of Clinical Child Psychology, 24,* 250–257.

*Funk, S. (1999). Risk assessment for juveniles on probation. *Criminal Justice and Behavior, 26,* 44–68.

Garrett, C. (1985). Effects of residential treatment on adjudicated delinquents: A meta-analysis. *Journal of Research in Crime and Delinquency, 22,* 287–308.

*Grenier, C. E., & Roundtree, G. A. (1987). Predicting recidivism among adjudicated delinquents: A model to identify high risk offenders. *Journal of Offender Counseling, Services and Rehabilitation, 12,* 101–112.

***Guerra, N., & Slaby, R. (1990). Cognitive mediators of aggression in adolescent offenders: Intervention. *Developmental Psychology, 26,* 269–277.

**Hagan, M., & Cho, M. (1996). A comparison of treatment outcomes between adolescent rapists and child sexual offenders. *International Journal of Offender Therapy and Comparative Criminology, 40,* 113–122.

*Hanson, C. L., Henggeler, S. W., Haefele, W. F., & Rodick, J. D. (1984). Demographic, individual, and family relationship correlates of serious and repeated crime among adolescents and their siblings. *Journal of Consulting and Clinical Psychology, 52,* 528–538.

Henggeler, S. (1999). Multisystemic therapy: An overview of clinical procedures, outcomes, and policy implications. *Child Psychology and Psychiatry Review, 4,* 2–10.

***Henggeler, S., Melton, G., Brondino, M., Scherer, D., & Hanley, J. (1997). Multisystemic therapy with violent and chronic juvenile offenders and their families: The role of treatment fidelity in successful dissemination. *Journal of Consulting and Clinical Psychology, 65,* 821–833.

***Henggeler, S., Melton, G., & Smith, L. (1992). Family preservation using multisystemic therapy: An effective alternative to incarcerating serious juvenile offenders. *Journal of Consulting and Clinical Psychology, 60,* 953–961.

*Hoge, R., Andrews, D., & Leschied, A. (1996). An investigation of risk and protective factors in a sample of youthful offenders. *Journal of Child Psychology and Psychiatry, 37,* 419–424.

*Jung, S., & Rawana, E. P. (1999). Risk and need assessment of juvenile offenders. *Criminal Justice and Behavior, 26,* 69–90.

**Kahn, T., & Chambers, H. (1991). Assessing reoffense risk with juvenile sexual offenders. *Child Welfare, 70,* 333–346.

*Katsiyannis, A., & Archwamety, T. (1997). Factors related to recidivism among delinquent youths in a state correctional facility. *Journal of Child and Family Studies, 6,* 43–55.

**Lab, S., Shields, G., & Schondel, C. (1993). Research note: An evaluation of juvenile sexual offender treatment. *Crime and Delinquency, 39,* 543–554.

Lee, R., Cottle, C., & Heilbrun, K. (2001, August). Predictors of recidivism in juvenile violent and sexual and violent offenders: A meta-analysis. Presented at the annual convention of the American Psychological Association, San Francisco.

Lipsey, M. (1992). Juvenile delinquency treatment: A meta-analytic inquiry into the variability of effects. In T. Cook, H. Cooper, S. Cordray, H. Hartmann, L. Hedges, R. Light, T. Louis, & F. Mosteller (Eds.), *Meta-analysis for explanation: A casebook.* New York: Russell Sage Foundation.

Lipsey, M. (1999). Can intervention rehabilitate serious delinquents? *Annals of the American Academy of Political and Social Sciences, 564,* 142–166.

Lipsey, M., & Wilson, D. (1998). Effective intervention for serious juvenile offenders: A synthesis of research. In R. Loeber & D. Farrington (Eds.), *Serious and violent juve-*

nile offenders: Risk factors and successful interventions (pp. 313–345). Thousand Oaks, CA: Sage.

*Minor, K. I., Hartmann, D. J., & Terry, S. (1997). Predictors of juvenile court actions and recidivism. Crime and Delinquency, 43, 328–344.

***Myers, W., Burton, P., Sanders, P., Donat, K., Cheney, J., Fitzpatrick, T., & Monaco, L. (2000). Project Back-on-Track at 1 year: A delinquency treatment program for early-career juvenile offenders. Journal of the American Academy of Child and Adolescent Psychiatry, 39, 1127–1134.

*Myner, J., Santman, J., Cappelletty, G., & Perlmutter, B. (1998). Variables related to recidivism among juvenile offenders. International Journal of Offender Therapy and Comparative Criminology, 42, 65–80.

*Niarhos, F. J., & Routh, D. K. (1992). The role of clinical assessment in the juvenile court: Predictors of juvenile dispositions and recidivism. Journal of Clinical Child Psychology, 21, 151–159.

*Putnins, A. (1984). Family structure and juvenile recidivism. Family Therapy, 11, 61–64.

**Rasmussen, L. (1999). Factors related to recidivism among juvenile sexual offenders. Sexual Abuse: A Journal of Research and Treatment, 11, 69–85.

*Repo, E., & Virkkunen, M. (1997). Young arsonists: History of conduct disorder, psychiatric diagnoses and criminal recidivism. Journal of Forensic Psychiatry, 8, 311–320.

Rosenthal, R. (1991). Meta-analytic procedures for social research. Newbury Park, CA: Sage.

**Smith, W., & Monastersky, C. (1986). Assessing juvenile sex offenders' risk for reoffending. Criminal Justice and Behavior, 13, 115–140.

*Stattin, H., & Magnusson, D. (1989). The role of early aggressive behavior in the frequency, seriousness, and types of later crime. Journal of Consulting and Clinical Psychology, 57, 710–718.

*Steiner, H., Cauffman, E., & Duxbury, E. (1999). Personality traits in juvenile delinquents: Relation to criminal behavior and recidivism. Journal of the American Academy of Child and Adolescent Psychiatry, 38, 256–262.

Stock, W. A. (1994). Systematic coding for research synthesis. In H. Cooper & L. Hedges (Eds.), The handbook of research synthesis (pp. 125–138). New York: Russell Sage Foundation.

*Towberman, D. (1994). Psychosocial antecedents of chronic delinquency. In N. J. Pallone (Ed.), Young victims, young offenders: Current issues in policy and treatment (pp. 151–164). Binghamton, NY: Haworth Press.

Whitehead, J. T., & Lab, S. P. (1989). A meta-analysis of juvenile correctional treatment. Juvenile Correctional Treatment, 26, 276–295.

*Wierson, M., & Forehand, R. (1995). Predicting recidivism in juvenile delinquents: The role of mental health diagnoses and the qualification of conclusions by race. Behaviour Research and Therapy, 33, 63–67.

Wilson, S., & Lipsey, M. (2000). Wilderness challenge programs for delinquent youth: A meta-analysis of outcome evaluations. Evaluation and Program Planning, 23, 1–12.

**Worling, J., & Curwen, T. (2000). Adolescent sexual offender recidivism: Success of specialized treatment and implications for risk prediction. Child Abuse and Neglect, 27, 965–982.

7

Davⁱᴅ C. Tate ᴀɴᴅ Richard E. Redding

Mental Health and Rehabilitative Services in Juvenile Justice

System Reforms and Innovative Approaches

Youth in the juvenile justice system have significant mental health needs, having prevalence rates of mental disorders far higher than those of other adolescents (see Cellini, 2001; Cocozza & Skowyra, 2000; Lexcen & Redding, 2002; Martinez, 2001; McGarvey & Waite, 2000; Teplin, Abram, McClelland, Dulcan, & Mericle, 2002). While an estimated 15 to 20% of youth who enter the juvenile justice system have a serious mental health problem, a much larger percentage of these youth experience *some* mental health problem (up to 80% in some studies) and thus require mental health services. In addition to higher rates of psychiatric problems, juvenile offenders often have experienced multiple problems, including physical abuse, sexual victimization, violent behavior, alcohol and substance abuse problems, and educational/learning difficulties (Dembo, Williams, & Schmeidler, 1993; Huizinga & Jakob-Chien, 1998; Morris et al., 1995).

If youth involved in the justice system often have mental health problems, the converse is also true: many youth being treated for emotional, behavioral, or mental health difficulties encounter problems with the law. Studies have consistently found substantial overlap between youth with mental health problems and those with juvenile justice involvement (see Rosenblatt, Rosenblatt, & Biggs, 2000; Shanok & Lewis, 1977). Quinn and Epstein (1998) reported that in their sample of emotionally disturbed or at-risk youth referred for services, 50% were on probation. Another recent study found that 66.5% of children with severe emotional and behavioral disturbances had some contact with police, 43.3% had been arrested at least once, and 34.4% were adjudicated delinquent (Greenbaum et al., 1998). In a multisite sample of 144 youth in mental health service systems, 61% had previous involvement with law enforcement, with an average of eight prior contacts (Duchowski, Hall, Kutash, & Friedman, 1998).

Thus, youth in the juvenile justice system need a range of rehabilitative and mental health treatment services. But the term "treatment" often carries different meanings in juvenile justice and mental health contexts. In juvenile justice, treatment often is a broader concept used interchangeably with "rehabilitation," meaning efforts to help delinquents modify their offending and antisocial behavior, with such efforts frequently involving standard mental health interventions (e.g., individual therapy, family therapy). Within a mental health framework, treatment is closely tied to the psychiatric or medical model aimed at alleviating symptoms. The distinction often reflects the functions of the systems themselves, rather than the needs of the youth they serve. In the juvenile justice system, "treatment" can refer to mental health intervention or the prevention of future delinquency. Thus, many interventions described as treatment programs may target additional or alternative problems, not only psychiatric or emotional difficulties. This is appropriate programmatically, given that adolescents in the juvenile justice system typically have multiple problems (Huizinga & Jakob-Chien, 1998). A service delivery system that addresses these needs in a comprehensive and systematic way should produce the greatest improvements in the child's overall functioning and prosocial behavior.

Current efforts to treat youth in the juvenile justice system can be understood in terms of historical trends in the treatment of delinquents, as well as system reforms occurring in both the children's mental health and juvenile justice systems. We first discuss reforms in, and changing conceptualizations of, the children's mental health and juvenile justice systems. We then review recent innovations in the delivery of mental health services within the juvenile justice system that have occurred in response to these reforms. We conclude with a discussion of the implications of these systems reforms and innovative treatment approaches for service delivery.

Children's Mental Health Services Reform

The recognition of the need for children's mental health services began as early as 1909 and 1930, when White House conferences recommended rights and programs for mentally disturbed children (Tuma, 1992). Calls for reform became more pronounced following the Joint Commission on Mental Health of Children's 1969 report, which found that children and adolescents with serious emotional and behavioral problems were underserved, receiving inappropriate or fragmented services in unnecessarily restrictive settings (Lourie, Stroul, & Friedman, 1998). Subsequent commissions and panels reached similar conclusions. Reforms were mandated in 1980, when a federal court ruling in the *Willie M. v. Hunt* (1981) class-action lawsuit required the state of North Carolina to develop a complete, integrated service system with a range of services to meet the needs of seriously disturbed and assaultive children—a group previously failed by extant service programs (Oswald & Singh, 1996).

Jane Knitzer's *Unclaimed Children* (1982) marked the beginning of real progress in the field of children's mental health services reform (Epstein, Kutash, & Duchnowski, 1998). The report highlighted gaps in services throughout the agencies and systems providing services to children and adolescents, including education, mental health, juvenile justice, and social services. Limitations in community-based services, case management, state and local leadership, and coordination across service agencies were cited as barriers to creating a system that meets the needs of children with serious emotional disturbance and their families (Knitzer, 1982). The report and other advocacy efforts led to the creation of the Child and Adolescent Service System Project (CASSP) in 1984. Funded by the National Institute of Mental Health, CASSP was intended to promote the development of community and state systems of care for children and adolescents with serious emotional disturbances.

The system-of-care concept was described more fully by Stroul and Friedman (1986). They defined it as a "comprehensive spectrum of mental health and other necessary services which are organized into a coordinated network to meet the changing needs of children and adolescents with severe emotional disturbances and their families" (p. iv) organized around eight major areas of service: mental health services, social services, educational services, health services, substance abuse services, vocational services, recreational services, and operational services, with a menu of specific services provided in each area. The system-of-care model provides a continuum of services to children and families. It does not correspond to a particular intervention or program, but models an ideal framework within which services should be delivered.

Evaluations of Systems of Care

An underlying assumption of the system-of-care concept is that improvement in the service systems and ways in which services are delivered will translate into better clinical and functional outcomes for children and families. But this assumption is difficult to test empirically, with system-of-care evaluations limited to particular system components, such as the characteristics of system users, organizational change, participant attitudes, and cost of services (Oswald & Singh, 1996). The largest, methodologically soundest attempt to evaluate the system-of-care approach is the "Fort Bragg study." It was designed "to test the efficacy of a Federal and State contract for providing a case management-based alternative delivery system of mental health services tailored to individual needs featuring the use of a full continuum of community-based services [and to] demonstrate that this continuum of services [would] result in improved treatment outcomes while the cost per client is decreased when compared to current CHAMPUS [Civilian Health and Medical Program of the Uniformed Services] costs" (Bickman et al., 1995, pp. 4–5). The study, which compared mental health care systems at two U.S. Army sites in North Carolina, has been described in detail by lead investigator Bickman and colleagues (Bickman, 1996; Bickman et al., 1995; Bickman, Heflinger, Lambert, & Summerfelt, 1996). Families in the Fort Bragg area (the demonstration site) received community-based nonresidential and residential service components, as well as a number of specially developed intermediate-level services, such as in-home therapy, afterschool services, day treatment, therapeutic homes, and 24-hour crisis management teams. These and other services were coordinated by case managers and interdisciplinary treatment teams, and the system followed Stroul and Friedman's (1986) model of an integrated, coordinated continuum of care. In contrast, families in the control site received typical CHAMPUS services consisting of outpatient, inpatient, and residential treatment.

A number of outcomes were measured at both sites, including mental health, child and family functioning, satisfaction with services, and cost utilization. In addition, the degree to which the demonstration site implemented a high-quality system of care was assessed. Results indicated that the continuum of care was successfully implemented at the demonstration site, which was characterized by reduced costs, greater consumer access, more client satisfaction, less restrictive treatment environments, and greater continuity of care—and clinical outcomes were comparable to those at the control site (Bickman, 1996). Bickman, Summerfelt, and Noser (1997) conducted another evaluation of a system-of-care model in Stark County, Ohio. In this study, 350 families were randomly assigned to either the experimental group, in which they gained access to a comprehensive, coordinated system of mental health and other necessary services, or the control group, in which they received the usual services in the community. At 6-month follow-up, there were no group differences in children's level of functioning or mental health symptoms, although there was greater access to care and more services received among families in the system-of-care program.

From these two relatively large-scale studies, Bickman and colleagues concluded that the impact of systems of care (and the attendant greater level of services) is limited to *systems-level outcomes* (e.g., cost of care, access to services) but does not appear to affect *clinical outcomes* (Bickman et al., 1997). The clinical outcome results were met with a wide range of reactions from the scholarly and system-of-care communities.[1] Critics have raised numerous questions about the interpretation of the results and whether the evaluation was a valid test of system-of-care principles. Concerns were also raised about the characteristics of the study population (Burchard, 1996; Friedman, 1996; Hoagwood, 1997); the nature and the integrity of the system-of-care and control-site treatment systems; the robustness of the treatment-control comparison (Feldman, 1997; Hoagwood, 1997); the nature of the clinical interventions (Henggeler, Schoenwald, & Munger, 1996; Weisz, Han, & Valeri, 1996); and the timing of the evaluation relative to the maturity of the system of care (Evans & Banks, 1996).

Many suggest that enhanced clinical outcomes will be detected with further research on the impact of systems of care. As Henggeler et al. (1996) argued, implementation of system-of-care principles (community-based care, family collaboration, individualized care, and interagency coordination) alone is insufficient to change clinical outcomes. But "pragmatic, skilled, and ecologically minded therapists who work in supportive systems of care will have higher success rates than their counterparts who work in disorganized, nonintegrated, family-blaming, and institution-reliant systems of care. Thus, the system of care may primarily impact clinical outcome as it facilitates or impedes the work of

1. For detailed discussions, see *American Psychologist*, 52(5), 536–565; and the *Journal of Child and Family Studies*, 5(2), 137–206.

therapists who are collaborating with families to provide effective clinical services" (pp. 180–181).

Importantly, research supports the multidetermined nature of juvenile delinquency and the effectiveness of treatment programs that target multiple risk factors in the environments in which they arise (see Henggeler, Schoenwald, Borduin, Rowland, & Cunningham, 1998b). Targeting the multiple risk factors present in the child's home, family, school, and neighborhood requires a system of care that provides a continuum of integrated and coordinated services across these systems.

Support for the development of system-of-care models has grown. Within ten years of its inception, CASSP's budget increased tenfold, with involvement in all 50 states (Stroul & Friedman, 1994). In addition, private organizations such as the Robert Wood Johnson Foundation and the Annie E. Casey Foundation have funded children's service delivery projects and other initiatives using a system-of-care approach that totaled more that $30 million (Epstein et al., 1998; Oswald & Singh, 1996).[2] In 1992, the CMHS established the Comprehensive Mental Health Services for Children and Their Families program, which has awarded numerous grants to communities across the nation; the budget for fiscal year 2002 was $96 million (see Center for Mental Health Services, 1999; Lourie et al., 1998).

Family Preservation and Community-Based Care

The second key reform in children's mental health services, linked to the system-of-care concept, is the shift from treatment in artificial or residential settings without substantial family involvement to community-based care that delivers services across the child's natural settings (e.g., home and family, school, neighborhood) and that actively involves families and significant others (e.g., extended family, teachers) as partners in treatment planning and services. By contrast, the traditional approach often viewed families as part of the problem, confined treatment to individual therapy for the child in the clinician's office or a residential treatment center, and did not involve parents and others in treatment planning (Knitzer, 1996; Osher & Osher, 2002).

The new approach, now perhaps the prevailing paradigm in children's mental health service delivery, views community-based care as the norm and residential placement as a last resort, emphasizes family preservation rather than out-of-home placement, involves families as active partners in treatment, provides services to the child and family in natural settings, and emphasizes collaboration and integration of treatment services across systems, agencies, and service providers (Knitzer, 1996).

2. CASSP has now been renamed the Planning and Systems Development Program, and is housed within the Child, Adolescent, and Family Branch of the Center for Mental Health Services (CMHS) of the Substance Abuse and Mental Health Service Administration (SAMHSA) at the U.S. Department of Health and Human Services.

Juvenile Justice System Reforms

Just as children's mental health services have been reconceptualized, so too has the juvenile justice system. An understanding of the historic trends and possible futures in juvenile justice system reform, especially regarding rehabilitation and treatment, provides the context within which to view modern mental health service delivery in the juvenile justice system.

Historical Trends in Juvenile Justice

At its inception in 1899 and for decades following, the juvenile justice system was based on the philosophy of *parens patriae*—the state as benevolent parent that protected and served the best interests of children (Dwyer & McNally, 1989; Fox, 1970). Because the system was designed to be informal and nonadversarial, few provisions were made for ensuring due process or procedural safeguards to protect juveniles' rights. Juvenile court judges were given ample discretion to make individualized dispositional decisions, because the treatment and rehabilitation of youth were the juvenile court's central missions (Fox, 1970; Ross, 1995). The early reformers (later referred to as the "child savers"), whose activism led to the establishment of a separate juvenile justice system, believed they could rescue children from criminal courts, jails, and even ineffective parents (Mahoney, 1987; Platt, 1977). The juvenile court's philosophical basis and informal structure went relatively unchallenged for 60 years. But by the 1960s, the social climate in the United States was one of distrust of government and those with discretionary power, and juvenile court judges applied justice quite variably (Orlando & Crippen, 1992). Moreover, the institutionalization of youth had increased and dispositions of incarceration were being made without due process. In 1966 the U.S. Supreme Court case of *Kent v. United States*, Judge Fortas proclaimed that "the child receives the worst of both worlds . . . he gets neither the protection afforded to adults, nor the solicitous care and regenerative treatment postulated for children" (p. 18). The trends—amidst concerns about civil rights—led to the Supreme Court case *In re Gault* (1967), which held that due process rights must be extended to juveniles in juvenile court (Fox, 1970).

In the 1970s and 1980s, growing concerns about youth violence and pressure on courts to restore law-and-order while containing costs led to a juvenile court system with reduced resources and an emphasis on the containment of delinquents (Grisso, 2001; Mahoney, 1987; Tonry & Moore, 1998). The court's apparent difficulty in serving the best interest of youth while also protecting society was accompanied by increasing cynicism about the system's ability to effectively rehabilitate youthful offenders and the perception that juvenile courts were far too lenient. Importantly, studies of treatment programs for offenders failed to substantiate their effectiveness, leading many to the conclusion that rehabilitation was not feasible—that "nothing works" (see Martinson, 1974). This led to reductions in therapeutic efforts and a shift toward control and incarceration. The public attitude toward delinquents became increasingly punitive, with "get tough" policies proliferating (Dwyer & McNally, 1989; Feld, 1999).

Indeed, the history of juvenile justice policy reflects diversity among political interest groups and waxing and waning ideological perspectives on handling juvenile offenders (Guarino-Ghezzi & Loughran, 1996). Often these perspectives created a tension between the punishment and rehabilitation functions of the juvenile justice system. Bernard (1992) described a predictable pattern—the "cycle of juvenile justice." Two opposing views drive the cycle. The first view is that delinquency represents a cry for help from youth in abusive or neglecting environments and that the justice system can address the problem by treating juveniles and their environments therapeutically. The second view is that juvenile offenders are criminals unconcerned about the rights of others, with the solution being harsher punishment and deterrence strategies. Bernard (1992) believed this pattern is likely to continue and that stable, reasonable policy will not be established unless the cycle can be broken. One way to break this cycle is for the juvenile justice system to adopt balanced policies that promote accountability as well as rehabilitation in juvenile offenders. We discuss two such approaches—*balanced and restorative justice* and *graduated sanctions*—in the next sections.

Possible Futures of the Juvenile Justice System

The future of the juvenile justice system is uncertain as it performs a rather complex balancing act with multiple goals that often seem in conflict. For example, the court must protect the public from dangerous youth while acting in the best interests of children, it must make youth accountable for their behavior while keeping in mind the unique circumstances of each child, and it must individualize dispositions while being fair and uniform across dispositions (Krisberg & Austin, 1993). Coates (1989) identified six apparent polarities that will shape the future of juvenile corrections: (a) rehabilitation versus punishment, (b) rehabilitation as a meaningful goal versus unattainable ideal, (c) use of institutions versus community-based treatment, (d) determinate versus indeterminate dispositions, (e) victim versus offender consideration, and (6) public versus private sector programming. The future of the juvenile justice system will be further complicated by three major social trends that require it to handle more deeply troubled adolescents: (a) an increasing number of youth are reared in poverty and have substance abuse problems, (b) cutbacks in funding for child welfare and programming to assist poor families will propel more children into the juvenile justice system (Krisberg & Austin, 1993), and (c) with the decline in the number of unskilled jobs available, undereducated youth are essentially locked out of the labor market and may instead enter the world of drug trafficking and crime.

Essentially, there are two possible futures for the juvenile justice system: abolition of the system or major system reforms. Some have questioned the need for a separate juvenile court given that sentencing in the juvenile court is increasingly punitive and procedural safeguards often are lacking, coupled with doubts that treatment services in the juvenile justice system will expand (Ainsworth, 1991; Feld, 1997). But abolition seems unlikely. Dismantling the system entirely would be difficult to do in practice and would mean discarding aspects of the system that *do* work well (Orlando & Crippen, 1992). Moreover, despite the recent "get tough" trend, sophisticated public opinion polls reveal that the public still favors early intervention, rehabilitation, and community-based treatment for juvenile offenders (Moon, Sundt, Cullen, & Wright, 2000). Grisso (2001) persuasively argued that the substantial financial and societal costs of punishing juveniles like adults, combined with a recent change in public attitudes in favor of rehabilitation, augers well for the long-term survival of the juvenile justice system. Many believe that the system can be reformed, reconceptualized, or rejuvenated, with several models of juvenile justice system reform gaining prominence.

Models of Juvenile Justice System Reform

Effective reform could begin by setting aside "either punishment or treatment" notions of juvenile justice. As Coates (1989) put it, "perhaps we would move further by directing our attention to what are appropriate societal responses to particular offenses or offenders, incorporating the need to punish and hold persons accountable for their acts while at the same time offering some long-term hope for restoration of the offender to the community" (p. 286). Contemporary reform models attempt to integrate what often seem to be competing demands to achieve the multiple goals of juvenile justice. Two leading models of systemic juvenile justice reform are balanced and restorative justice (BARJ) and graduated sanctions. The U.S. Justice Department's Office of Juvenile Justice and Delinquency Prevention (OJJDP) has funded efforts to demonstrate and implement both of these models to enhance the effective operation of the juvenile justice system (Ingersoll, 1997). The models emphasize community-based treatment and rehabilitation and integrated continua of care across agencies and service providers.

BALANCED AND RESTORATIVE JUSTICE (BARJ)

The BARJ model is centered around community-oriented responses to nonviolent crime wherein multiple stakeholders (e.g., victims, offenders, courts, corrections, police, schools, churches, community groups, youth advocacy groups) participate in the justice process (Bazemore, 1997; Bazemore & Walgrave, 1999; Guarino-Ghezzi & Loughran, 1996; Umbreit, 1995). Table 7.1 outlines the roles of the different participants in the BARJ system. Balanced and restorative justice entails a shift in organizational structure away from a bureaucratic, "top-down" system to one of community empowerment that embodies the concept of total quality management, requiring "every employee—from managers to line staff—to determine whether their operations and activities are helping to achieve the organization's mission" (English, 1993, p. 19). Through extensive interagency collaboration and citizen participation, decisions are made about how to intervene with juveniles, what steps are necessary to repair the damage that has been done, and how to minimize public safety risks. Unlike punishment-only and

TABLE 7.1 The Participants in a Balanced and Restorative Justice System

Crime victims
- Receive support, assistance, compensation, information, and services
- Receive restitution or other reparation from the offender
- Are involved and are encouraged to give input at all points in the system as to how the offender will repair the harm done
- Have the opportunity to face the offenders and tell their story
- Feel satisfied with the justice process
- Provide guidance and consultation to juvenile justice professionals on planning and advisory groups

Offenders
- Complete restitution to their victims
- Provide meaningful service to repay the debt to their communities
- Face the personal harm caused by their crimes by participating in victim–offender mediation or other victim awareness programs
- Complete work experience and active and productive tasks that increase skills and improve the community
- Are monitored by community adults as well as juvenile justice providers and supervised to the greatest extent possible in the community
- Improve decision-making skills and have opportunities to help others

Citizens, families, and community groups
- Are involved to the greatest extent possible in rehabilitation, community safety initiatives, and holding offenders accountable
- Work with offenders on local community service projects
- Provide support to victims
- Provide support to offenders as mentors, employers, and advocates
- Provide work for offenders to pay restitution to victims and service opportunities that allow offenders to meake meaningful contributions to the quality of community life
- Assist families to support the offender in obligation to repair the harm and increase competencies
- Advise courts and corrections and play an active role in disposition

Juvenile justice professionals
- Sanctioning: facilitate mediation, ensure restoration, develop creative or restorative community service options, engage community members, and educate the community on its role
- Rehabilitation: develop new roles for young offenders that allow them to practice and demonstrate competency, assess and build on youth and community strengths, and develop community partnerships
- Public safety: develop incentives and consequences to ensure offender compliance with supervision objectives, help school and family control and maintain offenders in the community, and develop prevention capacity of local organizations

Source: From "Restoring the Balance: Juvenile and Community Justice," (1997), by G. Bazemore and S. E. Day, *Juvenile Justice, 3*(1), pp. 9, 12. Reprinted with permission.

treatment-only models of juvenile justice, which are offender-driven, the balanced approach emphasizes the needs of victims, offenders, and communities throughout the process (Bazemore, 1997).

Three goals comprise the BARJ model: competency building, offender accountability, and public safety. Competency building involves helping youth build adaptive and prosocial bonds with peers and community. Accountability requires that the offenders take responsibility for their illegal behaviors and the harm they caused their victims, and this process typically includes victim confrontation and victim-offender mediation, restitution, community service, or other activities (Bazemore, 1997; Bazemore & Walgrave, 1999; Umbreit, 1995). Public safety relies primarily on prevention and intensive monitoring rather than incapacitation and incarceration. The intervention programs for youth represent the equilibrium of these diverse goals, and administrative structures ensure that funds are distributed equitably towards the achievement of each. One BARJ model, known as *family group conferencing*, has been widely implemented in Australia and New Zealand. In the family group conference, the offender and his family, the victim, and other concerned parties discuss the causes of the offense and determine an appropriate sanction (Levine, 2000; Levy, 1999; Morris & Maxwell, 1993).

Systems that adapt a BARJ model must be flexible, creative, accountable for decisions, aware of public safety risks, and oriented toward the community reintegration of offenders. Programmatically, these considerations may translate into (a) the need for a range of surveillance programs to monitor offenders, (b) a range of service programs that provide competence-building opportunities, (c) private sector involvement in designing and managing programs, (d) rational decision structures for making accountable placement decisions, and (e) programs that prepare youth for successful community reintegration (Guarino-Ghezzi & Loughran, 1996).

GRADUATED SANCTIONS/THE COMPREHENSIVE STRATEGY

The Office of Juvenile Justice and Delinquency Prevention's Comprehensive Strategy for Chronic, Serious, and Violent Offenders outlines a continuum of sanctions and services based on the seriousness and chronicity of offending (Krisberg & Howell, 1998; Wilson & Howell, 1995). Its goal is to increase program effectiveness and juvenile accountability while decreasing the cost of juvenile corrections by "improving the juvenile justice response to delinquent offenders through a system of graduated sanctions and a continuum of treatment alternatives that includes immediate intervention, intermediate sanctions, and community-based corrections sanctions, incorporating restitution and community service when appropriate" (Wilson & Howell, 1995, p. 37). Graduated sanctions means that the intensity of intervention and the restrictiveness of placement increases as offenses become more severe or repetitive, thus heightening the need for community protection. But regardless of the level, sanctions serve to stabilize the child's environment to permit efficacious treatment intervention for the required period of time.

The comprehensive strategy espouses the use of multiple interventions through interagency collaboration to address the multiple risk factors (at the individual, family, school, peer, and community levels) giving rise to delinquency. Early intervention is critical, with immediate sanctions applied to first-time offending youth or non-serious repeat-offending youth. Interventions for these groups include community-based, nonresidential services and an array of possible sanctions, such as diversion, restitution, informal probation, or community services. Intermediate sanctions are reserved for first-time serious or violent offenders or juveniles who did not respond to immediate sanctions. Intermediate sanctions are still community-based but may be residential or nonresidential, including intensive supervision, substance abuse treatment, electronic monitoring, day treatment, community-based residential treatment, and brief stays in confinement.

Finally, for the small percentage of offenders who are serious, chronic, and violent (see Snyder, 1998), secure confinement may be necessary, but even many of these youth could be placed in small, community-based facilities that provide intensive services. Incarceration in out-of-community placements is used only as a last resort, and community-based aftercare is a key component of postresidential treatment. By contrast, many states still place far too many youth in detention and correctional facilities when they could be placed safely in community-based programs (Mendel, 2000). Recent studies have shown that placement in residential facilities is far more costly than community placement and is associated with higher rates of postrelease recidivism (see Redding, 2003; Wooldredge, 1988).

Several notable programs have embraced many of the principles—community-based treatment, graduated sanctions, and balanced approaches—articulated in the BARJ and graduated sanctions models of system reform.

MASSACHUSETTS DIVISION OF YOUTH SERVICES (MDYS). Massachusetts has been recognized for its superior youth corrections systems. During the 1970s, the state underwent a process of deinstitutionalization, abandoning large training schools in favor of smaller, local, secure facilities (Krisberg & Austin, 1993). Only 15% of the juvenile offenders committed to the MDYS are now placed in high security programs; the vast majority are placed in non-secure facilities, including day treatment, foster care, group homes, and intensive supervision programs. These services are partially administered by the private sector at greatly reduced cost, with an estimated $11 million saved annually (Howell, Krisberg, & Jones, 1995). Many placement decisions are dictated by state legislation, a practice that minimizes judicial discretionary biases (Guarino-Ghezzi & Loughran, 1996). The MDYS system has recidivism rates comparable to or better than those of most other jurisdictions, and the effects have been sustained over a 2-year period (Howell et al., 1995).

THE HIGH POINT YOUTH VIOLENCE INITIATIVE. This community initiative uses the community-based and system-of-care treatment models, multiagency collaboration, and wraparound teams to provide rehabilitative treatment to juvenile offenders and their families, who are referred to the program after the youth has been adjudicated. A comprehensive intake assessment, emphasizing a strength-based approach to addressing risk factors, is conducted. Wraparound teams then work as partners with the family to develop a treatment plan. The team is unique for each family, as it may include the child's family, teachers, neighbors, and representatives from agencies and community resources. Service coordinators, trained in the system-of-care approach, work with the child and family on a daily basis. Preliminary program evaluations indicate that the program produced substantial reductions in delinquency, problem behavior, and mental health symptoms among juveniles (Frabutt, Arbuckle, & Campbell, 2002).

THE CITY OF JACKSONVILLE'S COMPREHENSIVE STRATEGY. The Jacksonville, Florida, Juvenile Justice Comprehensive Strategy is a particularly good example of multiagency collaboration to form a comprehensive and multifaceted set of interventions designed specifically to address the risk factors for juvenile crime existing in the local community (City of Jacksonville, FL, 2001). Jacksonville was chosen to be a pilot site for implementation of OJJDP's Comprehensive Strategy. First, as called for in the Comprehensive Strategy, an assessment was undertaken to determine the risk factors most prevalent in the Jacksonville area that should receive priority in interventions. Family management problems, lack of commitment to school, early academic failure, availability and use of firearms, and economic deprivation were identified as priority risk factors. Based on the assessment, a wide variety of intervention programs were developed and coordinated, involving a diverse array of agencies, community leaders, and service providers in the planning and implementation of a system of care to prevent juvenile offending and provide rehabilitative services. The local state attorney's and sheriff's offices were key players. Initiatives include comprehensive counseling, substance abuse, education, and leadership and mentoring programs. Also, as part of the program, Jacksonville instituted a faith-based initiative, a community education initiative, a truancy interdiction program, and a partnership for a drug-free community.

INTENSIVE AFTERCARE PROGRAM (IAP). This initiative was designed to help correctional agencies implement effective aftercare programs for chronic and serious juvenile offenders. Aftercare following residential placement is critical for ensuring continuity of care and the maintenance of positive behavioral changes. IAP addresses recognized shortcomings of institutional settings, including their failure to prepare youth adequately for return to community environments where the youths' problems originated and may continue to exist, and that improvements made while in correctional programs may be short-lived unless they are reinforced upon reentry into the community (Altschuler & Armstrong, 2001). The IAP model consists of three phases: "pre-release and preparatory planning during incarceration; structured transition that requires the participation of institutional and aftercare staff prior to and following community re-entry; and long-term, re-integrative activities that ensure adequate service delivery and the necessary level of social control" (Altschuler & Armstrong, 1996, p. 15). The program emphasizes the development of prosocial networks for the youth in the community, working with families and schools and blending treatment with surveillance through graduated sanctions, intensive supervision, case management, multiagency collaboration and service delivery, and a system of positive incentives (Altschuler, 1999; Wiebush, McNulty, & Le, 2000). The success of IAP has been attributed to the fact that it includes both strong surveillance and treatment components that intervene in the offender's home, community, and social network (Altschuler, Armstrong, & MacKenzie, 1999). The OJJDP IAP demonstration programs were completed at three sites and the results have been encouraging (see Meisel, 2001).

These initiatives are encouraging. Even more auspicious is the fact that the efficacy of community-based programs has now been established in a number of empirical studies (see Lipsey & Wilson, 1998). Yet relatively few juvenile justice programs are empirically evaluated and few evaluations use an experimental design (Roberts, 1989). Rigorous evaluation studies of programs are needed to build and refine the knowledge base surrounding effective interventions that satisfy public safety needs. But these model programs illustrate that the goals of public safety and holding young offenders accountable are fully compatible with community-based treatment and the best interests of children. Such programs provide "a balanced approach of accountability, public safety, and competency development. Politicians can endorse the comprehensive, integrated process and still stress the sanctions and accountability while noting the cost-effectiveness of early intervention and community-based strategies" (Merlo & Benekos, 2000, p. 155).

Innovative Mental Health Services in the Juvenile Justice System

Clearly, the mental health and juvenile justice systems have both reformed how they conceptualize and deliver services. Both systems have recognized the importance of providing a continuum of treatment options, emphasizing the development of a range of community-based services that may reduce the need for costlier residential placements. These services attempt to use multiagency collaborations that provide individualized treatments focusing on a variety of needs that go beyond mental health services (e.g., including familial, educational, recreational, and other services). In the next section, we highlight several noteworthy treatment initiatives that are designed for youth who may be served by both systems: multiproblem adolescents with serious emotional disturbances and juvenile justice involvement. These initiatives, all of which reflect community-based system-of-care philosophies, are wraparound services, multisystemic therapy, intensive family preservation, and therapeutic foster care.

Wraparound Services

"Wraparound services" that "wrap" services around youth and their families grew out of the system-of-care movement, which emphasized the need for flexible and highly individualized services for children. These services are characterized by strong interagency collaboration, flexible funding and care, individualized and family-centered care, and care when needed (Brown, Borduin, & Henggeler, 2001). They require all of the involved individuals and systems to come together and agree on what is needed for a particular child and his or her family (Burchard & Burns, 1998). Out of this needs-based assessment, an individualized service plan is developed, but "instead of having professionals try to fit the child into existing categorical services, the people who are most influential to the child and family tailor the services to fit the child and family" (Burchard & Burns, 1998, p. 364). At the systems level, wraparound is a process that brings state and local agencies together; at the intervention level, wraparound describes how individualized service plans are designed and implemented (VanDenBerg, 1999).

Wraparound Milwaukee is the best example of wraparound services designed to serve emotionally disturbed youth in the juvenile justice system (Goldman & Faw, 1999; Kamradt, 1998). The program began as a pilot project that used a wraparound approach to facilitate the return of youth in residential treatment centers to the community. By 1998, the program had expended to serve 610 severely emotionally disturbed youth in the child welfare and juvenile justice systems, funded through Medicaid, child welfare, the county delinquency program, and a CMHS federal grant. Families are court-ordered into the program, which utilizes care coordinators and mobile crisis teams to individualize services and help the family obtain whatever services they require from a network of 120 provider agencies. Care coordinators also facilitate the development of a team of resource people and natural supports for the family and the creation of crisis plans. The program has a strong commitment to training, quality assurance, and cultural competence.

Evaluations of Wraparound Milwaukee have shown it to be effective in reducing both the number of children in daily residential care and psychiatric hospitalizations, with preliminary data showing an 85% reduction in arrest rates (see Mendel, 2000). This has resulted in significantly reduced costs: the cost of placing youth in residential treatment ($4,800 per month) or in psychiatric hospital care ($15,000 per month) is much greater than the cost of wraparound services ($3,200 per month). In addition, stakeholder feedback suggests improved relationships among child welfare, juvenile justice, and mental health systems (Goldman & Faw, 1999). However, because there is relatively little research on the effectiveness of wraparound services (Brown et al., 2001), empirical support is not yet well established.

Multisystemic Therapy

Probably the leading and most promising new treatment approach to juvenile delinquency is multisystemic therapy (MST) (see Sheidow & Henggeler, ch. 12 in this volume). Consistent with a family preservation model of service delivery,

MST is an intensive, multimodel, family-based treatment approach that has been used to treat a number of challenging populations, including chronic and violent juvenile offenders, substance abusing/dependent delinquents, gang-affiliated youth of color, adolescent sex offenders, and youth at immediate risk for hospitalization due to suicidal, homicidal, or psychotic behaviors (see also Schoenwald, Borduin, & Henggeler, 1998). MST is grounded in family systems and social-ecological theories of behavior and is informed by research demonstrating the multidetermined nature of delinquent behavior. Accordingly, individualized services target problems and risk factors across the multiple systems in a child's life: family, peers, school, and neighborhood (Borduin, 1994). MST interventions are based on an individualized assessment of the factors contributing to the child's delinquency across all systems. Interventions are delivered in the home or other community settings to promote cooperation, enhance treatment generalization, and leave in place an indigenous support network for families so that behavioral changes can be maintained after treatment terminates (Schoenwald, Scherer, & Brondino, 1995). This contrasts markedly with traditional treatments, which focus only on one or two aspects of the youth's deficits, "remove youth from their natural environment, attempt to 'fix' the youth, and then return him or her to the same family, peer, school, neighborhood and community context." (Henggeler et al., 1996, p. 179).

As essential and vital resources, families participate collaboratively in the formation of treatment goals. To reach these goals, MST draws upon a variety of interventions and therapeutic modalities, including strategic and structural family therapies, behavioral parent training, cognitive-behavioral therapy, social skills training, recreational services, and effective school and community consultation. Specific goals common to MST treatments include improving parental discipline practices and family affective relations, decreasing the juvenile's association with delinquent peers, promoting the youth's involvement in prosocial activities, and improving school performance.

The efficacy of MST has been demonstrated in a growing number of rigorous outcome studies that have randomly assigned juvenile offenders to court-referred, traditional services (e.g., individual therapy, referral to social service agencies), or MST (see Borduin et al., 1995). Multisystemic therapy produced impressive 25 to 75% reductions in rearrest rates *beyond* the reductions achieved with traditional services and 47 to 64% reductions in out-of-home placements, decreased drug use, and improved family relations (see Henggeler, Michalic, Rone, Thomas, & Timmons-Mitchell, 1998a). Notably, substantial reductions in recidivism persisted for 5 years after treatment and were consistent across age, race, social class, and gender. Treatment completion rates were very high, but even dropouts had substantially lower rearrest rates (see Henggeler et al., 1998a). In one study of 96 youth at risk for out-of-home placement due to violent or chronic offending, youth who received MST had half as many arrests 59 weeks postreferral as youth who received the usual DYS services of institutional treatment followed by community probation and parole (Henggeler, Melton, & Smith, 1992). Multisystemic therapy has been found to be much more cost-effective than traditional sanctions, producing substantial savings to taxpayers through reduced recidivism and crime costs.

Intensive Family Preservation Services

Intensive family preservation services (IFPS) are short-term crisis intervention programs for families with children at-risk for out-of-home placement. The goal of IFPS is to stabilize families and improve family functioning by providing in-home services and linking families to ongoing sources of support (Brewer, Hawkins, Catalano, & Neckerman, 1995). One of the first successful IFPS programs was Homebuilders, established in Washington State in 1974. Homebuilders counselors work with families for 4 and 8 weeks, spending 8–10 hours per week in face-to-face contact with family members, and remain "on call" 24 hours a day. In addition to individual therapy, family therapy, and crisis intervention, Homebuilders counselors provide instrumental support, such as shopping, housecleaning, and transportation (Guarino-Ghezzi & Loughran, 1996). Family Ties, a New York program for juvenile offenders, is grounded in the Homebuilders model of IFPS. It is a 4- to 6-week program that provides an array of in-home services. Following program completion, if the judge finds the youth and family to have made significant progress, the out-of-home placement is averted and the youth is placed on probation (Soler, 1992). Evaluations of both programs found that they were effective in preventing out-of-home placements for up to 12 months, after which the effects dissipated (Borduin, 1994). The cost savings in the Family Ties program were substantial, however, with nearly $70,000 saved for each residential placement averted through participation in Family Ties (Schoenwald et al., 1995; Soler, 1992). Although the long-term efficacy of these programs has not been demonstrated, there is evidence that IFPS stabilizes families and reduces the number of costly out-of-home placements.

Treatment Foster Care

Treatment foster care (TFC), a treatment approach grounded in social learning theory and designed to address several risk factors for delinquency (e.g., harsh discipline, poor supervision, negative peer influence), is a promising alternative to institutionalization for emotionally and behaviorally disturbed youth in the juvenile justice system (Chamberlain, 2003). TFC uses community families that are carefully selected, trained, and supervised to provide temporary placements for adolescents for an average of about 6 months. It is based on the premise that foster parents can serve as primary providers of therapy via their daily interactions with the child in a natural home setting (Redding, Fried, & Britner, 2000). Foster parents are trained to implement a behavioral management system that provides a therapeutic environment for youth, while family therapy frequently is provided to the youth and his family of origin. TFC includes eight components (Chamberlain, 1996): (a) preservice training for TFC parents; (b) ongoing support and supervision for foster parents; (c) daily management in the home and community using an individualized behavioral program; (d) individual child treatment, including weekly sessions and on-call crisis intervention; (e) promotion of contact with the family of origin when possible; (f) case management services; (g) school programming and consultation; and (h) psychiatric consultation.

Several studies have found that when compared to incarceration or alternative diversion programs, serious and chronic juvenile offenders in TFC have substantially fewer subsequent arrests and spend less time incarcerated, with one study finding a sevenfold reduction in rearrest rates (Chamberlain & Moore, 1998; Chamberlain & Reid, 1998). Treatment foster care offers an appealing alternative to restrictive residential placements, which are more costly and increase a juvenile's exposure to deviant peers (Chamberlain, 1996; Schoenwald et al., 1995). Economic analyses show that TFC produced $14 in taxpayer savings per dollar spent (Aos, Phipps, Barnoski, & Lieb, 1999). TFC and similar programs, such as the Teaching Family Model (see Fizsen & Blase, 1993), require further evaluation, but their promise has led to their widespread adoption (Schoenwald et al., 1995).

Implications of System Reforms and Innovative Approaches for Systems of Care for Juvenile Offenders

Systems of Care

The ascendancy of systems of care has been a major development in the children's mental health service system and, more recently, the juvenile justice system. Systems of care are appealing for many reasons. First, their values and principles make intuitive sense and depict an ideal picture of how services should be delivered. Second, families have greater access to a broader array of services, which may translate into greater levels of family satisfaction. In addition, agencies that once were characterized by disconnection and turfism may develop better relations with one another. Finally, several evaluation studies of system-of-care services have reported the cost effectiveness of these services. Legislators and taxpayers may be happy with the "bottom line." In the past, systems of care have been targeted mainly to children with severe emotional disturbances, but as system-of-care models for serving mentally disordered youth in the juvenile justice system continue to grow, they should be guided by the following goals and principles:

- Juvenile justice service systems should be consistent with system-of-care values and principles, including a child-centered focus with family involvement; provision of services that are community-based, culturally competent, integrated, and coordinated; and case management.
- Active coordination with other agencies and systems (including mental health, child welfare, and education) can be achieved if agencies allocate time and resources for developing and maintaining an understanding about (a) the nature of the other agencies, (b) the ways in which agencies may collaborate, (c) common goals for the youth they serve, and (d) provisions for collecting and sharing information. Casey, Keilitz, and Hafemeister (1992) identified ways to enhance

and evaluate interagency communications, collaboration, and service delivery.

- Interagency collaborations should include interagency service agreements and integrated planning, multiagency budgets, comprehensive assessment and referral centers, team approaches to assessment and case management, and staff cross training (Cocozza & Skowyra, 2000).
- A balanced continuum of care within a juvenile justice context should contain not only a continuum of treatment options (including specialized treatments for offender subgroups, such as sex offenders or substance abusers) but also a range of supervision levels (from secure placements to nonresidential services) (Guarino-Ghezzi & Loughran, 1996).
- Special attention should be given to the transition period from secure to community-based facilities, ensuring that both surveillance and treatment services are provided.
- Systems of care must implement rigorous quality assurance protocols that provide comprehensive measurement of processes and outcomes linked to a system of continuous quality improvement (Bickman, 1999).
- Continued effectiveness research to evaluate juvenile justice service systems is imperative. System developers and researchers must find comparison groups to study, using random assignment to groups when possible.
- Evaluations should examine whether coordinated interagency efforts will improve outcomes, the specific factors identified as effective components of interagency partnerships, the specific aspects of case management that make interagency provision of services more effective, and the cost-effectiveness of interagency services (Soler, 1992).

Beyond Systems of Care: Model Programs

The most recent, thorough, and methodologically rigorous system-of-care evaluations have found that the improved organization and integration of services alone are not enough to affect clinical outcomes (Bickman, 1996; Bickman et al., 1997). If the individual services or interventions themselves are not effective, then it follows that changing how they are organized will not increase their effectiveness (Henggeler et al., 1996). Although many past interventions with violent, delinquent, and multiproblem youth were not effective, over the last several decades effective approaches have been developed, even for serious and violent juvenile offenders (Tate, Reppucci, & Mulvey, 1995). MST is perhaps the best example. Lipsey and Wilson's (1998) seminal meta-analysis of 200 studies of treatment programs for serious and violent juvenile offenders found that, on average, interventions reduced recidivism by 6%, with the more effective programs reducing recidivism an average of 15 to 20%.

Although it is unlikely that any single approach will ever be "the silver bullet," the most successful approaches have certain common elements. They:

- Address the multiple social contexts in which youth are embedded
- Deliver services in youths' natural environments
- Are flexible and individualized
- Emphasize treatment goals and methods that are practical, problem-focused, and action-oriented
- Hold staff accountable for therapeutic outcomes (Borduin, 1994)

Juvenile delinquents are a heterogenous group. Youth with certain symptomatic or delinquent profiles may respond differently to interventions than do others (Rosenblatt & Furlong, 1998). In addition, youth with specific demographic or cultural backgrounds may have unique needs. Girls in the juvenile justice system, for example, have different constellations of problems than do boys, including more contact with the court for status offenses and a greater likelihood of prior sexual victimization (Dembo et al., 1993). More gender-specific programs and practices should be developed, as well as gender-specific and culturally sensitive crisis intervention protocols (Prescott, 1997, 1998).

But regardless of the groups served, effective programs share common characteristics. They target criminogenic risk factors (e.g., truancy, association with delinquent peers, substance abuse) amenable to intervention, and they are (a) individualized; (b) family-based and delivered in community settings; (c) multimodal, with a behavioral, cognitive-behavioral, or social skills orientation; and (d) based on a particular treatment model having demonstrated effectiveness. They also (e) have a high level of fidelity to the treatment model along with good program and client monitoring; (f) have highly trained and well-supervised staff; (g) are of at least 6 months' duration; and (h) provide aftercare (Corbett & Petersilia, 1994; Lipsey, 1999; Lipsey & Wilson, 1998; McGuire & Priestley, 1995).

Beyond Model Programs: Day-to-Day Practice

Although the results from model programs offer hope that "something works" for youth in the juvenile justice system, translating model programs into community practice often is quite difficult, a problem seen with clinical interventions generally (see Weisz, Donenberg, Han, & Kauneckis, 1995a; Weisz, Donenberg, Han, & Weiss, 1995b). "We seem generally incapable of translating demonstration treatment approaches into operating pieces of the existing service delivery system" (Mulvey, 1989, p. 13). It is wrongly assumed that, if properly trained, mental health and juvenile justice professionals are equally adept at executing an intervention (Mulvey, 1989). Programs for institutionalized offenders that use mental health rather than criminal justice personnel to administer treatment have comparatively lower rates of recidivism (Lipsey & Wilson, 1998). This finding raises an interesting question for the justice system: what functions should be carried out by which professionals? Mulvey (1989) suggested that mental health practitioners limit their activities to addressing mental health problems and that juvenile justice personnel focus on providing a useful daily structure and activities for the youth. It may, however, be useful for personnel from both systems to receive cross-training to learn the relevant knowledge and skills of the other's culture, an understanding necessary for the effective collaboration required of systems of care and to better integrate correctional and rehabilitative functions. Juvenile justice professionals can learn how their supervision of youth could be more therapeutic. Mental health professionals can learn how juvenile justice systems operate and about the barriers to cross-system collaboration, how to tailor their services to best fit juvenile justice contexts, and how best to advocate for programs and policies (Needleman & Needleman, 1997).

Needleman and Needleman's (1997) suggestions for improving practice for social workers in juvenile justice systems are applicable:

- *Appropriate training:* The skills necessary to function effectively within the juvenile justice system go beyond mental health treatment and include program evaluation, community analysis, legal research, and organizational change techniques.
- *Better networking:* Practitioners in the court system have much to gain by fostering relationships with practitioners outside of the court system and by developing a more sophisticated knowledge base of the services available in the community.
- *Community analysis:* The community context of youth and families in the system must be understood by practitioners. This includes knowing how parents and youth feel about the justice system, how parents understand delinquency, and how other systems (such as schools) respond to delinquent youth and their families. In working with diverse groups and organizations; this knowledge helps practitioners bridge the gaps in perspectives held by different stakeholders.

Conclusion

Like most large systems, the juvenile justice system is slow to change. Alternative, progressive models are promising, but it will take time before they are adopted on a broad scale. Positive evaluation findings must be publicized to policy-makers and the public at large, because the media accounts of high-profile incidents of juvenile crime are seized on and often drive policy decisions more forcefully than data (see Shepherd, 1999). Large-scale system reforms that may be initially unpopular can lead to positive developments, as evidenced by the reforms in Massachusetts. Innovative models, such as balanced and restorative justice, may hold the best hope of winning public confidence that the juvenile justice system can achieve goals of both community protection and rehabilitation and that the provision of systems of care (particularly mental health services) to juvenile offenders is not being soft on crime, but rather is a reform that will reduce juvenile crime and enhance public safety.

References

Ainsworth, J. E. (1991). Re-imagining childhood and re-constructing the legal order: The case for abolishing the juvenile court. *North Carolina Law Review, 69*, 1083–1133.

Altschuler, D. M. (1999). Issues and challenges in the community supervision of juvenile offenders. *Southern Illinois University Law Journal, 23*, 469–483.

Altschuler, D. M., & Armstrong, T. L. (1996). Aftercare not afterthought: Testing the IAP model. *Juvenile Justice, 3*(1), 15–22.

Altschuler, D. M., & Armstrong, T. L. (2001). Reintegrating high-risk juvenile offenders into communities: Experiences and prospects. *Corrections Management Quarterly, 5*(3), 72–88.

Altschuler, D. M., Armstrong, T. L., & MacKenzie, D. L. (1999). *Reintegration, supervised release, and intensive aftercare.* Washington, DC: US Department of Justice, Office of Justice Programs, Office of Juvenile Justice and Delinquency Prevention.

Aos, S., Phipps, P., Barnoski, R., & Lieb, R. (1999). *The comparative costs and benefits of programs to reduce crime: A review of national research findings with implications for Washington state.* Olympia, WA: Washington State Institute for Public Policy.

Bazemore, G. (1997). What's "new" about the balanced approach? *Juvenile and Family Court Journal*, 1–22.

Bazemore, G., & Day, S. E. (1997). Restoring the balance: Juvenile and community justice. *Juvenile Justice, 3*(1), 3–13.

Bazemore, G., & Walgrave, L. (Eds.). (1999). *Restorative juvenile justice: Repairing the harm of youth crime.* Monsey, NY: Criminal Justice Press.

Bernard, T. (1992). *The cycle of juvenile justice.* New York: Oxford University Press.

Bickman, L. (1996). A continuum or care: More is not always better. *American Psychologist, 51*, 689–701.

Bickman, L. (1999). Practice makes perfect and other myths about mental health services. *American Psychologist, 54*, 965–978.

Bickman, L., Guthrie, P., Foster, E. W., Summerfelt, W. T., Breda, C., & Heflinger, C. A. (1995). *Managed care in mental health: The Fort Bragg experiment.* New York: Plenum.

Bickman, L., Heflinger, C. A., Lambert, E. W., & Summerfelt, W. T. (1996). The Fort Bragg managed care experiment: Short term impact on psychopathology. *Journal of Child and Family Studies, 5*, 137–160.

Bickman, L., Summerfelt, W. T., & Noser, K. (1997). Comparative outcomes of emotionally disturbed children and adolescents in a system of services and usual care. *Psychiatric Services, 48*, 1543–1548.

Borduin, C. M. (1994). Innovative models of treatment and service delivery in the juvenile justice system. *Journal of Clinical Child Psychology, 23*(Supplement), 19–25.

Borduin, C. M., Mann, B. J., Cone, L., Henggeler, S. W., Fucci, B. R., Blaske, D. M., et al. (1995). Multisystemic treatment of serious juvenile offenders: Long-term prevention of criminality and violence. *Journal of Consulting and Clinical Psychology, 63*, 569–578.

Brewer, D. D., Hawkins, J. D., Catalano, R. F., & Neckerman, H. J. (1995). Preventing serious, violent, and chronic juvenile offending: A review of evaluations of selected strategies in childhood, adolescence, and the community. In J. C. Howell, B. Krisberg, J. D. Hawkins, & J. J. Wilson (Eds.), *Sourcebook on serious, violent, and chronic juvenile offenders* (pp. 61–141). Thousand Oaks, CA: Sage.

Brown, T. L., Borduin, C. M., & Henggeler, S. W. (2001). Treating juvenile offenders in community settings. In J. Ashford, B. Sales, & W. Reid, *Treating adult and juvenile offenders with special needs* (pp. 445–464). Washington, DC: American Psychological Association.

Burchard, J. D. (1996). Evaluation of the Fort Bragg managed care experiment. *Journal of Child and Family Studies, 5,* 173–176.

Burchard, J. D., & Burns, E. J. (1998). The role of the case study in the evaluation of individualized services. In M. H. Epstein, K. Kutash, & A. Duchnowski (Eds.), *Outcomes for children and youth with emotional and behavioral disorders and their families: Programs and evaluation best practices* (pp. 363–383). Austin, TX: PRO-ED, Inc.

Casey, P., Keilitz, I., & Hafemeister, T. L. (1992). Toward an agenda for reform of justice and mental health systems interactions. *Law and Human Behavior, 16,* 107–128.

Cellini, H. R. (2001). Mental health concerns of adjudicated adolescents—a challenge for the juvenile justice system. In G. Landsberg & A. Smiley (Eds.), *Forensic mental health: Working with offenders with mental illness* (pp. 34-2–34-14). Kingston, NJ: Civil Research Institute.

Center for Mental Health Services. (1999). *Annual report to Congress on the evaluation of the Comprehensive Community Mental Health Services for Children and Their Families program, 1999.* Atlanta, GA: ORC Macro.

Chamberlain, P. (1996). Community-based residential treatment for adolescents with conduct disorder. In T. H. Ollendick & R. J. Prinz (Eds.), *Advances in clinical child psychology* (Vol. 18, pp. 63–89). New York: Plenum.

Chamberlain, P. (2003). *Treating chronic juvenile offenders: Advances made through the Oregon multidimensional treatment foster care model.* Washington, DC: American Psychological Association.

Chamberlain, P., & Moore, K. (1998). A clinical model for parenting juvenile offenders: A comparison of group care versus family care. *Clinical Child Psychology and Psychiatry, 3,* 375–386.

Chamberlain, P., & Reid, J. B. (1998). Comparison of two community alternatives to incarceration for chronic juvenile offenders. *Journal of Consulting and Clinical Psychology, 66,* 624–633.

City of Jacksonville, FL. (2001). *Juvenile justice comprehensive strategy.* Available at www.ojjdp.ncirs.org.

Coates, R. B. (1989). The future of corrections in juvenile justice. In A. R. Roberts (Ed.), *Juvenile justice: Policies, programs, and services* (pp. 281–297). Chicago: Dorsey Press.

Cocozza, J. J., & Skowyra, K. R. (2000). Youth with mental disorders: Issues and emerging responses. *Juvenile Justice, 7*(1), 3–13.

Corbett, R. P., & Petersilia, J. (1994). What works with juvenile offenders: A synthesis of the literature and experience. *Federal Probation, 58*(4), 63–67.

Dembo, R., Williams, L., & Schmeidler, J. (1993). Gender differences in mental health service needs among youth entering a juvenile detention center. *Journal of Prison and Jail Health, 12,* 73–101.

Duchowski, A. J., Hall, K. S., Kutash, K., & Friedman, R. M. (1998). The alternatives to residential treatment study. In M. H. Epstein, K. Kutash, & A. Duchnowski (Eds.), *Outcomes for children and youth with emotional and behavioral disorders and their families: Programs and evaluation best practices* (pp. 55–80). Austin, TX: PRO-ED, Inc.

Dwyer, D. C., & McNally, R. B. (1989). Juvenile justice: Reform, retain, and reaffirm. In A. R. Roberts (Ed.), *Juvenile justice: Policies, programs, and services* (pp. 319–327). Chicago: Dorsey Press.

English, T. R. (1993). TQM and all that jazz: Reinventing juvenile justice. *Juvenile Justice, 1,* 16–22.

Epstein, M. H., Kutash, K., & Duchnowski, A. (1998). *Outcomes for children and youth with emotional and behavioral disorders and their families: Programs and evaluation best practices.* Austin, TX: PRO-ED, Inc.

Evans, M. E., & Banks, S. M. (1996). The Fort Bragg managed care experiment. *Journal of Child and Family Studies, 5,* 169–172.

Feld, B. C. (1999). The honest politician's guide to juvenile justice in the twenty-first century. *Annals of the American Academy of Political and Social Science, 564,* 10–27.

Feld, B. C. (1997). Abolish the juvenile court: Youthfulness, criminal responsibility and sentencing policy. *Journal of Criminal Law and Criminology, 88,* 68–136.

Feldman, S. (1997). The Fort Bragg demonstration and evaluation. *American Psychologist, 52,* 560–561.

Fizsen, D. L. & Blase, K. A. (1993). Creating new realities: Program development and dissemination. *Journal of Applied Behavior Analysis, 26,* 597–615.

Fox, S. J. (1970). Juvenile justice reform: A historical perspective. *Stanford Law Review, 22,* 1187–1239.

Frabutt, J. M., Arbuckle, M. B., & Campbell, D. (2002, June/July). Youth violence and juvenile justice: Using a system of care to support youth and families. *Juvenile Justice, 8*(3), 1–2, 14.

Friedman, R. M. (1996). The Fort Bragg study: What can we conclude? *Journal of Child and Family Studies, 5,* 161–168.

Goldman, S. K., & Faw, L. (1999). Three wraparound models as promising approaches. In B. J. Burns & S. K. Goldman (Eds.), *Promising practices in wraparound for children with serious emotional disturbance and their families.* Systems of care: Promising practices in children's mental health, 1998 series (Vol. IV). Washington, DC: Center for Effective Collaboration and Practice, American Institutes for Research.

Greenbaum, P. E., Dedrick, R. F., Friedman, R. M., Kutash, K., Brown, E. C., Lardieri, S. P., et al. (1998). National Adolescent and Child Treatment Study (NACTS): Outcomes for children with serious emotional and behavioral disturbance. In M. H. Epstein, K. Kutash, & A. Duchnowski (Eds.), *Outcomes for children and youth with emotional and behavioral disorders and their families: Programs and evaluation best practices* (pp. 21–54). Austin, TX: PRO-ED, Inc.

Grisso, T. (2001). Why juvenile justice will survive its centennial. In R. Bonnie & L. Frost (Eds.), *The evolution of mental health law* (pp. 167–180). Washington, DC: American Psychological Association.

Guarino-Ghezzi, S., & Loughran, E. J. (1996). *Balancing juvenile justice.* New Brunswick, NJ: Transaction Publishers.

Henggeler, S. W., Melton, G. B., & Smith, L. A. (1992). Family preservation using multisystemic therapy: An effective alternative to incarcerating serious juvenile offenders. *Journal of Consulting and Clinical Psychology, 60,* 953–961.

Henggeler, S. W., Michalic, S. F., Rone, L., Thomas, C., & Timmons-Mitchell, J. (1998a). Multisystemic therapy. In D. Elliott (Ed.), *Blueprints for violence prevention* (Book 6). Boulder, CO: Institute of Behavioral Science, University of Colorado.

Henggeler, S. W., Schoenwald, S. K., Borduin, C. M., Rowland, M. D., & Cunningham, P. B. (1998b). *Multisystemic treatment for antisocial behavior in youth.* New York: Guilford Press.

Henggeler, S. W., Schoenwald, S. K., & Munger, R. L. (1996). Families and therapists achieve clinical outcomes, systems of care mediate the process. *Journal of Child and Family Studies, 5,* 177–183.

Hoagwood, K. (1997). Interpreting nullity: The Fort Bragg experiment—A comparative success or failure? *American Psychologist, 52,* 546–550.

Howell, J. C., Krisberg, B., & Jones, M. (1995). Trends in juvenile crime and youth violence. In J. C. Howell, B. Krisberg, J. D. Hawkins, & J. J. Wilson (Eds.), *Sourcebook
on serious, violent, and chronic juvenile offenders* (pp. 1–35). Thousand Oaks, CA:
Sage.

Huizinga, D., & Jakob-Chien, C. (1998). The contemporaneous co-occurrence of serious
and violent juvenile offending and other problem behaviors. In R. Loeber &
D. P. Farrington (Eds.), *Serious and violent juvenile offenders: Risk factors and successful interventions* (pp. 47–67). Thousand Oaks, CA: Sage.

In re Gault, 387 U.S. 1 (1967).

Ingersoll, S. (1997). The National Juvenile Justice Action Plan: A comprehensive response to a critical challenge. *Juvenile Justice, 3*(2), 11–20.

Kamradt, B. J. (1998). The 25 kid project: How Milwaukee utilized a pilot project to
change their system of care. *A TA brief from the National Resource Network*. Washington, DC: Office of Juvenile Justice and Delinquency Prevention, U.S. Department of Justice.

Kent v. United States, 383 U.S. 541 (1966).

Knitzer, J. (1982). *Unclaimed children*. Washington, DC: Children's Defense Fund.

Knitzer, J. (1996). Children's mental health: changing paradigms and policies. In
E. F. Zigler, S. L. Kagan, & N. W. Hall (Eds.), *Children, families, and government:
Preparing for the twenty-first century*. New York: Cambridge University Press.

Krisberg, B., & Austin, J. F. (1993). *Reinventing juvenile justice*. Newbury Park, CA: Sage.

Krisberg, B., & Howell, J. C. (1998). The impact of the juvenile justice system and
prospects for graduated sanctions in a comprehensive strategy. In R. Loeber & D. P.
Farrington (Eds.), *Serious and violent juvenile offenders: Risk factors and successful
interventions* (pp. 346–366). Thousand Oaks, CA: Sage.

Levine, M. (2000). The family group conference in the New Zealand children, young
persons, and their families act of 1989 (CYPYF): Review and evaluation. *Behavioral
Sciences and the Law, 18*, 517–556.

Levy, K. S. (1999). The Australian juvenile justice system: Legal and social science dimensions. *Quinnipiac Law Review, 18*, 521–572.

Lexcen, F., & Redding, R. E. (2002). Mental health needs of juvenile offenders. *Juvenile
Correctional Mental Health Report, 3*(1), 1–16.

Lipsey, M. W. (1999, July). Can intervention rehabilitate serious delinquents? *Annals of
the American Academy of Political and Social Science, 564*, 142–166.

Lipsey, M. W., & Wilson, D. B. (1998). Effective intervention for serious juvenile offenders: A synthesis of research. In R. Loeber & D. P. Farrington (Eds.), *Serious and violent juvenile offenders: Risk factors and successful interventions* (pp. 313–345). Thousand Oaks, CA: Sage.

Lourie, I., Stroul, B., & Friedman, R. M. (1998). Principles of a community-based system
of care. In M. Epstein, K. Kutash, & A. Duchnowski (Eds.), *Outcomes for children
and youth with emotional & behavioral disorders and their families: Programs and
Evaluation Best Practices* (pp. 3–20). Austin, TX: PRO-ED.

Mahoney, A. R. (1987). *Juvenile justice in context*. Boston: Northeastern University Press.

Martinez, O. L. (2001, Sept./Oct.). Building a juvenile correctional mental health system.
Juvenile Correctional Mental Health Report, 1(6), 81–83, 91–93.

Martinson, R. (1974). What works? Questions and answers about prison reform. *Public
Interest, 10*, 22–54.

McGarvey, E. L., & Waite, D. (2000). Mental health needs among juveniles committed
to the Virginia Department of Juvenile Justice. *Developments in Mental Health Law,
20*, 1–24.

McGuire, J., & Priestley, P. (1995). Reviewing "what works": Past, present, and future. In J. McGuire (Ed), *What works: Reducing reoffending: Guidelines from research and practice* (pp. 3–34). New York: Wiley.

Meisel, J. S. (2001). Relationships and juvenile offenders: The effects of intensive after-care supervision. *Prison Journal, 81*(2), 206–245.

Mendel, R. A. (2000). *Less hype, more help: Reducing juvenile crime, what works—and what doesn't*. Washington, DC: American Youth Policy Forum.

Merlo, A. V., & Benekos, P. J. (2000). *What's wrong with the criminal justice system: Ideology, politics and the media*. Cincinnati, OH: Anderson Publishing.

Moon, M. M., Sundt, J. L., Cullen, F. T., & Wright, J. P. (2000). Is child saving dead? Public support for juvenile rehabilitation. *Crime and Delinquency, 46*, 38–60.

Morris, A., & Maxwell, G. M. (1993, March). Juvenile justice in New Zealand: A new paradigm. *Australia & New Zealand Journal of Criminology, 26*, 72–90.

Morris, R. E., Harrison, E. A., Knox, G. W., Tromanhauser, H., Marquis, D. K., & Watts, L. L. (1995). Health risk behavioral survey from 39 juvenile correctional facilities in the United States. *Journal of Adolescent Health, 17*, 334–344.

Mulvey, E. P. (1989). Scenes from a marriage: How can juvenile justice and mental health go together? *Forensic Reports, 2*, 9–24.

Needleman, C., & Needleman, M. L. (1997). Social work with juvenile offenders. In A. R. Roberts (Ed.), *Social work in juvenile and criminal justice settings* (pp. 221–249). Springfield, IL: Thomas Books.

Orlando, F. A., & Crippen, G. L. (1992). The rights of children and the juvenile court. In I. Schwartz (Ed.), *Juvenile justice and public policy: Toward a national agenda* (pp. 89–100). New York: Lexington.

Osher, T. W., & Osher, D. M. (2002). The paradigm shift to true collaboration with families. *Journal of Child and Family Studies, 11*(1), 47–60.

Oswald, D. P., & Singh, N. N. (1996). Emerging trends in child and adolescent mental health services. In T. H. Ollendick & R. J. Prinz (Eds.), *Advances in Clinical Child Psychology* (Vol. 18, pp. 331–365). New York: Plenum.

Platt, A. M. (1977). *The child savers* (2nd ed.). Chicago: University of Chicago Press.

Prescott, L. (1997). Adolescent girls with co-occurring disorders in the juvenile justice system. Report prepared for the National GAINS Center, Delmar, NY.

Prescott, L. (1998). *Improving policy and practice for adolescent girls with co-occurring disorders in the juvenile justice system*. Report prepared for the National GAINS Center, Delmar, NY.

Quinn, K. P., & Epstein, M. H. (1998). Characteristics of children, youth, and families served by local interagency systems of care. In M. H. Epstein, K. Kutash, & A. Duchnowski (Eds.), *Outcomes for children and youth with emotional and behavioral disorders and their families: Programs and evaluation best practices* (pp. 81–114). Austin, TX: PRO-ED, Inc.

Redding, R. E. (2003). The effects of adjudicating and sentencing juveniles as adults: Research and policy implications. *Youth Violence and Juvenile Justice, 1*, 128–155.

Redding, R. E., Fried, C., & Britner, P. A. (2000). Predictors of placement outcomes in residential foster care: Implications for foster parent selection and service delivery. *Journal of Child and Family Studies, 9*(4), 425–447.

Roberts, A. (1989). National survey and assessment of 66 treatment programs for juvenile offenders: Model programs and pseudomodels. In A. R. Roberts (Ed.), *Juvenile justice: Policies, programs, and services* (pp. 299–307). Chicago: Dorsey Press.

Rosenblatt, J. A., & Furlong, M. J. (1998). Outcomes in a system of care for youth with emotional and behavioral disorders: An examination of differential change across clinical profiles. *Journal of Child and Family Studies, 7,* 217–232.

Rosenblatt, J. S., Rosenblatt, A., & Biggs, E. E. (2000). Criminal behavior and emotional disorder: Comparing youth served by the mental health and juvenile justice systems. *Journal of Behavioral Health Services and Research, 27*(2), 227–237.

Ross, C. J. (1995). Disposition in a discretionary regime: Punishment and rehabilitation in the juvenile justice system. *Boston College Law Review, 36,* 1037–1060.

Schoenwald, S. K., Borduin, C. M., & Henggeler, S. W. (1998). Multisystemic therapy: Changing the natural service ecologies of adolescents and families. In M. H. Epstein, K. Kutash, & A. Duchnowski (Eds.), *Outcomes for children and youth with emotional and behavioral disorders and their families: Programs and evaluation best practices* (pp. 485–511). Austin, TX: PRO-ED, Inc.

Schoenwald, S. K., Scherer, D. G., & Brondino, M. J. (1995). Effective community-based treatments for serious juvenile offenders. In S. W. Henggeler & A. B. Santos (Eds.), *Innovative approaches for difficult-to-treat populations* (pp. 65–82). Washington, DC: American Psychiatric Press.

Shanok, S., & Lewis, D. (1977). Juvenile court versus child guidance referral: Psychosocial and parental factors. *American Journal of Psychiatry, 134,* 1130–1133.

Shepherd, R. E. (1999). Film at eleven: The news media and juvenile crime. *Quinnipiac Law Review, 18,* 687–700.

Snyder, H. N. (1998). Appendix: Serious, violent, and chronic juvenile offenders—an assessment of the extent and trends in officially recognized serious criminal behavior in a delinquent population. In R. Loeber & D. P. Farrington (Eds.), *Serious juvenile offenders: Risk factors and successful interventions* (pp. 428–444). Thousand Oaks, CA: Sage.

Soler, M. (1992). Interagency services in the juvenile justice systems. In I. Schwartz (Ed.), *Juvenile justice and public policy: Toward a national agenda* (pp. 134–150). New York: Lexington.

Stroul, B. A., & Friedman, R. M. (1986; rev. ed. 1994). *A system of care for children and youth with severe emotional disturbances.* Washington DC: Georgetown University Child Development Center.

Tate, D. C., Reppucci, N. D., & Mulvey, E. P. (1995). Violent juvenile delinquents: Treatment effectiveness and implications for future action. *American Psychologist, 50,* 777–781.

Teplin, L. A., Abram, K. M., McClelland, G. M., Dulcan, M. K., & Mericle, A. A. (2002). Psychiatric disorders in youth in juvenile detention. *Archives of General Psychiatry, 59,* 1133–1143.

Tonry, M. H., & Moore, M. H. (Eds.). (1998). *Youth violence.* Chicago, IL: University of Chicago Press.

Tuma, J. M. (1992). Mental health services for children: The state of the art. *American Psychologist, 44,* 188–199.

Umbreit, M. S. (1995). The development and impact of victim-offender mediation in the United States. *Mediation Quarterly, 12*(3), 263–276.

VanDenBerg, J. (1999). History of the wraparound process. In B. J. Burns & S. K. Goldman (Eds.), *Promising practices in wraparound for children with serious emotional disturbance and their families.* Systems of care: Promising practices in children's mental health, 1998 series (Vol. IV). Washington, DC: Center for Effective Collaboration and Practice, American Institutes for Research.

Weisz, J. R., Donenberg, G. R., Han, S. S. & Kauneckis, D. (1995a). Child and adolescent psychotherapy outcomes in experiments versus clinics: Why the disparity? *Journal of Abnormal Child Psychology, 23,* 83–106.

Weisz, J. R., Donenberg, G. R., Han, S. S., & Weiss, B. (1995b). Bridging the gap between laboratory and clinic in child and adolescent psychotherapy. *Journal of Consulting and Clinical Psychology, 63,* 688–701.

Weisz, J. R., Han, S. S., & Valeri, S. M. (1996). What we can learn from Fort Bragg? *Journal of Child and Family Studies, 5,* 185–190.

Wiebush, R. G., McNulty, B., & Le, T. (2000). Implementation of the intensive community-based aftercare program. *Juvenile Justice Bulletin.* Washington, DC: U.S. Department of Justice, Office of Juvenile Justice and Delinquency Prevention.

Wilson, J. J., & Howell, J. C. (1995). Comprehensive strategy for serious, violent, and chronic juvenile offenders. In J. C. Howell, B. Krisberg, J. D. Hawkins, & J. J. Wilson (Eds.), *Sourcebook on serious, violent, and chronic juvenile offenders* (pp. 35–46). Thousand Oaks, CA: Sage.

Willie M. v. Hunt, 657 F.2d 55 (1981).

Wooldredge, J. D. (1988). Differentiating the effects of juvenile court sentences on eliminating recidivism. *Journal of Research in Crime and Delinquency, 25,* 264–300.

8

DEBORAH A. CHAPIN AND PATRICIA A. GRIFFIN

Juvenile Diversion

This chapter examines juvenile justice diversion as an alternative to formal juvenile justice adjudication and juvenile placement, particularly residential placement. Juvenile diversion is based on the premise that youths' exposure to the justice system may be more harmful than beneficial (Shelden, 1999). It has been argued that the diversion of low-risk, nonviolent misdemeanor offenders from the justice system into community-based treatment and interventions will reduce the likelihood of future delinquent behavior (Whitehead & Lab, 2001). In this chapter, we discuss the various definitions of juvenile diversion; its purpose, relevant history, and goals; types of diversion; and the various rationales for this process that have been offered. We next describe the key elements in the diversion process and then turn to a discussion of the relevant research on the characteristics of youth and programs that have been associated with juvenile diversion. Finally, we discuss the implications of these arguments, theories, and data for diversion in the context of the larger juvenile justice system.

Definitions of Diversion

For the purposes of this chapter, we define juvenile diversion as "an attempt to divert, or channel out, youthful offenders from the juvenile justice system" (Bynum & Thompson, 1996, p. 430), through the official halting or suspension of formal criminal or juvenile justice proceedings (Wood-Westland, 2002). Others have also provided definitions/descriptions of diversion. For instance, Lemert's idea of diversion as a process in which problems typically addressed in the context of delinquency and official action are defined and handled by other means, with "minimal penetration" into the juvenile justice system (Lemert, 1981, p. 36), has also been a well-used definition of diversion. Another characterization of diversion is when youth are referred to some community alternative that provides appropriate services (Lemert, 1981).

Diversion can also refer to "the use of a wide range of interventions as alternatives to either initial or continued formal processing" (Kammer, Minor, & Wells, 1997, p. 51). It can stress the difference between a youth's experiences of formal justice processing and diversion (Osgood & Weichselbaum, 1984) or "the process of channeling a referred juvenile from formal juvenile court processing to an alternative forum for resolution of the matter and/or a community-based agency for help" (Kurlychek, Torbet, & Bozynski, 1999, in Griffin & Torbet, 2002, p. 49). Griffin and Torbet (2002) observed that diversion is a loose term — and is often practiced loosely, with many youthful offenders never officially charged and the arresting officer often releasing the child with a verbal warning or to parents with a promise of no further delinquent behavior. This kind of informal practice, in which the juvenile is let go with a promise of good behavior, but without supervision, referrals, obligations, sanctions, or services of any kind, may be appropriate in some situations, and is certainly widespread, but is not diversion in the sense it was originally intended (Kurlychek et al., 1999).

Wood-Westland (2002) also offered a useful definition of a *diversion program* (a continuum of requirements a juvenile must complete in order to earn the dismissal, or its equivalent, of an offense and avoid increased involvement in the juvenile justice system). This definition is used throughout this chapter.

Purposes of Juvenile Diversion

Diverting youth from the juvenile justice system has a number of potential benefits to youth, community, and society (Whitehead & Lab, 2001). It has been argued that diversion can lessen the load on the juvenile courts, reduce juvenile justice system costs, lessen the degree of social control exercised by the juvenile justice system, and diminish the stigma attached to justice involvement (McCord, 1999; Shelden, 1999; Whitehead & Lab, 2001). For many years, labeling theorists assumed that when youth came into contact with the juvenile justice system, increased youth delinquency would result, from both intensive contact with delinquent peers and internalization of stigmatizing labels (Kammer et al., 1997; McCord, 1999; Shelden, 1999; Whitehead & Lab, 2001). From a labeling theory perspective, diversion involves avoiding any sanction or treatment imposed by official or unofficial individuals involved with juvenile justice; more often, diversion means referral to services and implies that youth are removed from the justice system and placed in alternative programs.

Lemert (1981) has also argued that diversion corrects a variety of shortcomings in juvenile justice. These include (a) the denial to juveniles of civil rights or fair treatment, (b) backlogs in the courts, making for inefficiency, (c) labeling and stigmatization of youth, (d) the failure of the juvenile justice system to reduce recidivism, and (e) the failure of communities to assume responsibility for solving youths' problems. More positive justifications for diversion involve reducing the cost of processing delinquency cases and promoting needed funding for youth services (Lemert, 1981).

The practice of juvenile diversion has been frequently criticized for its failure to meet its expressed goals, including the reduction of delinquency and stigmatization, the enhancement of social control over youth, and the increase of rights and due process safeguards (Gensheimer, Mayer, Gottschalk, & Davidson, 1986). Other critical comments have focused on the definitional ambiguity of "diversion," the overrepresentation of minority and poor groups among youth who are diverted, the failure to obtain clear empirical support for effectiveness, and poorly established rationale, funding, and implementation (Dunford, Osgood, & Weichselbaum, 1982; Gensheimer et al., 1986).

History of Diversion Efforts

Diversion was an important aspect of the original justifications for the establishment of a separate juvenile court. This justification was twofold: (a) to intervene with youth (rehabilitation) and (b) to keep them out of the adult criminal court and prison systems (diversion) (Gensheimer et al., 1986; Zimring, 2000). Indeed, Zimring (2000) argued that the latter justification has consistently been regarded as the more important of these two.

The President's Commission on Law Enforcement and Administration of Justice was formed in 1967 to consider crime and delinquency and make recommendations for national policy (Gensheimer et al., 1986). The Commission focused a good deal of attention on juvenile justice, describing the use of formal sanctions and involvement in the juvenile justice system as "a last resort for dealing with delinquency" (Whitehead & Lab, 2001, p. 268). The Commission also suggested a diminished role for the juvenile court and used the term "diversion" to describe a process involving referring youth to community treatment programs.

After the Commission issued its report, the number of diversion programs in the United States increased sharply (Gensheimer et al., 1986). The Juvenile Task Force of the President's Crime Commission may have been particularly influential in promoting this increase. This Task Force advocated the creation of Youth Service Bureaus and focused on increased limitation of the scope of the juvenile court's role. In 1973, youth diversion was one of the recommendations of the National Advisory Commission on Criminal Justice Standards and Goals; shortly thereafter, its implementation was facilitated through federal and state funding from a variety of sources (Lemert, 1981).

The proliferation of juvenile diversion programs continued in the 1970s and early 1980s as a means for dealing with low-risk, nonviolent status offenders and delinquent youth (Dunford et al., 1982). Such diversion programs offered the potential for reducing delinquency and recidivism at a time when the juvenile justice system seemed decreasingly effective in meeting these goals (Kammer et al., 1997; Whitehead & Lab, 2001). In a broader sense, Palmer and Lewis (1980) summarized five goals common to most diversion programs: (a) to avoid labeling, (b) to reduce social control and coercion, (c) to reduce costs, (d) to reduce recidivism, and (e) to provide services.

Types of Diversion

Whitehead and Lab (2001) noted that the President's Commission failed to carefully define its meaning of diversion. Thus, a variety of diversion programs were developed and diversion was defined according to the overall goals of each program. They suggested several different types: (a) *true diversion*, in which law enforcement handle youth informally, (b) *referral, service, and follow-up*, as a system in which youth are referred before adjudication to a non–justice-related treatment source, (c) *minimization of penetration*, in which the youth is limited in his or her contact with the justice system, and (d) *channeling to non-court institutions*, in which the youth is moved into some intervention without being processed by the courts (Whitehead & Lab, 2001).

Frazier and Cochran (1986) noted that "pure" diversion involves no intervention imposed on the juvenile, either officially or unofficially. This is consistent with one premise of labeling theory—that delinquent behavior is often transitory and that official intervention may encourage rather than discourage youth from further offending. They also observed, however, that a second view of diversion—that in which services are provided—is also prevalent. Indeed, diversion efforts have more often been of the second type (Rojek & Erikson, 1982).

Rationale for Diversion

The most commonly cited justifications for diversion include labeling theory, deterrence, net widening, and balanced and restorative justice. We discuss each briefly.

Labeling

The basic perspective provided by labeling theory is that juvenile delinquency may be strengthened, and the risk of subsequent offending increased, by assigning the label of "juvenile delinquent." In this way, the individual is forced to join a deviant group (Matza, 1964) and has reduced legitimate opportunities and possibly a more negative self-image (Erikson, 1962) in the larger social context in which our society places delinquency (Rausch, 1983).

Deterrence

A commonly cited justification for criminal sanctions with adults, deterrence can also be applied to youthful offenders. It involves the assumption that a "risk-benefits" analysis by the potential offender will keep the individual from offending when the risk of apprehension and sanctions outweighs the benefits of the delinquent behavior (Rausch, 1983).

Net Widening

For some time, there has been concern that diverting youthful offenders from the juvenile justice system would expand the boundaries of social control over these youth, offering services to more youth than would normally have occurred without diversion services. This is referred to as "net widening." Binder and Geis observed that "It is widely proclaimed by critics that an inauguration of a diversion program will extend the bite of social control to youngsters who otherwise would have escaped its jaws" (1984, p. 627). Youth without the diversion option might have received only limited sanctions, or in some cases none whatsoever. Consistent with this, Nejelski (1976) warned of the danger of expanding coercive interventions into the lives of children and families without concern for their rights, while Blomberg (1983) noted that diverting youth into interventions (diversion programs) when they would otherwise have been diverted from the juvenile system with no further justice involvement is inconsistent with the original goal of diversion—reducing the number of youth coming into contact with the juvenile justice system.

Balanced and Restorative Justice

One of the questions regarding the juvenile justice ystem has always been what role it should play in the rehabilitation and retribution involving youthful offenders (Office of Juvenile Justice and Delinquency Prevention [OJJDP], 1998). Beginning as a national initiative of the OJJDP in 1993, the *balanced and restorative justice model* (BARJ) attempts to balance offender accountability with the needs of the victim, the offender, and the community. Crime is considered as "an act against the victim and the community" (OJJDP, 1998, p. 1). This approach strives to involve the victim, the offender, and the community in reparation for the offense, geographic, religious, economic protection and due process" (OJJDP, 1998, p. 5).

The BARJ has three components: accountability, competency development, and community safety. Accountability involves having the youthful offender take responsibility for delinquent actions and make efforts to repair any harm. Youth are expected to gain an understanding of the effects of their choices and behavior on their victims, act to repair the harm done, and change behaviors and attitudes to prevent delinquent behavior in the future (OJJDP, 1998).

Competency is "the capacity to do something well that others value" (OJJDP, 1998, p. 19). All adolescents need to develop into competent young adults. To allow youth to rehearse newly developed skills, youthful offenders are given opportunities to work in the community and demonstrate their competency. Key competencies in the BARJ model include the acquisition of educational and vocational skills; achievement of adequate communication, decision-making, and problem-solving skills; and an understanding of good health and citizenship (OJJDP, 1998).

Community safety in this model encompasses both immediate and long-term safety. It "is achieved when community members live in peace, harmony, and mutual respect and when citizens and community groups feel that they personally can prevent and control crime" (OJJDP, 1998, p. 27). Under the auspices of community safety, juvenile justice specialists match the severity of the offense with the level of supervision, respond swiftly to breaches of safety conditions, engage the community in protecting itself, and assist the community with methods for the development of strategies involving youth and adults in collaborative problem solving (OJJDP, 1998).

Key Elements in Diversion

Several scholars have provided suggestions regarding the important elements in diversion programs. Griffin and Torbet (2002) described the following: (a) guidelines that are firm enough to assist decision-makers but sufficiently flexible to allow the use of discretion; (b) a mechanism for allowing victim input; (c) a written diversion agreement specifying the conditions under which the case will be diverted, which is the product of a meeting involving the juvenile, his/her parent(s) or guardian(s), and the intake officer and obtained with the informed consent of the parent/guardian and the assent of the juvenile; and (d) programs that are positive and address victim and community concerns, requiring restitution and letters of apology and promoting other prosocial actions, such as participation in community activities and support and education groups (Griffin & Torbet, 2002).

A somewhat different perspective on the key elements of diversion is provided by Kelley, Schulman, and Lynch (1976). They offered seven fundamentals of successful diversion:

1. Doing something—justice-involved youth should be referred to a community-based service provider or rehabilitating agency rather than threatened, warned, and released
2. Noncoercion—diversion alternatives should be voluntary
3. Support by the availability of effective community services
4. Inclusion of follow-up, research, and evaluation
5. Provision of formal guidelines or criteria for diversion, although allowing the intake officer some discretion
6. Quick response to the youthful offender
7. Allowance of adequate time to make the decision regarding diversion

There are certain key areas that are both potentially amenable to treatment/rehabilitation and function as a risk factor for juvenile offending. When such deficits are identified, they may form the basis for individual or programmatic decisions regarding diversion. We now turn to mental health and substance use problems, which are two such areas.

Mental Health and Substance Use Screening and Assessment

It has been estimated that approximately 20% of children and adolescents in the United States have a mental or emotional disorder (Costello, 1989). This prevalence appears even higher among youth in the juvenile justice system (Kazdin, 2000; Otto, Greenstein, Johnson, & Friedman, 1992). More than 1 million youth come in contact with the juvenile justice system each year, according to one estimate (Cocozza, 1997); of these, as many as 20% have serious mental health problems and 50 to 75% also have a co-occurring substance use disorder (Cocozza & Skowyra, 2000). Other estimates of the prevalence of mental health disorders in youth processed in the juvenile justice system are even higher (e.g., 40%; see Teplin, Abram, McClelland, Dulcan, & Mericle, 2002). Clearly, therefore, it is very important to administer mental health and substance use screening and assessment instruments to juveniles in order to determine the extent to which they need appropriate services.

Screening is a brief process designed to identify youth who are at increased risk of having disorders that warrant immediate attention, intervention, or more comprehensive review (Grisso & Barnum, 2000). It is the first in a sequence of intervention strategies, conducted to identify youth who may require additional attention, monitoring, immediate treatment, facility programming, or more comprehensive assessments (Grisso & Barnum, 2000). Screening may occur at a number of points along the juvenile justice processing continuum and should include the use of a standardized screening instrument. One such screening instrument is the MAYSI-2 (Massachusetts Youth Screening Instrument-2), which has been used and researched on juvenile justice youth (Grisso, Barnum, Fletcher, Cauffman, & Peuschold, 2001). The MAYSI-2 is designed "to assist non-clinical personnel in collecting information quickly, efficiently, and cheaply, for use in making decisions about emergency intervention or professional consultation" (Grisso, 1999, p. 148).

Screening may trigger further assessment if potential problems are indicated. This may include mental health and substance use assessment in particular that is more comprehensive and individualized, examining psychosocial needs and other problems as identified during the initial screen. This includes the type and extent of mental health and substance abuse disorders and deficits associated with the disorders, as well as recommendations for treatment services intervention. There is a variety of standardized tools and procedures that are appropriate for such assessment with juveniles (Hoge, 1999). These include instruments that have been developed to assess psychiatric disorders, symptoms and problem behaviors, family and community characteristics, and youth and family strengths (Grisso, 1999). Such instruments provide alternatives to the informal and unstructured procedures frequently employed in these systems; adopting them for specific assessment needs should promote more effective, better informed decision making for youth (Hoge, 1999).

Risk Assessment

One of the more compelling needs at present in the juvenile system involves "focusing the resources of the juvenile justice system . . . to effectively address crime committed by low-risk juvenile offenders who are best served by remaining in the community" (Matthews & Larkin, 1999, p. vii). In many instances, juvenile justice activity and attention is focused on the more serious offender. However, only a minority of delinquent youth consists of serious, violent, or chronic offenders. The process of risk assessment is valuable in distinguishing lower risk from higher risk juveniles, using risk factors (those causally related to criminal activity) that are scored to "determine the likelihood of recidivism for that individual based on a group of persons with similar characteristics" (Ashford & LeCroy, 1988, p. 141). Risk assessment can be useful in linking risk of reoffending to needed services and interventions "because it allows an agency to allocate resources so that the low-risk cases receive the least supervision and the high-risk cases receive the most supervision" (Ashford & LeCroy, 1988, p. 141).

Researchers (Heilbrun et al., 2000; Hoge & Andrews, 1996) have stressed the need for specialized risk assessment tools in determining the risk levels for youth at various stages in juvenile justice processing. These instruments guide decision making with the goal of deterring youth from committing future crimes (Hoge & Andrews, 1996). Risk/needs tools such as the Youth Level of Service/Case Management Inventory (YLS/CMI) are useful in "all phases of the juvenile justice and corrections process, including decisions about . . . pretrial diversion" and are "particularly relevant to case planning in community and institutional settings" (Hoge, 2001, p. 25). One of the key issues for diversion programs involves matching the client with a program fitting his/her needs. This can be facilitated by the formal assessment of risk, need, and responsivity (Andrews & Bonta, 1998).

Informal Intake

One important innovation in the juvenile justice system has been the development of informal intake, one goal of which is to screen and divert individuals to available community resources (Kelley, Schulman, & Lynch, 1976). This process is particularly useful in managing the number of cases for adjudication and serving as a conduit for diversion services. It can also function as a (potentially) less harmful approach to the alternative of standard, formal sanctions in identifying and diverting low risk juveniles (Kelley et al., 1976).

Community-Based Interventions

In a meta-analysis of 80 programs (Andrews et al., 1990), appropriate services were defined as those that "target high-risk individuals; address criminogenic needs such as substance abuse or anger management; and use styles and modes of treatment (e.g., cognitive and behavioral) that are matched with client needs and learning styles" (Greenwood, 1994, p. 64). In another study of 400 programs

(Lipsey, 1991), it was found "that positive effects were larger in community rather than institutional settings" (Greenwood, 1994, p. 65).

Matthews and Larkin (1999) identified 12 community-based programs for lower risk juvenile offenders. They reported that most intervention programs contained some or all of the following:

- Emphasis on reintegration and reentry services
- Enriched educational and vocational programming
- A variety of forms of individual, group, and family counseling matched to the needs of youth
- Opportunities for success and development of a positive self-image
- Youth bonding to program-social adults and institutions
- Program components adapted to the needs of individual youth
- Simultaneous, systemic focus on all aspects of youths' lives

Relevant Research on Participants and Outcomes

According to the OJJDP Juvenile Court Statistics series, U.S. juvenile courts handled 1,757,400 delinquency cases in 1998 (Stahl, 2001). Twenty-four percent (429,300) of the cases were processed informally, with youth voluntarily agreeing to a disposition such as probation (Butts, Buck, & Coggeshall, 2002). Frazier and Cochran (1986) considered whether youth would be as involved in intervention when diverted as through standard justice processing. They reported that diverted youth were in the system longer, whether the outcome was time in the justice system, time involved in prosecution and subsequent processing, or time in the intake stage. They concluded that youth diverted to this project experienced as much official intervention in their lives as did nondiverted youth, if not more.

Programs

Kelley et al. (1976) conducted an evaluation of a decentralized intake diversion approach in Wayne County (Detroit), Michigan, to assess the impact of this type of diversion on subsequent behavior. The intake officers followed the fundamentals of diversion described earlier in this chapter. A control group was obtained from youth outside of the geographical area of the target group but who otherwise could have been selected for the program. The following data were gathered from the treatment and control groups: (a) official court contacts (number and type of complaints filed with the juvenile court), (b) official petitions (number of complaints headed for adjudication), (c) official delinquents (number of youth having violated the Michigan Juvenile Code), (d) probation and placement dispositions (number of youth on probation or in a correctional facility), and (e) type and seriousness of offense. The results appeared to support the notion that using certain criteria could result in a successful diversion program. The treatment group (those youth within the target area) had significantly fewer official court contacts, fewer officially adjudicated delinquents, more case dismissed dispositions, and fewer institutional commitments. Also, treatment group youth who either refused or dropped out of service had significantly more official court contacts than the treatment group youth successfully completing at least 90 days of service (Kelley et al., 1976).

Quay and Love (1977) studied the Juvenile Services Program in Pinellas County, Florida. The program handled 12- to 16-year-old youth referred from informal sources such as community agencies and school, children in need of supervision (CINS), and other youth adjudicated as delinquent. Services were provided in the areas of individual and group counseling, educational assistance, and vocational training and counseling. A control group, similar in composition, was formed from a random selection of all youth eligible for the program. The investigators considered rates and types of rearrest, both during and following the program, for the experimental and control groups. The Juvenile Services Program reduced the rearrest rate of program participants after successful termination from the program significantly, relative to the control group (32% participants vs. 45% control group). Furthermore, youth informally referred to the program had fewer rearrests (25%) than informally referred youth in the control group (64%). However, CINS youth and youth adjudicated delinquent had a rearrest rates similar to those of the control groups (Quay & Love, 1977).

Bohnstedt (1978) reported an evaluation of 11 California diversion projects, obtaining data on the number of youth diverted, the amount of money saved, and the extent to which the program reduced recidivism. A total of 51% of these justice-involved youth were diverted from the system. Savings as a result of the lack of further processing were substantial, although the total cost of the diversion projects was slightly more than the savings (Bohnstedt, 1978). Recidivism was defined by the project managers as rearrest within 6 months of referral to the diversion project. For three counties (projects), the reduction in recidivism was statistically significant compared to the comparison group. Of these counties, one provided service brokerage that included counseling and school-related services, another provided counseling and individual contact, and the third used Conjoint Family Therapy, developed by Virginia Satir, in a juvenile hall setting (Bohnstedt, 1978).

The Youth Services Program was developed as a skills-training program for youth as a part of the Dallas Police Department's Youth Section (Collingwood & Genthner, 1980). Police officers and civilians staffed the 6-month program, which served first time offending youth committing moderate to severe offenses. Youth not on probation but with prior arrests for less serious offenses could also be allowed into the program. The program team had received training in interpersonal and problem-solving skills to enhance interaction with youth. Youth received primarily skills training. These training efforts included interpersonal skills such as listening, attending, and responding, with an emphasis on using these skills with parents and teachers. Studying and learning skills and physical fitness skills were also taught, and there was a particular focus on decision making. Youth eligible for the program but who preferred other services served as the control group, raising the possibility of sampling bias. The authors reported that the Youth Services Program had significantly fewer recidivist youth than did the comparison group (24% vs. 43%, respectively). They also reported that reoffending among program youth was less serious than that among youth in the control group (Collingwood & Genthner, 1980).

Palmer and Lewis (1980) surveyed the 74 Law Enforcement Alliance of America (LEAA)-funded diversion programs in California in 1974, with 15 representative programs chosen for follow-up study. These projects were operated by various police and community agencies and provided direct assistance to youth. The investigators considered the number of youth being diverted, whether recidivism was reduced, and the cost of the diversion program. Half of these youth were referred with some criminal offense and the others were referred with status offenses; approximately two thirds were first-time offenders. Palmer and Lewis reported that of all justice system and non–justice-system referrals combined, a total of 51% had been diverted from initial or further processing within the justice system. However, they also indicated that 49% of combined referrals would not have been processed within the traditional justice system, so had the diversion projects not existed, these youth would not have received services or been placed under diversionlike controls. A total of 25% of the diverted youth and 31% of the comparison group had been arrested at 6-month follow-up across all 11 projects, a statistically significant difference. However, in 8 of the 11 projects, there were no significant differences in the recidivism rates between diverted clients and comparisons. In the 3 more successful projects, by contrast, the differences between groups in these recidivism rates ranged from 33 to 56%. The average cost per case in these 3 projects was nearly twice as large in the 3 "successful" projects as it was in the 8 "unsuccessful" ones. In addition, the successful projects had more contacts with youth than the unsuccessful projects and worked with youth who had the largest number of prior arrests (Palmer & Lewis, 1980).

Osgood (1983) studied three U.S. diversion programs (one in the Midwest, the second in the upper South, and the third in the lower South) to consider the relationship between offense history and program effectiveness. The midwestern site consisted of two programs: one was operated by the city police department and offered short-term crisis intervention, and the second was administered by the city and provided longer term case management. The upper South site involved a private, nonprofit organization housing the diversion project. The project received youth from juvenile court intake and served as a brokering agency. Youth were interviewed to determine service placements; the diversion project staff monitored services offered by various community agencies. Youth received services such as family and individual counseling, educational and vocational services, and recreational services. The lower South site was also operated by a private nonprofit agency, and it brokered services as well. Each client was contracted for a specific amount and type of service, particularly recreational, and depending only on the service agency chosen. Analyses indicated that there were no significant interactions between prior arrests and treatment condition. There was also evidence that these diversion programs were less oriented to social control and coercion, and more oriented to serving clients' needs, than were justice agencies. The author suggested that these benefits could be obtained only if diversion programs were used as an alternative to formal dispositions in the justice system (Osgood, 1983).

The Connecticut Deinstitutionalization of Status Offenders project (Rausch, 1983) was designed to compare court- and community-based interventions, each under minimum or maximum intervention conditions. No differences were found in the recidivism rates between status offenders in court-based versus community-based programs.

The Adams County Juvenile Diversion Project in Colorado was designed to reduce court caseloads, lower recidivism rates, avoid widening the net of social control, and lend itself to rigorous evaluation (Pogrebin, Poole, & Regoli, 1984). Using treatment and control groups, the project targeted first- and second-time nonviolent offenders. Youth in the control group received a warning and release, regardless of offense. Youth in the treatment group were asked if they would like to participate and were interviewed extensively on school and other background information for the development of a services plan. The program lasted 6 months, during which the youth attended counseling and other services determined by the Multidisciplinary Diversion Team. The investigators reported that court filings did decrease over time, although it was not clear whether this could be attributed to the Juvenile Diversion Project. The recidivism rate for diverted clients was lower than that of the control group, although it increased following termination of services. The main variables used in this study were services participation and recidivism rates. Since there was no assessment of potentially mediating variables (e.g., relevant skills), the authors could not draw any conclusion regarding why this diversion program reduced recidivism (Pogrebin et al., 1984).

Regoli, Wilderman, and Pogrebin (1985) evaluated the effectiveness of six state-funded, community-based, voluntary juvenile diversion programs in the Denver, Colorado, area using recidivism rate as their outcome measure. Four of the diversion programs (North Denver Youth Services, Inc., Northeast Denver Youth Services System, Southeast Denver Youth Service Bureau, and Southwest Denver Youth Service Bureau) brokered services as well as provided direct services to youth referred by police, juvenile court, schools, parents, and others. The fifth program, Police-to-Partners, was a direct service mentoring agency for youth referred by the police or the four programs mentioned above. The sixth program was Project New Pride, a program for postadjudication, lower SES, inner-city delinquents. The investigators first obtained recidivism rates for the youth in each of these programs and compared them with the rates of a matched sample of nondiverted youth involved with the Denver juvenile justice system. They also obtained recidivism rates for youth in each of these programs. Across four of the programs, recidivism was reduced by a total of 26%. Police-to-Partners and the Southwest Denver Youth Services Bureau failed to reduce recidivism significantly, but did reduce recidivism for adolescent girls. The investigators concluded that there was a trend toward reduced recidivism based on diversion services, but could not draw a clear conclusion about the more specific mechanism(s) that lowered such rates.

One particular program that has been evaluated is the Memphis-Metro

Youth Diversion Project. This program, which serves Memphis and Shelby County, Tennessee, was initially funded as a research and demonstration project through OJJDP (Whitaker, Severy, & Morton, 1984). Program goals included reduction in the number of youth processed by the justice system, reallocation of existing community resources to provide more cost-effective services, reduction in juvenile recidivism, and concentration of limited resources on those youth at highest risk for reoffending. Youth were randomized into one of three groups: (a) diversion with services, in which the youth and family were informed of the project; if participation was desired, the youth would be diverted to some community service; (b) diversion without services, in which the youth and family were informed of the project but told that further action would not take place as they had the ability to resolve their problems; and (c) penetration, in which youth went through the justice system and traditional processing (Whitaker et al., 1984). Success for this project was defined as the effective collaboration of the participating service providers, such as recreation, individual and family counseling, substance abuse counseling, and school interventions. Youth were diverted to targeted agencies and evaluation processes were developed for service delivery record-keeping. Both of these strategies reportedly improved case management and accountability (Whitaker et al., 1984). Recidivism rates in the three groups were not significantly different at either 6- or 12-month follow-up.

When recidivism rates were considered as a function of services provided, it was apparent that recidivism occurred more often in youth needing family counseling and individual counseling, while smaller recidivism rates were seen in the group needing other types of services (Whitaker & Severy, 1984). Also, the extent of service delivered was significantly associated with recidivism at 12 months. It was beneficial to receive between 60 and 100% of the projected service plan, but less beneficial when one received less or more than what was originally identified as necessary. These findings suggested that the types of youth needs, the type of agency in which the youth was placed, and the percentage of proposed service that was actually delivered were each related to recidivism patterns. Youth needing social adjustment or educational assistance were less likely to recidivate than those needing family or individual counseling. Further, youth service agencies responded more quickly, provided more services, followed through with a greater percentage of the proposed service cycle, and in general had more success than did the mental health centers. Additionally, youth who received approximately 80 to 100% of projected services apparently derived the greatest benefit and were least likely to recidivate (Whitaker & Severy, 1984).

Another study using behavioral contracting and advocacy diversion strategies yielded similar results (Davidson, Redner, Blakely, Mitchell, & Emshoff, 1987). Davidson et al. (1987) developed a set of five conditions within which to divert youth referred from the local juvenile court. The conditions included (a) behavioral contracting and child advocacy to provide interventions for the multitude of problem areas within the youth's life, (b) behavioral contracting with youth and family members only, (c) supervision plus treatment, (d) relationship building with student volunteers, a placebo condition in which student volunteers were not trained, and (e) a control condition in which youth were returned to the court for processing. All conditions occurred in the youth's "natural environment" (p. 70). Analysis indicated that the behavioral contracting and child advocacy conditions and the relationship-building condition (with a volunteer) were statistically significant in their reduction of recidivism relative to the control (Davidson et al., 1987). It should be noted that these conditions used highly supervised staff members, so the generalizability of these findings may be limited accordingly. However, the three treatment conditions did focus on "positive rather than pathological processes or punishment" (Davidson et al., 1987, p. 74), approaches prognostic of potential success with this group of youth.

Sturges (2001) studied the 19 Youth Commissions in Westmoreland County, Pennsylvania, covering 59 municipalities. The Commissions were composed of volunteers from the community and endorsed the philosophy of Balanced and Restorative Justice. Youth between the ages of 10 and 17 who were first-time, nonviolent offenders were handled by the Commissions. The youth had to accept responsibility for his or her actions and agree to the conditions set forth by the Commission. No comparison group was used. Data analysis consisted of frequency distributions and cross tabulations that described participating youth and their progress in the program. The modal length of supervision was 6 months, with 3 months being the second most frequent duration of supervision. Youth were accountable for their actions to the victims, as well as to the victims' families and the community. Curfews and community service work were employed; skills were developed through essay writing, counseling, and school activities to encourage better grades. Program completion rates were found to be 91%. Different completion rates were seen based upon guardianship: youth with the father present in the home completed the program more often than those who lived with single-parent mothers. Youth living with guardians other than natural parents had the lowest completion rates. Youth with longer supervision times had lower completion rates than youth with shorter supervision periods. There were no recidivism rates drawn from this study. The program did lower costs for the juvenile justice system because the 444 youth were supervised by community volunteers (Sturges, 2001).

Discussion

As may be seen, the results of research on the effectiveness of diversion are mixed. The most frequently used outcome has involved recidivism, either from self-report or from official sources. It is not yet possible to say whether diversion is a viable concept upon which policy should be based. Yet some of the data from these studies suggest that there is considerable promise for certain approaches to diversion. Deciding whether youth need a particular court service appears to be a function of available alternatives, which vary over time and across jurisdictions (Whitaker & Severy, 1984). Existing research is limited because of small sample sizes, the tendency toward single-site sampling, the failure in some studies to operationalize variables, and the insensitivity of recidivism as an exclusive outcome measure. Research that has fewer of these limitations and is closer to the jurisdiction in question in terms of sample characteristics and available community resources is most likely to be generalizable for the purposes of policy decisions and program development.

Some, however, have argued that diversion is both inevitable and desirable, serving system goals better than formal judicial processing under some circumstances (Griffin & Torbet, 2002). There are several examples of such circumstances. First, the stigmatization of adjudication can cause needless harm to some youth. Channeling youth into services and corrective action without formal adjudication can prevent such damage. Second, programs often include strategies such as restitution to the community and accountability to the victim, while traditional juvenile adjudication is more likely to leave out these other involved parties.

Third, diversion programs lighten the load on the juvenile court system when fewer youth are formally adjudicated. Diversion may also be significantly faster and less costly than formal adjudication. In addition, court and probation caseloads can be reduced so that resources can be allocated to more serious offenders. Finally, the option of an informal response to youth delinquent behavior is appropriate because the majority of youth referred to juvenile court do not return (Griffin & Torbet, 2002).

There are also ways in which diversion programs can strengthen families and communities, consistent with the BARJ model. Typically diversion requires the consent of the parent(s) or guardian(s), promoting improved familial relationships. Also, using the BARJ framework, diversion programs strive to interrupt the disconnection between community members, youth, and their parent(s)/guardian(s), while holding youth accountable for their offenses (Wood-Westland, 2002).

There is growing awareness of the importance of fair procedures in improving attitudes, increasing outcome satisfaction, and reducing recidivism in working with juvenile offenders, particularly those who are low risk and first offenders (Logalbo & Callahan, 2001). Diversion research has yielded only mixed results, making it difficult to describe diversion as empirically supported. For a variety of reasons, however, diversion retains significant promise as a mechanism for managing youth outside the formal contours of the juvenile justice system.

References

Andrews, D. A., & Bonta, J. (1998). *The psychology of criminal conduct* (2nd ed.). Cincinnati, OH: Anderson.

Andrews, D. A., Zinger, I., Hoge, R. D., Bonta, J., Gendreau, P., & Cullen, F. T. (1990). Does correctional treatment work? A clinically-relevant and psychologically-informed meta-analysis. *Criminology, 28,* 369–404.

Ashford, J. B., & LeCroy, C. W. (1988). Predicting recidivism: An evaluation of the Wisconsin Juvenile Probation and Aftercare Risk Instrument. *Criminal Justice and Behavior, 15,* 141–151.

Binder, A., & Geis, G. (1984). *Ad populum* argumentation in criminology: Juvenile diversion as rhetoric. *Crime and Delinquency, 30,* 624–647.

Blomberg, T. G. (1983). Diversion's disparate results and unresolved questions: An integrative evaluation perspective. *Journal of Crime and Delinquency, 20*(1), 24–38.

Bohnstedt, M. (1978). Answers to three questions about juvenile diversion. *Journal of Research in Crime & Delinquency, 15*(1), 109–114.

Butts, J. A., Buck, J., & Coggeshall, M. B. (2002). *The impact of teen court on young offenders.* The Urban Institute, Washington, DC: U.S. Department of Justice, Office of Juvenile Justice and Delinquency Prevention, National Institute for Juvenile Justice and Delinquency Prevention.

Bynum, J. E., & Thompson, W. E. (1996). *Juvenile delinquency: A sociological approach* (3rd ed.). Needham Heights, MA: Allyn & Bacon.

Cocozza, J. J. (1997). Identifying the needs of juveniles with co-occurring disorders. *Corrections Today, 59*(7), 146–149.

Cocozza, J. J., & Skowyra, K. R. (2000). Youth with mental health disorders: Issues and emerging responses. *Juvenile Justice Journal, 7*(1).

Collingwood, T. R., & Genthner, R. W. (1980). Skills training as treatment for juvenile delinquents. *Professional Psychology, 11*, 591–598.

Costello, E. (1989). Developments in child psychiatry epidemiology. *Journal of the American Academy of Child and Adolescent Psychiatry, 28*, 836–841.

Davidson, W. S., Redner, R., Blakely, C. H., Mitchell, C., & Emshoff, J. G. (1987). Diversion of juvenile offenders: An experimental comparison. *Journal of Consulting and Clinical Psychology, 55*, 68–75.

Dunford, F. W., Osgood, D. W., & Weichselbaum, H. F. (1982). *National evaluation of diversion projects: Executive summary.* Washington, DC: U.S. Department of Justice, Office of Juvenile Justice and Delinquency Prevention, National Institute for Juvenile Justice and Delinquency Prevention.

Erikson, K. (1962). Notes on the sociology of deviance. *Social Problems, 9*, 307–314.

Frazier, C. E., & Cochran, J. K. (1986). Official intervention, diversion from the juvenile justice system, and dynamics of human services work: Effects of a reform goal based on labeling theory. *Crime and Delinquency, 32*, 157–176.

Gensheimer, L. K., Mayer, J. P., Gottschalk, R., & Davidson, W. S. II. (1986). Diverting youth from the juvenile justice system: A meta-analysis of intervention efficacy. In S. J. Apter & A. P. Goldstein (Eds.), *Youth violence: Programs and prospects.* Pergamon General Psychology Series (Vol. 135, pp. 39–57). Elmsford, NY: Pergamon Press.

Greenwood, P. W. (1994). What works with juvenile offenders: A synthesis of the literature and experience. *Federal Probation, 58*, 63–67.

Griffin, P., & Torbet, P. (Eds.). (2002). *Desktop guide to good juvenile probation practice.* Washington, DC: Office of Juvenile Justice and Delinquency Prevention, National Center for Juvenile Justice.

Grisso, T. (1999). Juvenile offenders and mental illness. *Psychiatry, Psychology and Law, 6*, 143–151.

Grisso, T., & Barnum, R. (2000). *Massachusetts Youth Screening Instrument-2: User's manual and technical report.* Worchester, MA: University of Massachusetts Medical School.

Grisso, T., Barnum, R., Fletcher, K. E., Cauffman, E., & Peuschold, D. (2001). Massachusetts Youth Screening Instrument for the mental health needs of juvenile justice youths. *Journal of the American Academy of Child and Adolescent Psychiatry, 40*(5), 541–548.

Heilbrun, K., Brock, W., Waite, D., Lanier, A., Schmid, A., Witte, G., et al. (2000). Risk factors for juvenile criminal recidivism: The postrelease community adjustment of juvenile offenders. *Criminal Justice and Behavior, 27*, 275–291.

Hoge, R. D. (1999). An expanded role for psychological assessments in the juvenile justice system. *Criminal Justice and Behavior, 26*, 251–266.

Hoge, R. D. (2001). A case management instrument for use in juvenile justice systems. *Juvenile and Family Court Journal, 52*, 25–32.

Hoge, R. D., & Andrews, D. A. (1996). *Assessing the youthful offender: Issues and techniques.* New York: Plenum.

Kammer, J. J., Minor, K. I., & Wells, J. B. (1997). An outcome study of the Diversion Plus Program for juvenile offenders. *Federal Probation, 61*, 51–56.

Kazdin, A. (2000). Adolescent development, mental disorders, and decision making of delinquent youths. In T. Grisso, & R. Schwartz (Eds.), *Youth on trial: A developmental perspective on juvenile justice.* Chicago: University of Chicago Press.

Kelley, T. M., Schulman, J. L., & Lynch, K. (1976). Decentralized intake and diversion: The juvenile court's link to the youth service bureau. *Juvenile Justice, 27*(1), 3–11.

Kurlychek, M., Torbet, P., & Bozynski, M. (1999). Focus on accountability: Best practices for juvenile court and probation. *JAIBG bulletin.* Washington, DC: Office of Juvenile Justice and Delinquency Prevention.

Lemert, E. M. (1981). What hath been wrought. *Journal of Research in Crime and Delinquency, 18*(1), 34–36.

Lipsey, M. W. (1991). Juvenile delinquency treatment: A meta-analytic inquiry into the variability of effects. In T. D. Cook, H. Cooper, D. S. Corday, H. Hartmann, L. V. Hedges, R. J. Light, et al. (Eds.), *Meta-analysis for explanation: A casebook.* New York: Russell Sage Foundation.

Logalbo, A. P., & Callahan, C. M. (2001). An evaluation of teen court as a juvenile crime diversion program. *Juvenile and Family Court Journal, 52*(2), 1–11.

Matthews, S. A., & Larkin, G. (1999). *Guide to community-based alternatives for low-risk juvenile offenders.* Topeka, KS: Koch Crime Institute.

Matza, D. (1964). *Delinquency and drift.* New York: Wiley.

McCord, J. (1999). Interventions: Punishment, diversion, and alternative routes to crime prevention. In A. Hess & I. Weiner (Eds.), *The handbook of forensic psychology* (pp. 559–579). New York: Wiley.

Nejelski, P. (1976). Diversion: The promise and the danger. *Crime and Delinquency, 22*, 393–410.

Office of Juvenile Justice and Delinquency Prevention. (1998). *Guide for implementing the balanced and restorative justice model.* Washington, DC: U.S. Department of Justice, Office of Justice Programs, Office of Juvenile Justice and Delinquency Preventions.

Osgood, D. W. (1983). Offense history and juvenile diversion. *Evaluation Review, 7*, 793–806.

Osgood, D. W., & Weichselbaum, H. F. (1984). Juvenile diversion: When practice matches theory. *Journal of Research in Crime and Delinquency, 21*, 33–56.

Otto, R., Greenstein, J., Johnson, M., & Friedman, R. (1992). Prevalence of mental health disorders among youth in the juvenile justice system. In J. J. Cocozza (Ed.), *Responding to the mental health needs of youth in the juvenile justice system* (pp. 7–48). Seattle, WA: National Coalition for the Mentally Ill in the Criminal Justice System.

Palmer, T. B., & Lewis, R. V. (1980). A differentiated approach to juvenile diversion. *Journal of Research in Crime and Delinquency, 17*, 209–227.

Pogrebin, M. R., Poole, E. D., & Regoli, R. M. (1984). Constructing and implementing a model juvenile diversion program. *Youth and Society, 15,* 305–324.

Quay, H. C., & Love, C. T. (1977). The effect of a juvenile diversion program on rearrests. *Criminal Justice and Behavior, 4,* 377–396.

Rausch, S. (1983). Court processing versus diversion of status offenders: A test of deterrence and labeling theories. *Journal of Research in Crime and Delinquency, 1,* 39–54.

Regoli, R., Wilderman, E., & Pogrebin, M. (1985). Using an alternative evaluation measure for assessing juvenile diversion programs. *Children and Youth, 7,* 21–38.

Rojek, D. G., & Erikson, M. O. (1982). Reforming the juvenile justice system: The diversion of status offenders. *Law and Society Review, 16,* 241–264.

Shelden, R. G. (1999). *Detention diversion advocacy: An evaluation.* Washington, DC: U.S. Department of Justice, Office of Justice Programs, Office of Juvenile Justice and Delinquency Prevention.

Stahl, A. L. (2001). *Delinquency cases in juvenile courts, 1998.* Washington, DC: U.S. Department of Justice, Office of Justice Programs, Office of Juvenile Justice and Delinquency Prevention.

Sturges, J. E. (2001). Westmoreland County Youth Commissions: A diversionary program based on balanced and restorative justice. *Juvenile and Family Court Journal, 52*(3), 1–9.

Teplin, L. A., Abram, K. M., McClelland, G. M., Dulcan, M. K., & Mericle, A. A. (2002). Psychiatric disorders in youth in juvenile detention. *Archives of General Psychiatry, 59,* 1133–1143.

Whitaker, J., Severy, L., & Morton, D. (1984). A comprehensive community-based youth diversion program. *Child Welfare, 63,* 175–181.

Whitaker, J. M., & Severy, L. J. (1984). Service accountability and recidivism for diverted youth: A client- and service-comparison analysis. *Criminal Justice and Behavior, 11,* 47–74.

Whitehead, J. T. & Lab, S. P. (2001). *Juvenile justice: An introduction* (3rd ed.). Cincinnati, OH: Anderson.

Wood-Westland, S. (2002). *Nebraska juvenile pretrial diversion guidelines and resources.* Lincoln, NE: Nebraska Commission on Law Enforcement and Criminal Justice.

Zimring, F. E. (2000). The common thread: Diversion in juvenile justice. *California Law Review, 88,* 2477–2495

9

Randy K. Otto and Alan M. Goldstein

Juveniles' Competence to Confess and Competence to Participate in the Juvenile Justice Process

Forensic clinical psychology can trace its roots to the juvenile courts and the juvenile justice system, as it was in that venue that psychologists first came to regularly assist judges and attorneys in their decision making (Otto & Heilbrun, 2002). Since establishment of the first juvenile court in Chicago over 100 years ago (Grisso, 1998b), psychologists have continued to demonstrate a strong presence in juvenile proceedings and provide assistance to the juvenile justice system as well as the youth involved in it.

A special court and justice system for juveniles was established, in part, in response to recognition that adolescents, while clearly showing greater cognitive, emotional, and behavioral capacities than their younger counterparts, did not possess many of the abilities that were manifested by adults and relevant to legal decision making and criminal responsibility (Otto & Borum, 2004). As a result, the juvenile court was to consider the criminal behavior of minors within its developmental context, with a greater emphasis on rehabilitation and a diminished focus on punishment (Zimring, 2000).

Since the juvenile court was to focus on rehabilitation rather than punishment, constitutional protections were considered to be neither appropriate nor required. Consequently, in juvenile court, the rights to legal representation granted under the Sixth Amendment and due process protection granted under the Fourteenth Amendment were traditionally not available to youth. However, dramatic changes occurred in the juvenile justice landscape in 1966 and 1967, altering forever the denial of constitutional protections for juveniles. In its decisions in *Kent v. United States* (1966) and *In re Gault* (1967) the U.S. Supreme Court questioned whether the rehabilitative ideal of the juvenile court had been supplanted by a focus on punishment and incapacitation and granted juveniles most of the rights guaranteed their adult counterparts in criminal proceedings.

Although juveniles were provided many of the same constitutional protections afforded adults, infrequently was attention paid to or concern expressed about whether a specific juvenile actually met the required legal competence

constructs. Juveniles' cases were heard in a setting in which the goal was to provide treatment and rehabilitation, and worst case scenarios involved commitment of juveniles adjudicated delinquent to secure detention facilities of some
type. However, when the youth reached the age of maturity (defined differently
by each state), he or she was released. Frequently, plea agreements were struck,
requiring some kind of psychological intervention or a finding of "adjudication
contemplating dismissal." Attorneys, advocating for the best interests of their
young clients, were reluctant to challenge this process or delay "justice" by raising questions regarding the client's possible lack of legal competence. Yet, when
still another dramatic change in the juvenile justice system occurred in the
1990s, attorneys and the courts took notice.

In response to the perception of an increase in serious juvenile offending,
the public and politicians called for "less coddling" of juvenile offenders. As described by Grisso and Schwartz (2000), state laws were enacted or modified that
increased the severity of sanctions in the juvenile system and made it easier to
transfer or waive juveniles accused of violent crimes to adult court, where they
faced more punitive and longer sanctions. The clear trend was away from rehabilitation toward a punitive model of juvenile justice (Griffin, Torbet, & Szymanski, 1998; Grisso, 1996; Larson & Goldstein, 2003). With the potential for
harsher dispositions in juvenile court, lawyers representing youth in these proceedings began to focus more on youths' capacities to understand and participate in the legal process, and how they might be affected by developmental factors, from the time of their detention and arrest through their disposition.

The varying abilities of minors, of course, should be considered throughout
their involvement in the legal system. Developmental differences are of importance from the time of their detention and arrest through their disposition via
either the juvenile court and the juvenile justice system or the criminal court
and the criminal justice process (for further discussion of the issues involved in
transfer or waiver of juveniles to criminal court, see Mulvey, ch. 10 in this volume). In this chapter we review the legal and psychological literatures focused
on the capacities of minors to participate in the juvenile justice process from the
time of their arrest and detention through the adjudicatory process. First, however, it is essential to understand how developmental factors affect youth and
their involvement in the juvenile justice system, as such developmentally related
abilities should always be taken into account.

Maturity, Development, and Juveniles' Capacity to Participate in the Justice Process

The physical, cognitive, social, and emotional capacities of children and adolescents are continually evolving. It is this constant and ongoing change, as well as
differences in capacities, that differentiate adolescents from adults (Griffin & Torbet, 2002; Grisso, 1998b, 2003b; McCord, Spatz-Widom, & Crowell, 2001; Otto &
Borum, 2004; Rosado, 2000). Too frequently, judgments about adolescents' matu-
ration are based on their age or physical development and characteristics or the

nature and severity of the delinquent acts they are accused of committing. These factors, however, are not reliable indicators of the capacities that are most relevant to understanding their behavior (Grisso, 1996, 1998b; Otto & Borum, 2004; Steinberg & Schwartz, 2000; Woolard, Reppucci, & Redding, 1996).

Although developmental psychology allows us to predict the development of youth and the emergence of physical, cognitive, and emotional capacities and characteristics as a function of their age, there is considerable variability among youth in the age and rate at which these different capacities develop (Grisso, 1996; Steinberg & Cauffman, 1996, 1999). Thus, children of similar ages may have very different capacities. Also complicating our understanding of adolescents' development and how it may affect their involvement in the juvenile and criminal justice systems is that the modal, age-based estimates of physical, cognitive, and emotional development that are provided are often based on research and study of middle class children from the White majority. These developmental markers and timelines are likely to be less applicable to the many youth in the juvenile justice system who are disproportionately drawn from minority populations and, as a group, show limitations in a variety of important areas, including socioeconomic status, physical development, language skills, cognitive and intellectual capacity, problem-solving abilities, and emotional and behavioral functioning (Graffam Walker, 1999; Grisso, 1996, 1998b, 2003a; Otto & Borum, 2004). Thus, the "average" trajectories and development of many youth in the juvenile justice system may be quite different from that portrayed in textbooks.

All relevant capacities do not develop uniformly within a particular child, so a youth's development in one arena (e.g., physical development) does not necessarily suggest his or her level of functioning in another arena (e.g., emotional maturity). Moreover, for any one child, physical, cognitive, emotional, and social capacities may develop at different rates and independently of one another. Although laypersons may assume that a physically mature adolescent has experienced similar progression and development in other important spheres, research makes clear that such assumptions are unfounded (Cauffman & Steinberg, 2000a). And although it is most obvious and perhaps easiest to assess, physical development is a poor indicator of psychosocial maturity (Steinberg & Schwartz, 2000).

It is also problematic to make judgments about a youth's development and maturity based on the offense that he or she is accused of committing ("If you're old enough to do the crime, you're old enough to do the time"). The use of adult sanctions and dispositions with juveniles who commit more serious offenses is based, in part, on the assumption that adolescents and other children who commit more serious offenses are more mature in their cognitive, social, and emotional functioning, thereby justifying and necessitating adult punishment (see also Redding & Mrozoski, ch. 11 in this volume, and Otto & Borum, 2004). Yet the severity of the index offense is not a good predictor of recidivism, nor is it a reliable sign of a youth's cognitive, emotional, or social functioning and maturity (Cauffman & Steinberg, 2000a).

What factors, then, should psychologists and the courts consider in attempting to understand an adolescent's delinquent or criminal behavior? Cauffman and Steinberg (2000a) stressed the importance of considering a juvenile's psychosocial maturity as it relates to legally relevant decision making and identified four developmental capacities of particular importance in the juvenile justice context: responsibility, time perspective, interpersonal perspective, and temperance (Cauffman & Steinberg, 2000a; Steinberg & Schwartz, 2000). Responsibility encompasses the youth's ability to be self-reliant, independent, and not overly influenced by external pressures or influence when making decisions. Time perspective refers to the youth's ability to appreciate and consider both long- and short-term implications of behaviors and decision making, while interpersonal perspective is concerned with the youth's ability to adopt and understand others' perspectives and differing points of view. Temperance refers to the youth's emotional and behavioral controls, and it focuses on the ability to exercise self-restraint and control impulses. Oberlander, Goldstein, and Ho (2001) offered recommendations for how such considerations may affect the evaluation process itself.

Forensic psychologists and others evaluating youth in the juvenile justice system should assess these capacities since they are most relevant to psychosocial maturity; they should not simply infer these capacities from other characteristics or factors that actually may not be related, such as those described above. Considering and presenting forensic issues in a developmental context will facilitate a more sophisticated, relevant juvenile forensic psychological examination (Grisso, 1998b; Oberlander et al., 2001).

For example, a few years ago the first author evaluated a 16-year-old who had been transferred to adult court and was charged with felony murder, which carried a 25-year minimum sentence. Because the evidence against the defendant was considerable and included a confession, fingerprints, and eyewitness testimony, his attorney recommended that he accept the state's offer of a 17-year sentence in exchange for a guilty plea. In response to the 16-year-old's refusal to consider the plea and demand that they go to trial, the defense attorney requested that this teenager's competence to proceed[1] be assessed. The examinee was of low average intelligence and had no history of significant emotional, behavioral, or substance abuse difficulties. Discussion with the examinee indicated that his decision making regarding the plea agreement and his insistence to go forward with a trial was significantly affected by his consideration of the 17-year sentence in light of his own age, and he specifically stated that the sentence was for a period of time longer than he had lived. Thus, although this 16-year-old "knew" that he faced a minimum of 25 years in prison if he was convicted, and he understood that a conviction was highly likely, his decision making was affected by

---

1. We use the term "competence to proceed" rather than "competence to stand trial" since (a) minors, in many jurisdictions, do not participate in trials in juvenile court, but rather adjudicatory hearings; (b) the issue of competence is important throughout the process, including such decisions as entering a plea; and (c) like their adult counterparts, the majority of minors appearing in juvenile court do not go to trial, but rather enter pleas.

his age and appreciation of time and was likely quite different than the decision making and appreciation of a 32-year-old male who might find himself in the same predicament.

Competence to Confess/Waive *Miranda* Rights

Legal Framework

CONSTITUTIONAL CONTOURS

British common law prohibited those individuals accused of crimes from being forced to testify against themselves at trial. This concept, incorporated into the Fifth Amendment, was gradually broadened to include prohibitions against forcing those under arrest to provide inculpatory statements that could be admitted at trial—in a sense introducing self-incriminating statements through witnesses, such as police interrogators (see Melton, Petrila, Poythress, & Slobogin, 1997, for a more complete discussion of the principle underlying the Fifth Amendment).

In *Brown v. Mississippi* (1936), the U.S. Supreme Court reviewed a case in which a confession was obtained after the suspect was whipped and hung from a tree. The Court held that "The rack and torture chamber may not substitute for the witness stand," ruling that physical brutality would no longer be tolerated as a method by which confessions could legally be obtained.

In 1959, the Supreme Court held in *Spano v. New York* (1959) that psychological pressure may also represent a form of coercion and is therefore illegal. The Court found that the suspect's confession occurred at a time when his "will was overborne by official pressure, fatigue and sympathy falsely aroused." However, the more recent trend in U.S. Supreme Court decisions over the last two decades has allowed interrogators wider latitude in techniques that may be used to obtain confessions. The Court has broadened the range of interrogation situations in which confessions have been deemed voluntary (e.g., *Arizona v. Fulminante*, 1991; *Colorado v. Connelly*, 1986; *Davis v. United States*, 1994; *Moran v. Burbine*, 1986; *Oregon v. Elstad*, 1985; *Rhode Island v. Innis*, 1980).

In *Escobedo v. Illinois* (1964) a defendant's requests to speak with an attorney were denied until a confession was provided. The Court ruled that "the purpose of the interrogation was to 'get him' to confess his guilt despite his constitutional right not to do so" and determined this to be a denial of his Sixth Amendment rights. The Court indicated that "the right to counsel would indeed be hollow if it began at a period when few confessions were obtained." Further, the Court recognized the marked disadvantage of suspects who are questioned by trained interrogators, unaware of their constitutional protections: "No system of criminal justice can, or should, survive if it comes to depend for its continued effectiveness on the citizens' abdication through unawareness of their constitutional rights."

These cases set the stage for the Court's landmark decision *Miranda v. Arizona* (1966). When first questioned by police about his suspected involvement in a sexual assault and kidnapping, Miranda denied involvement. But, after 2 hours

of interrogation, he confessed. Noting that Miranda did not allege any miscon-
duct or coercion on the part of police, the Court emphasized the disadvantage
for suspects questioned in an unfamiliar setting, isolated from friends and family,
and under the stress of criminal accusations. The Court ruled that ". . . the
modern practice of in-custody interrogation is psychological rather than physically oriented" and went on to note that "Privacy results in secrecy and this in
turn results in a gap in our knowledge as to what in fact goes on in the interrogation rooms." Commenting that police interrogators are well trained in techniques to elicit confessions, the Court required, to "level the playing field," that
suspects under arrest be reminded of their constitutional rights. More specifically, they must be informed of their right to remain silent, that any statements
made can be used as evidence in court against them, that they have a right to an
attorney before and during interrogation, and that they have the right to a court-
appointed attorney if indigent. The exact wording of these warnings varies across
legal jurisdictions, however, and the warnings may differ in sentence length,
vocabulary, reading level, and complexity.

Confessions obtained from a defendant who has not been "Mirandized" are
considered inadmissible as evidence. However, exposure to and a simple understanding of the rights is not enough. Waiver of one's rights must be done knowingly, intelligently, and voluntarily. This suggests that juveniles (and adults) must
understand the function of rights in the interrogation situation, including
the possible consequences of waiving or asserting these rights and the intended
functions of the rights (Larson, 2003).

More recently, in Dickerson v. United States (2000), the Supreme Court
reaffirmed Miranda. A challenge to the Miranda holding arose based upon a
1968 law passed by Congress (18 U.S.C. 3501) requiring that confessions must be
obtained without coercion and eliminating the knowingly and intelligently criteria. Miranda warnings would have been unnecessary in federal cases, returning
interrogation procedures to the pre-Miranda era. That is, confessions would
have been considered legally obtained, and therefore admissible in court, if they
were voluntarily provided. The Court held that "Miranda, being a constitutional
decision of this court, may not be in effect overruled by an Act of Congress, and
we decline to overrule Miranda ourselves." Further, the Court emphasized that
"Miranda has become embedded in routine police practice to the point where
the warnings have become part of our national culture."

In considering whether a waiver of the Miranda rights was made knowingly,
intelligently, and voluntarily, judges typically consider "the totality of the circumstances" (also see discussion of Fare v. Michael C., 1979, below). That is, any
and all factors related to the characteristics of the defendant (e.g., age, level of
education, intelligence, personality, influence of alcohol or drugs, prior experience with the police) and the nature of the interrogation process itself (e.g., time
of day, length, number of interrogators, methods of interrogation, physical
conditions, provision of food, drink, and/or medical care) are to be considered in
determining the validity of the waiver (Coyote v. United States, 1967; see also
Frumkin, 2000; Grisso, 1998b, 2003a; Oberlander, 1998; Oberlander & Goldstein, 2001; Oberlander, Goldstein, & Goldstein, 2003).

OPERATIONALIZATION OF THE LEGAL REQUIREMENT

Initially, *Miranda* applied only to adult suspects. Prior to the 1960s, the sole Supreme Court case holding that coerced confessions provided by juveniles could not be admitted as evidence was *Haley v. Ohio* (1948). In this case, police questioned a 15-year-old from midnight until 5:00 a.m., during which time he was not permitted to speak with counsel or any adult. The Court noted that although adults might be capable of resisting or succumbing to police pressure, because of immaturity a juvenile might be an "easy victim of the law." The Court stated that police tactics and the interrogation itself ". . . can overawe and overwhelm a lad in his early teens."

KNOWING, INTELLIGENT, AND VOLUNTARY WAIVER. In *People v. Lara* (1967), the Supreme Court of California attempted to distinguish between "knowing" and "intelligent" waivers. *Knowing* refers to the suspect's understanding of the words used in the warnings (i.e., vocabulary, reading ability if the rights were read by the suspect, language in which the rights were written or read, ability to hear the spoken word or lip-read), whereas the term *intelligent* requires a higher level of comprehension, most typically the ability to consider the advantages and disadvantages of a waiver, to weigh those considerations, and to apply the rights to the interrogation situation. *Voluntary* is typically considered to refer to freedom from police coercion in making the waiver.

TOTALITY OF THE CIRCUMSTANCES. In a case involving a 16-year-old defendant, *Fare v. Michael C.* (1979), a confession was given without a waiver having been obtained. The adolescent had asked to speak with his probation officer rather than an attorney. In considering this case, the Court extended the "totality of circumstances" approach to adolescent cases. Although the Court ruled that adolescent status does not, by itself, automatically invalidate a *Miranda* waiver (*People v. Lara*, 1967; *West v. United States*, 1968; *Fare v. Michael C.*, 1979), it noted that, as a class, adolescents are at greater risk for deficits in intelligence and functioning and these deficits are relevant to their competence to make a valid wavier (Grisso, 1998b; see Feld, 2000, for a comprehensive review of legal cases related to juveniles' waiver of *Miranda* rights).

THE INTERESTED ADULT. A number of cases address the role of the "interested adult" in assisting the adolescent in deciding whether or not to waive *Miranda* rights. The requirement of an interested adult was designed to reduce the likelihood of invalid waivers and untrustworthy confessions among juveniles (Grisso, 1981, 1998b). Many state legislatures and courts provide juveniles with more protections during interrogation than are provided to their adult counterparts (Oberlander et al., 2003). For example, some states require law enforcement officers to provide the juvenile the opportunity to contact a parent, guardian, or other adult before beginning the interrogation process and at least 13 states exclude statements given by juveniles when not provided the opportunity to speak with an interested adult (Larson, 2003).

In *Gallegos v. Colorado* (1962), the U.S. Supreme Court held that an adviser or an adult relative, friend, or attorney might serve to reduce the effects of adolescent suggestibility and immaturity, ensuring the voluntariness of the juvenile's confession, building on the decision in *Haley v. Ohio* (1948). Although the interested adult is not empowered to make legal decisions for the minor, it is expected that he or she will serve as an advisor and reduce the coercive aspect of the interrogation environment (Larson & Goldstein, 2003). Some states have no requirement that an interested adult be contacted before interrogation, noting that such a requirement may restrict the prosecution of the sophisticated or repeat youthful offender (Grisso, 1981).

Most states that employ an interested adult rule have established a threshold age for requiring the adult's presence, typically set between 14 and 16 years of age (Oberlander et al., 2003). For adolescents under the age of 13, courts are more likely to find an insufficient level *Miranda* comprehension generally (Oberlander & Goldstein, 2001). Older adolescents are seen as relatively mature and consequently having little or no need for consultation with an adult (Oberlander et al., 2003). Age limits cited by courts, are not, per se, a reason to invalidate a *Miranda* waiver. For example, in *Commonwealth v. King* (1984), a waiver by a young adolescent was considered valid because, despite his chronological age and lack of parental consultation, the juvenile was "capable and mature . . ." and competent to make a knowing, intelligent, and voluntary waiver.

Courts have generally been reluctant to invalidate waivers based upon the quality or type of information provided by the adult (Oberlander et al., 2003). In *Commonwealth v. Philip S.* (1993), the Supreme Court of Massachusetts ruled that a parent who fails to advise the child to remain silent, who advises the juvenile to tell the truth, or who fails to obtain immediate legal assistance is *not* a "disinterested adult."

EXPERIENCE WITH THE JUVENILE JUSTICE SYSTEM.   Prior experience with the juvenile justice system is considered by many courts as relevant to *Miranda* comprehension (Oberlander & Goldstein, 2001, see, e.g., *In re Morgan*, 1975, and *State v. Prater*, 1970). As reviewed in more detail, however, research conducted by Grisso (1981) indicated there is no simple relationship between youths' prior experience with the juvenile justice system and their comprehension of *Miranda* rights.

FALSE CONFESSIONS BY JUVENILES.   Juveniles in particular may be at risk for making false confessions (Goldstein et al., 2001). In *Miranda v. Arizona* (1966), the U.S. Supreme Court expressed concern that police practices in obtaining confessions might not only violate constitutional rights, but also increase the likelihood of obtaining untruthful confessions from young, susceptible suspects. Similarly, in *Crane v. Kentucky* (1986), the Supreme Court distinguished between legal issues addressed at a hearing related to the validity of a *Miranda* waiver and expert testimony at trial regarding the truthfulness of a confession. The Court held that defendants have a constitutional right to introduce evidence at trial related to the trustworthiness of their confession. This decision indicated that "such evidence might assist the trier of fact in deciding how much weight to give a confession in its deliberations" (Oberlander et al., 2003, p. 349).

As noted above, judges ruling on the validity of a juvenile's *Miranda* waiver consider the totality of circumstances. In order to properly address factors falling under the totality of circumstances umbrella, judges must be made aware of relevant empirical research in order to promote balance and fairness when considering these factors.

Research Relevant to Miranda Comprehension of Juveniles

Research on juveniles' comprehension of the *Miranda* warnings has focused primarily on those factors cited in case law as relevant to the totality of the circumstance. That is, researchers have studied such variables as juveniles' age, intelligence, level of education, socioeconomic status, experience with the juvenile justice system, and the presence of an interested adult as they relate to the knowing and intelligent criteria necessary to establish a valid waiver of *Miranda* rights (Oberlander et al., 2003). Because of the inherent problems in defining, establishing, and corroborating that physical or psychological coercion was a factor in obtaining a confession, considerably less research has been conducted that focuses on variables related to the voluntariness requirement. Only recently has a self-report instrument been developed relating voluntariness to a number of juvenile variables and its relationship to the likelihood of juveniles' providing false confessions (Goldstein et al., 2001).

AGE AND JUVENILES' *MIRANDA* COMPREHENSION

Grisso's (1981) research examining juveniles' comprehension of *Miranda* rights serves as the basis for much of the research that has followed over the last 30 years. In a series of studies, Grisso examined the competence-related abilities of four groups of subjects: adults with a history of contact with the criminal justice system, adults with no history of contact with the criminal justice system, adolescents with a history of contact with the juvenile justice system, and adolescents with no history of contact with the juvenile justice system.

Grisso (1981) reported that although 42% of adults refused to talk in interrogation settings, only 9% of juveniles exercised their right to silence. According to Grisso, "Refusal to talk was virtually non-existent below age 15, and occurred in about 12–14% of interrogations involving 15- and 16-year-olds . . . " (1981, p. 37). Grisso found that youth, ages 12 and younger, lacked meaningful comprehension of their rights. By age 13, age, by itself, was limited as a predictor of *Miranda* comprehension. Above 13 years of age, "age was a better predictor of understanding when it was combined with level of intelligence" (Oberlander et al., 2003, p. 342). For 16-year-olds, Grisso found that despite better understanding, a high degree of variability remained. He reported that comprehension was sufficient for approximately 75% of those juveniles aged 16 to 19. As assessed by one instrument (Comprehension of Miranda Rights), the scores of 16-year-olds were not significantly different from those obtained by 17- to 22-year-olds. However, their scores were significantly lower than those obtained by subjects 23 years of age and older. When comparing adults' with juveniles' understanding, Grisso (1981) reported that "most of the differences . . . occurred on Warning II (use of incriminating information in court) and Warning III (right to counsel before and during interrogation)" (p. 100).

DEVELOPMENTAL COGNITIVE MATURITY AND JUVENILES' *MIRANDA* COMPREHENSION

Recently, the professional literature has identified *cognitive developmental maturity* as a factor that affects the capacity of juveniles to meaningfully participate in the juvenile justice process (Barnum, 2000; Bonnie & Grisso, 2000; Grisso, 1997, 1998b, 2000, 2003; Grisso & Schwartz, 2000; Scott, 2000; Scott, Reppucci, & Woolard, 1995). Although much of what has been written addresses the impact of developmental maturity on the trial competence and decision making of youth, it is the position of the authors of this chapter that developmental maturity may be involved in the decision making of juveniles to exercise or waive their *Miranda* rights as well. That is, some youth, because of cognitive developmental immaturity, may be too quick to trust interrogators, suspend judgment in the face of reality, underestimate the seriousness of the charges, and minimize the impact of inculpatory statements on future plea negotiation and trial strategy. The functional ability required to make an informed decision as to whether to waive *Miranda* rights may not yet be fully developed because of cognitive immaturity. While no specific research has been published on this topic, cognitive developmental maternity may explain, in part, Grisso's findings that age, by itself, is a poor predictor of *Miranda* comprehension, accounting for some of the variability he reports.

INTELLIGENCE AND JUVENILES' *MIRANDA* COMPREHENSION

Grisso (1981) found that almost all juveniles who obtained IQ scores below 75 demonstrated a lack of comprehension of their rights. Although Grisso acknowledged that courts rightfully considered juveniles' intellectual abilities when considering the validity of a *Miranda* waiver, his results suggested that courts may overestimate the comprehension abilities of juveniles with IQs between 75 and 80. Grisso noted that only between 40 and 50% of 14- to 16-year-olds who obtained IQ scores between 80 and 100 demonstrated adequate understanding. Osman and colleagues (2002) reported that the *Miranda* comprehension of adolescent offenders participating in special education programs was significantly lower than that of those not qualifying for special education.

EXPERIENCE WITH THE JUVENILE JUSTICE SYSTEM AND
JUVENILES' *MIRANDA* COMPREHENSION

As noted earlier, courts have often assumed that greater understanding of one's rights results from more extensive contact with the juvenile justice system (*In re Morgan*, 1975; *State v. Prater*, 1970). With such youth, judges sometimes believe that a thorough review of issues related to waivers is of little importance (Oberlander et al., 2003). However, Grisso's (1981) research suggested that there is no simple relationship between one's experience with the legal system and one's understanding of one's *Miranda* rights. His findings led him to hypothesize that although repetitions of the warnings accompanying repeat arrests may increase *familiarity* with the warnings, familiarity does not equal comprehension.

Citing data indicating that there is sometimes a negative relationship between a juvenile's arrest history and *Miranda* comprehension, Oberlander and Goldstein (2001) suggested that some juveniles, when previously arrested for less serious charges, may simply be admonished by police and sent on their way. In these minor arrests, other evidence may have been sufficient, with no need for obtaining a confession, and the police may have anticipated that a trial would not be necessary and little significance was given to the *Miranda* warnings. However, when arrested on more serious charges, these juveniles may become confused by "Competing and, sometimes, incompatible roles of *state as parent* and *state as adversary* in juvenile proceedings . . . [affecting] reasoning about the need to exercise rights" (Oberlander & Goldstein, 2001, p. 466). As such, some juvenile offenders may inappropriately believe their *Miranda* rights to be irrelevant or inconsequential—a belief that may have been true during prior arrests—and fail to recognize their increased potential legal significance and the protections they afford in their current, more serious cases.

THE INTERESTED ADULT AND JUVENILES' *MIRANDA*
COMPREHENSION

A number of state legislatures have enacted interested adult requirements in cases involving interrogation of juveniles, based on the assumption that the adult will provide assistance to enable the juvenile to make an informed and voluntary decision regarding waiver of *Miranda* rights. However, research indicating that adolescents who are provided with an interested adult are no less likely to waive their *Miranda* rights suggests that the presence of an interested adult does not necessarily fulfill this expectation (Grisso, 1998b). Oberlander et al. (2003) suggested that the adult may be fearful, anxious, or mentally incapacitated at the time of the consultation and therefore unable to provide meaningful advice. Other parents may assume an authoritative or disciplinary role in the presence of law enforcement authorities and direct the minor to waive his or her rights. As such, they do not fulfill the role expectation of serving as legal advocate for the juvenile; that is, they do not safeguard youths' constitutional protections (Grisso, 1998b; Grisso & Ring, 1979; Oberlander et al., 2003).

Parents often believe that they should pressure their arrested child to tell the truth and accept responsibility for their illegal actions, a poor strategy for a legal defense (Grisso, 1981; Grisso & Ring, 1979). In their study of parent–juvenile interactions in arrest settings, 70% of the parents offered no advice to their children, and there was simply silence in a majority of cases (66%). Moreover, when advice was provided, the interested adult favored waiving rights and speaking to the police about the crime without benefit of an attorney three times more often than advising the youth to remain silent.

REVISION OF THE GRISSO *MIRANDA* COMPREHENSION INSTRUMENTS

In recent years, Grisso (1998a) has criticized the *Miranda* comprehension instruments that he developed during the course of his (1981) research. Three major sources of concern have focused on (a) the specific language of the *Miranda* warnings employed by Grisso, which served as his test stimuli; (b) the possibility that the norms obtained by Grisso regarding competence-related abilities of juveniles and adults in the late 1970s are outdated and unrepresentative; and (c) speculation that today's youth are more legally sophisticated and better informed about their rights than was true in the 1970s, when the original data were collected.

Goldstein, Oberlander, and Geier (2002) revised Grisso's assessment instruments to include language more commonly found in *Miranda* warnings administered throughout the United States, and new norms are in the process of being established. The investigators found that the simplified language used in some *Miranda* warnings does not appear to result in improved comprehension of their constitutional rights by juveniles (Goldstein, Condie, Kalbeitzer, Osman, & Geier, 2003). In addition, juveniles in the new normative sample demonstrated an understanding and appreciation of constitutional rights that was similar to that of subjects who formed the basis for Grisso's earlier work. Consistent with Grisso's data from 20 years ago, both age and verbal IQ were independently related to *Miranda* comprehension in this more contemporary sample. The authors concluded that " . . . adolescent offenders' *Miranda* comprehension in the early 21st century is similar to the levels of understanding of delinquent boys in the 1970's" (Goldstein et al., 2003, p. 366).

JUVENILES' SUGGESTIBILITY AND FALSE CONFESSIONS

Confessions are one of the most powerful sources of evidence in determining guilt (Driver, 1968; Kassin & Neumann, 1997). The finding that juveniles are more suggestible than adults (Richardson, Gudjonsson, & Kelly, 1995) raises questions regarding the likelihood that they may be at increased risk of providing false confessions in response to real or imagined police coercion. Feld (2000) indicated that juveniles' "social status relative to adult authority figures such as police also render them more susceptible than adults to the coercive pressures of interrogation" (p. 115). Consequently, questions arise as to the likelihood that youthful offenders might offer false confessions to police in response to the pressures and stress of interrogation.

Oberlander, Goldstein, and Grisso (in preparation) developed a self-report instrument of the likelihood of providing false confessions when various police interrogation techniques were applied to them in hypothetical situations. Using an earlier version of this tool, male juveniles (aged 13 to 18 years) residing in a postadjudication, juvenile justice facility were assessed (Goldstein et al., 2001). Twenty-four percent of the juveniles indicated they would offer false confessions in at least one of the interrogation situations, and 42% reported that they "leaned toward" offering a false confession in at least one of the interrogation conditions. However, when age, verbal IQ, and *Miranda* comprehension were controlled, only age significantly predicted the self-reported likelihood of false confessions, leading the researchers to recommend that forensic evaluators, police officers, and courts be especially aware of the potential for false confessions in juveniles aged 15 and younger.

In their conclusions, the investigators noted that, because participation in a research study is less stressful than that in a true criminal interrogation, the research results may underestimate the likelihood that juveniles may provide false confessions. Reports by others (Gudjonsson, Rutter, & Clare, 1995; Hansdottir, Thorsteinsson, Kristinsdottir, & Ragnarsson, 1990) indicating that suggestibility increases during times of anxiety also raise some concern about the possibility that a juvenile would provide a false confession under the stress of interrogation (also see Oberlander et al., 2003, for a discussion of the topic of false confessions and relevant assessment methodology).

Evaluation of Juveniles' Competence to Confess/Waive Miranda Rights

Analyses of peer-reviewed articles in forensic psychology journals, professional presentations, and chapters published in professionally recognized forensic psychology texts indicate that a standard of care for conducting assessments of *Miranda* waivers can be identified (Frumkin, 2000; Goldstein, 1994, 2003; Grisso, 1981, 1986, 1998b, 2003a; Heilbrun, 2001; Heilbrun, Marczyk, & DeMatteo, 2002; Larson, 2003; Oberlander, 1998; Oberlander & Goldstein, 2001; Oberlander et al., 2003, in preparation; Shapiro, 1991; Wulach, 1981). There is a high degree of consistency across sources of information and authors, suggesting that these evaluations should follow Grisso's (2003a) model for conducting forensic assessments.

Steps in conducting these assessments involve the identification of the relevant legal competency construct (the ability to make a knowing, intelligent, and voluntary waiver of *Miranda* rights). Since these criteria for *Miranda* waiver are legal terms, they must be "operationalized" (Grisso, 1986, 2003a) or translated into concepts that psychologists and other mental health professionals can assess. Multiple sources of information must by accessed, since some information relevant to the competence question is not available via interview with the examinee. Such third party information also is helpful with respect to the assessment of the examinee's response style (Rogers & Bender, 2003; Rogers, Salekin, Sewell, Goldstein, & Leonard, 1998; Rogers, Sewell, & Goldstein, 1994). In addition, the use of multiple sources of data serves to provide information consistent with the totality of circumstance requirement delineated by the courts.

Various steps in the evaluation are outlined in Table 9.1. As may be seen, the first step in the assessment process is to obtain relevant records, including the juvenile's signed *Miranda* waiver form and any description or documentation of the circumstances under which the waiver was obtained. If videotape of the administration of the warnings was made, this and the juvenile's statement should be reviewed as well. Because the language of the warnings differs from jurisdiction to jurisdiction, the evaluator must obtain, if possible, the *exact* wording that was presented to the juvenile to conduct a relevant assessment of comprehension (Frumkin, 2000; Grisso, 1998b; Oberlander et al., 2003). Hearing or deposition transcripts of the arresting officers' testimony frequently contain information regarding the number of times the warnings were administered, where they were provided, and when they were administered (Frumkin, 2000). Other relevant documentation includes school records; scores on measures of intelligence and academic achievement; records documenting the need for special educational services; mental heath and medical records; and records of prior contact with the juvenile justice system, including prior placements and services received.

As in all forensic evaluations, the juvenile should be informed about the nature and purpose of the assessment, how it will be used, and the limits of confidentiality. The process by which notification was made and informed consent or assent was obtained, including language used by the evaluator, the need to clarify and simplify the information presented, and the juvenile's comprehension of what was explained should be carefully documented, as it may prove relevant in testimony. The process of obtaining consent or assent is similar to that employed by interrogators in obtaining a *Miranda* waiver, and as such, questions may arise during testimony related to the ability of the juvenile to provide informed consent.

The juvenile should be interviewed for historical information, with specific attention to those factors that may be relevant to the case (Frumkin, 2000; Grisso, 1981, 1998b; Oberlander et al., 2003). This interview has a number of purposes, including (a) acquiring relevant background information, (b) identifying independent sources of third party information necessary to verify what the juvenile has claimed (Heilbrun, Warren, & Picarello, 2003), (c) assessing the juvenile's present psychological functioning, (d) obtaining the juvenile's version of what transpired before and during the interrogation, and (e) specifically evaluating the juvenile's comprehension of *Miranda* rights at the time of the interrogation and reasons for confessing (Frumkin, 2000; Grisso, 1998b; Oberlander, 1998; Oberlander & Goldstein, 2001; Oberlander et al., 2003).

Psychological assessment instruments are usually selected on the basis of reasonable hypotheses concerning a juvenile's specific reported or suspected impairments (Oberlander et al., 2003). Most *Miranda* waiver assessments include traditional tests of intellectual functioning and educational achievement be-

TABLE 9.1 Outline for Competence to Waive *Miranda* Rights Evaluation

Preevaluation
　Access and review relevant third-party information
　　Juvenile's *Miranda* waiver form and related documentation of the waiver
　　Medical records
　　Academic records
　　Mental health records
　　Juvenile justice records
　　Interviews/depositions of teachers, therapists, "interested adults," arresting and
　　　interrogating police officers (if available)

Evaluation
　Notification
　Interview with parent or guardian regarding relevant history
　Interview with youth
　　Social history
　　Family history
　　Developmental history
　　Medical history
　　Academic history
　　Substance use and mental health history
　　Juvenile justice history
　Assessment of understanding and appreciation of *Miranda* rights
　　Via interview
　　　Spontaneous recollection of the rights that should have been provided
　　　Designated inquiry into meaning of specific warnings
　　　Circumstances before and during interrogation
　　　Juvenile's recollection of what was said by police and how rights were administered
　　　Juvenile's recollection of thoughts and feelings at the time of interrogation
　　　Juvenile's explanation for speaking to the police
　　　Assessment of postconfession knowledge related to warnings
　　Psychological testing
　　　Intelligence testing
　　　Achievement testing
　　　Neuropsychological testing (if indicated)
　　　Personality testing (if indicated)
　　　Grisso's *Miranda* comprehension measures

cause of their direct relationship to vocabulary, reasoning, and comprehension. Case-specific information may suggest the need for tests of neuropsychological deficits or underlying emotional disturbances that may have affected the validity of the *Miranda* waiver.

Grisso's measures of *Miranda* comprehension (1981, 1998a) serve as forensic assessment instruments that provide data directly relevant to the ability of a juvenile to make a knowing, intelligent waiver of his or her rights and to understand the impact of those rights on both the interrogation situation and the juvenile justice system in general. Grisso (1998a) provided guidelines for the administration, scoring, and interpretation of these instruments and presented data on their reliability and internal and external validity. Grisso's measures consist of the following:

- *Comprehension of Miranda Rights* (CMR) assesses general comprehension by presenting each of the four St. Louis County, Missouri, warnings to the juvenile, who is then asked to paraphrase each.
- *Comprehension of Miranda Rights–Recognition* (CMR-R) provides information about whether juveniles can recognize the meaning of each right. It requires the defendant to determine whether each of four statements is the same as or different from each of the four elements of the warning.
- *Comprehension of Miranda Vocabulary* (CMR-V) requires the juvenile to define six words contained in the warnings to assess whether confusion about the rights may have originated with vocabulary difficulties.
- *Function of Rights in Interrogation* (FRI) provides information about whether the juvenile understands the function of the right to silence, the right to counsel, and the adversarial nature of the justice system in the context of an arrest and interrogation. Examinees are presented with a series of four pictures and accompanying vignettes and asked questions involving the application of rights to hypothetical situations.

Lally (2003) surveyed 64 forensic psychologists who were board certified by the American Board of Professional Psychology (ABPP) to determine what psychological tests they considered acceptable to use in a number of psycholegal contexts. He found that in conducting assessments of an individual's ability to make a valid waiver of *Miranda* rights, "the majority of the diplomates rated as acceptable Grisso's Instruments for Assessing Understanding and Appreciation of *Miranda* Rights (Grisso instruments)" (p. 495). Among the traditional and forensic assessment instruments surveyed, only Grisso's measures and the WAIS-III were recommended by the majority of ABPP board-certified forensic psychologists.

New norms for updated revisions of these instruments are being compiled at this time (Oberlander et al., in preparation). Interviewing parents, teachers, therapists, and police officers who conducted the interrogation (if available) may provide additional, relevant information. Often youth do not know important information about their health, medical, and academic histories. Accessing such information through knowledgeable third parties also allows the examiner to assess the youth's response style. Information regarding the nature and conditions of the interrogation can sometimes be provided by these third parties. If the juvenile had an interested adult with whom he or she consulted around the time of the interrogation, an interview with this person may shed additional light on the juvenile's initial comprehension of the warnings and how a decision to waive the rights was reached. Finally, knowledge of the youth's functioning, as observed by others, can provide the expert with useful, appropriate examples of situations in which the juvenile had previously encountered difficulty comprehending instructions, questions, or directions or instances in which the juvenile acquiesced to authority figures.

As noted earlier, an integral part of any forensic assessment is the evaluation of the examinee's response style. The juvenile's recollections of what occurred at the time of interrogation and his or her rendition of understanding of each of the warnings at that time may be distorted. Reasons for inaccurate reporting include, among other things, the intentional effort to deceive with the expectation that the confession will ultimately be excluded from trial. Thus, the examiner should make an explicit attempt to assess the youth's response style in a number of ways, including via corroboration of accounts offered by the examinee, along with use of specific measures that assess response style, when appropriate.

It is important to note that this forensic evaluation involves the youth's comprehension of his or her rights at the time of the interrogation, not at the time of the evaluation. The examiner, therefore, is required to make inferences about the youth's ability at the time of interest, using all available, relevant data. In interpreting the data, "the evaluator considers whether the full range of evaluation data support a connection between impairments in the defendant's functioning and deficits in *Miranda* comprehension" (Oberlander et al., 2003, p. 346). If interview data, performance on intelligence and achievement tests, school records, and other records, and third party interviews are consistent with data relevant to *Miranda* comprehension, a descriptive explanation of the juvenile's poor performance may prove helpful to the court. These sources of information usually help establish reasons for the juvenile's impairments. The deficits in *Miranda* comprehension, as revealed during the interview and as assessed by Grisso's measures, should be described with both clarity and specificity. It is not unusual for a defendant to comprehend some warnings, but not understand others. "Providing data-based information in a scientifically sound but descriptive format enhances the likelihood that the fact finder will find the report data useful, necessary, and relevant to the legal determination about the validity waiver" (Oberlander et al., 2003, p. 346).

Competence to Proceed

Legal Framework

The requirement that a defendant be capable of assisting in his or her defense and participating in the legal process can be traced to at least the 14th century, when courts refused to proceed against defendants considered incompetent as a result of a mental disorder or mental defect (Poythress, Bonnie, Monahan, Otto, & Hoge, 2002; Stafford, 2003). This requirement is considered to serve multiple purposes, including promoting dignity, accuracy, and autonomy (Otto & Borum, 2004; Poythress et al., 2002). Trying those whose impairment prevents them from assisting in their defense or limits their awareness of the nature and purpose of the proceedings challenges conceptions about the fundamental fairness of the legal process (Goldstein & Burd, 1990). Additionally, the defendant's and the legal system's investment in accurate judicial outcomes precludes prosecution of those who are significantly impaired, insofar as a defendant's ability to provide information helpful to his or her defense and challenge the state's allegations may be compromised by an underlying mental disorder. Finally, the law's requirement that it is ultimately the accused who must make decisions about legal strategies and decisions (with the assistance of his or her attorney) requires that the defendant have the capacity to do so.

CONSTITUTIONAL CONTOURS

The Constitution requires that defendants be competent to participate in the criminal justice process. In *Dusky v. United States* (1960) the U.S. Supreme Court ruled that a defendant must have ". . . sufficient present ability to consult with his lawyer with a reasonable degree of rational understanding . . . [and have a] rational as well as factual understanding of the proceedings against him." Although the Court in *Dusky* only identified the constitutional minimum, most states have adopted some variant of the *Dusky* language and approach (Grisso, 2003b).

While some of the Court's language in *Dusky* is vague and ambiguous, authorities have reached a consensus regarding the standard and what it requires (Grisso, 2003b; Poythress et al., 2002; Stafford, 2003). Although the *Dusky* standard does not identify any predicate conditions that must be present and result in any observed deficits in capacity (e.g., mental illness, mental retardation, normal "limitations" associated with youth), essentially all state statutory schemes refer to incapacity resulting from some type of mental impairment (i.e., mental illness, mental retardation, or other cognitive impairment). Some states, in addition, allow adjudication of incompetence based on developmental factors (e.g., Virginia Code Annotated Section 16.1-356, 2003).

References to "sufficient" ability and a "reasonable" degree of understanding in the *Dusky* standard suggest that the defendant's capacities need not be complete and without impairment. The reference to "present" ability indicates that the focus is on the defendant's competence-related abilities as they exist at present and in the immediate future. Use of the term "capacity" suggests that a lack of knowledge about the proceedings or process, or an unwillingness to participate in the proceedings, do not render someone incompetent to proceed. Finally, reference to both a "factual " and "rational" understanding of the process indicates that the defendant must possess more than a simple knowledge of facts and factors relevant to the proceedings. They also must possess an ability to appreciate and consider the proceedings and case facts that is not significantly impaired by mental disorder. In *United States v. Duhon* (2000), a U.S. District Court found that mere rote learning of answers related to questions designed to evaluate trial competence was not sufficient to establish fitness for trial. The court offered that the hospital's determination that the defendant was competent remained in question given the staff's failure to address the defendant's ability to assist in his defense. In this case, the defendant, a mentally retarded man, had been adjudicated incompetent to stand trial, was committed to a forensic hospital, and was enrolled in a Competence Restoration Group. The court opined that the forensic examiner's report describing the defendant as competent to proceed provided no support for the claim that simply repeating factual information until a mentally retarded defendant can repeat it provides little information about the issue of the defendant's competence. The court asked the rhetorical question, "What exactly does Duhon actually understand?" and concluded that, despite rote learning, he still failed to meet the *Dusky* standard necessary to establish trial competence. Goldstein and Burd (1990) drew a distinction between a defendant's merely answering "factual" questions regarding the nature of the charges and the role of various courtroom personnel and the ability of the defendant to more meaningfully and actively assist in his or her own defense.

Authorities also agree that competence is a function of not only the defendant's capacity, but also the case-specific demands (Poythress et al., 2002; Roesch, Zapf, Golding, & Skeem, 1999). Thus, a defendant might be incompetent to proceed on one charge (e.g., an allegation of complicated security fraud) and, at the same time, be competent to proceed with another (e.g., a simple charge of driving with a suspended license).

Although it articulated in *Dusky* the capacities that adult defendants must possess when participating in criminal proceedings, the Supreme Court has never addressed the question of whether juveniles who are participating in delinquency proceedings must be competent and, if so, what specific capacities are required of them. Indeed, with the exception of the past 10 years, the issue of juveniles' capacity to proceed has received little attention from either legal or mental health commentators. As noted above, this may be due, in part, to the fact that the juvenile justice system has historically been less adversarial and punitive than the adult system and more focused on rehabilitation efforts. We also observed earlier, however, that as the juvenile justice system has diminished its emphasis on rehabilitation and become more focused on retribution, the issue of juvenile competence has received more attention (Grisso, 2003a, 2003b; Otto & Borum, 2004).

Thirty-four states and the District of Columbia specifically address the issue of competence in juvenile proceedings, and most of these states have simply adopted *Dusky*-like criteria that are employed in adult proceedings (Grisso, 1998b, 2003a; see Redding & Frost, 2001, for a detailed review of these 26 state statutes). Although some courts have ruled that the capacity required of a respondent in a juvenile proceeding can be no less than the capacity demanded of an adult in a criminal proceeding (e.g., *In the Matter of the Welfare of DDN* [1998]), others have suggested that the *Dusky* standard may be conceptualized differently in juvenile proceedings. For example, in *Ohio v. Settles* (1998), the court, in considering that state's competence standard for minors, ruled that "juveniles are assessed by juvenile rather than adult norms," and in the case *In re Causey* (1978) the court held that even nonimpaired juveniles may not demonstrate the same abilities as adults with respect to rationally understanding the proceedings or working and consulting with their attorneys. At least one court (Oklahoma), however, has determined that juveniles need not be competent to participate in delinquency proceedings, as the juvenile justice process is not considered punitive in nature (*G.J.I. v. State*, 1989). In describing this decision, Redding and Frost (2001) noted the date of the case (1989) and queried whether a similar decision would occur in contemporary times, given the changing landscape of the juvenile court and juvenile justice system.

Given the developmental differences between adults and juveniles that are described above, adoption of competence standards and criteria used with adults, while relatively easy, may prove problematic. For example, many states require that findings of incompetence be due to mental illness or mental retardation, with the result that juveniles whose capacity to participate in the process due to normal developmental or maturational "limitations" cannot be found incompetent to proceed (Redding & Frost, 2001).

OPERATIONALIZATION OF THE LEGAL REQUIREMENT

In an attempt to provide attorneys, judges, and examiners with more direction, some jurisdictions, legal authorities, and mental health commentators have attempted to operationalize and further delineate the general competence standard enunciated in *Dusky* and adopted by many states. Consideration of some of these efforts provides more insight into the competence standard more broadly.

The Competency to Stand Trial Assessment Instrument (CAI; Laboratory of Community Psychiatry, 1973), an instrument which structures clinical assessment of trial competence, was developed by an interdisciplinary group of mental health and legal professionals based on their clinical and courtroom experience and their review of appellate cases and the legal literature. The CAI structures the competence evaluation and directs the examiner to assess the defendant's (a) appraisal of available legal defenses; (b) behavior as it might affect participation in the trial or interactions with others; (c) ability to relate to and interact with his or her attorney; (d) ability to deliberate and consider legal strategies with his or her attorney; (e) understanding of the roles of the main actors in the process, including defense counsel, the prosecutor, the judge, the jury, the defendant, and witnesses; (f) understanding of court procedure; (g) appreciation of the charges; (h) appreciation of the range and nature of possible penalties; (i) appraisal of likely case outcomes; (j) ability to disclose pertinent facts surrounding the offense including his or her behavior at and around the time of interest; (k) capacity to challenge adverse witnesses; (l) capacity to testify relevantly; and (m) motivation to act in his or her own best interests during the proceedings.

Consistent with the above, the Florida legislature, in its attempt to operationalize the competence standard and provide some direction to judges, attorneys, and mental health professionals, requires mental health professionals evaluating adults and juveniles on matters of competence to assess the examinee's (a) appreciation of the charges and allegations; (b) appreciation of the range and nature of possible penalties or dispositions; (c) understanding of the legal process and its adversarial nature; (d) capacity to disclose to his or her attorney facts pertinent to the proceedings; (e) ability to manifest appropriate courtroom behavior; and (f) ability to testify relevantly, as well as any other factors considered by the examiner to be relevant in the case at hand (Florida Statutes

916.12(3), 2000; Florida Rules of Juvenile Procedure 8.095 (d)(1)(B), 2003). Thus, both professional authorities and state legislatures have provided some direction to forensic psychologists called on to evaluate those whose competence to proceed with the legal process is questioned, and guidance has been offered by way of attempts to operationalize the general competence standard delineated in *Dusky*.

DISPOSITION OF JUVENILES ADJUDICATED INCOMPETENT

After a juvenile has been adjudicated incompetent to proceed, the state has the authority to direct the juvenile to undergo those treatments or interventions necessary to "restore" him or her to competence. Most state statutes demonstrate a preference for less restrictive (and the least expensive) treatment in community settings, and the states have been more successful in attaining this goal with their juvenile incompetent populations than with their adult incompetent populations (McGaha, McClaren, Otto, & Petrila, 2001; Redding & Frost, 2001).

In *Jackson v. Indiana* (1972) the Supreme Court made clear that the Constitution requires that the state detain as incompetent only those defendants who show a reasonable likelihood of attaining competence with treatment or other interventions. Thus, juveniles determined to be incompetent and "unrestorable" cannot be detained or committed by the state as incompetent to proceed, although they may be subject to other dispositions (e.g., civil commitment, dependency), provided they meet the requisite and appropriate criteria. Some states provide for dismissal of charges upon a judicial finding of "incompetence" and "unrestorability," while others allow the prosecutor to stay the charges with the expectation that they could be reinstituted at some point in the future if the juvenile were to attain competence.

Research Regarding the Competence-Related Abilities of Juveniles

Just as the issue of juvenile competence was neglected by the legal community until a decade ago, psychologists devoted little attention to the study of juveniles' psycholegal capacities until recently (see Grisso, 1997, 2000, for reviews). Some investigators (e.g., Savitsky & Karras, 1984) assessed age-related differences in knowledge of the legal process, while others (e.g., Cowden & McKee, 1995; McKee & Shea, 1999) have assessed the capacities of minors referred for competence evaluations and compared them to their adult counterparts, and others have investigated differences between adults and juveniles with respect to how they interact and work with their attorneys (Schmidt, Reppucci, & Woolard, 2003).

As might be expected, researchers have documented a relationship between age and psycholegal capacity, with children below the age of 12 showing considerably more limited abilities than those aged 15 and older and children between the ages of 12 and 14 showing transitional abilities (Cooper, 1997; Grisso, 2000). Consistent with what we know about development more generally, researchers have also documented considerable variability among comparably aged children.

Research indicates that elementary school children can provide some information about the legal process (e.g., the role of the judge, the purpose of a trial) and, by the age of 13, most children can offer basic descriptions of the key figures involved in and the purpose of legal proceedings (Grisso, 2000; Peterson-Badali & Abramovitch, 1992; Peterson-Badali, Abramovitch, & Duda, 1997; Warren-Leubecker, Tate, Hinton, & Ozbeck, 1989). Research also suggested a relationship between intelligence and the competency-related abilities of minors, with those who have been adjudicated incompetent to proceed showing greater rates of mental retardation/borderline intellectual functioning diagnoses and placement in special classes than those adjudicated competent to proceed (McKee & Shea, 1999). Mental retardation, in fact, appears to be a more integral factor in the competence-related abilities of minors than of adults. McGaha et al. (2001) reported that as many as two thirds of a sample of over 400 juveniles adjudicated incompetent in Florida courts and ordered to undergo restoration had a diagnosis of mental retardation, whereas fewer than 10% of adults adjudicated incompetent to proceed and ordered to undergo treatment for restoration typically receive a diagnosis of mental retardation.

Perhaps the most comprehensive data regarding the competence-related abilities of juveniles were provided by a research study funded by the MacArthur Research Network on Adolescent Development and Juvenile Justice. Grisso et al. (2003) examined the competence-related abilities of 927 adolescents and 466 young adults using a standardized measure of competence to proceed (the MacArthur Competence Assessment Tool-Criminal Adjudication, or MacCAT-CA; Poythress et al., 1999) and a measure that assesses psychosocial influences on legal decision making (the MacArthur Judgment Evaluation, or MacJEN; Grisso et al., in press). Adolescents, ranging in age from 11 to 17, were sampled from both the community and juvenile justice facilities, and young adults, ranging in age from 18 to 24, were sampled from the community and jails.

On all three subscales of the MacCAT-CA (understanding, reasoning, and appreciation) there was a significant effect for age, with 11- to 13-year-olds performing more poorly than 14- to 15-year-olds, who performed more poorly than 16- to 17-year-olds and young adults. Consistent with previous research, the competence-related abilities of 16- to 17-year-olds, as measured by the MacCAT-CA, were no different than those of the young adults aged 18 to 24. Based on criteria established when using the MacCAT-CA with various samples of adults offenders (Otto et al., 1998; Poythress et al., 1999), approximately one third of the 11- to 13-year-olds, and one fifth of the 14- to 15-year-olds, showed deficits via assessment with the MacCAT-CA that were similar to adult defendants with severe and persistent mental illness who had been adjudicated incompetent to proceed. Juveniles between the ages of 11 and 13 were more than three times as likely as young adults between the ages of 18 and 24 to show evidence of serious competence-related deficits, and those 14 to 15 years of age were twice as likely as young adults to show such serious deficits in psycholegal capacity based on their MacCAT-CA performance. Consistent with previous research, these investigators also found a relationship between IQ and competence-related abilities as assessed by the MacCAT-CA. Also of interest was the finding that MacCAT-CA performance was not related to prior experience in the juvenile or adult justice systems for those subjects who were in detention or jail.

In addition to more limited psycholegal capacities surrounding understanding, reasoning, and appreciation, subjects aged 15 and below also employed different decision-making processes, as assessed by the MacJEN (Grisso et al., in press). Relative to their older counterparts, younger subjects were less likely to identify the risks associated with various choices in the justice process (e.g., agreeing to be interrogated, entering a plea), more likely to comply with requests made by authority figures (e.g., police, attorneys), and less likely to identify and consider the long-term consequences of their behavior and choices in the juvenile justice context. Thus, the impact of development on competence-related abilities is well established, suggesting that those evaluating the competence-related abilities of juveniles consider the potential limitations that may result from immaturity as well as from emotional/behavioral disorders or cognitive limitations.

Evaluation of Juveniles' Competence to Proceed

The challenge facing the mental health professional assessing a juvenile's competence to proceed can be broken down into three tasks. First, the examiner must assess and describe the juvenile's capacity to understand and participate in the legal proceedings. Second, the examiner should identify and describe any mental disorders, impairments, or limitations, broadly defined, that may be responsible for any observed incapacities. Finally, the examiner must identify the causes of any limitations in psycholegal abilities that are observed and identify those that may be remedied and those that may not be remedied with appropriate intervention. For those that may be remedied, the examiner should make specific treatment or rehabilitation recommendations, and in those cases in which the underlying disorder cannot be treated or otherwise rehabilitated, the examiner should make clear to the court the likely enduring nature of the incapacity so alternative dispositions can be considered.

Although a detailed description of the competence evaluation process is not offered (see Grisso, 1998, as well as Otto & Borum, 2004, and Stafford, 2003, for such discussion, and Table 9.2 for a recommended evaluation format; and see Oberlander et al., 2001, for a review of developmental considerations as they affect the competence evaluation process), a few important issues are reviewed. First, as noted above, the test of competence is one of *capacity*, as distinguished from knowledge or willingness. Thus, juveniles who are simply ignorant about their charges, possible penalties, or the legal system and its operation are not incompetent to proceed, provided they have the ability to incorporate and utilize such information in their decision-making process when it is made available. When an examinee professes a lack of knowledge about important information, the examiner should impart such knowledge and later assess the examinee's ability to retain and utilize the information.

Second, an important corollary is that simple rote knowledge does not equate to capacity (*United States v. Duhon*, 2000). Some juveniles with limited

TABLE 9.2 Outline for Competence to Proceed With Evaluation

Preevaluation
    Access and review relevant third-party information
        Medical records
        Academic records
        Mental health records
        Arrest reports and delinquency petition
    Interview with defense attorney

Evaluation
    Notification
    Interview with parent or guardian regarding relevant history
    Interview with youth
        Social history
        Family history
        Developmental history
        Medical history
        Academic history
        Substance use and mental health history
        Juvenile justice history
    Competence inquiry
        Understanding of the legal process and its adversarial nature
        Understanding and appreciation of charges and allegations
        Understanding and appreciation of possible sanctions dispositions
        Capacity to work with attorney and provide relevant information
        Ability to testify relevantly
        Ability to manifest appropriate courtroom behavior
    Assessment of mental status/current clinical functioning
    Psychological testing (if indicated)
        Intelligence testing
        Achievement testing
        Neuropsychological testing
        Personality testing

intellectual abilities may answer questions about the legal system correctly but may still show no true or meaningful understanding or appreciation of the topic at hand. Similarly, juveniles who exhibit disordered thought content (i.e., delusional thinking) may be able to offer organized factual accounts and depictions, but their appreciation of the same factors may be limited by specific delusions (Goldstein & Burd, 1990).

Third, juveniles who are capable of working with their attorneys or otherwise participating in the legal process, but choose not to do so for reasons other than those attributed to mental disorder, mental retardation, other impairment, or developmental limitations, have the capacity to participate. The examiner must focus on describing *capacity* and identifying factors that may limit it, rather than simply referencing the examinee's willingness to participate in the process.

Finally, it is important that the examiner considers juveniles' capacities in context. Examiners should not only assess the degree to which a juvenile may be affected by mental disorder or cognitive impairment, but also consider developmental factors such as responsibility, time perspective, interpersonal perspective, and temperance (Cauffman & Steinberg, 2000b) and how these factors affect understanding of, and decision making in, the justice process.

A number of forensic assessment instruments have been developed to assess adult defendants' competence to participate in the criminal process, but their utility with juvenile populations remains to be determined (see Grisso, 2003a, Melton et al., 1997, Roesch et al., 1999, and Stafford, 2003, for reviews of these instruments). None of the instruments that employ norms or cut scores (e.g., MacArthur Competence Adjudication Tool-Criminal Adjudication, Poythress et al., 1999; Competency Screening Test, Laboratory of Community Psychiatry, 1973; Georgia Court Competency Test, Wildman et al., 1978) have juvenile norms or data available. However, the large-scale study of juveniles' competence-related abilities funded by the MacArthur Research Network on Adolescent Development and Juvenile Justice and employing the MacArthur Competence Adjudication Tool-Criminal Adjudication (Poythress et al., 1999) may facilitate the development of juvenile norms for this measure in the near future. Perhaps of more potential value in juvenile contexts at present are those competence assessment tools that simply structure the clinical inquiry (e.g., Interdisciplinary Fitness Interview, Golding, Roesch, & Schreiber, 1984; Competence to Stand Trial Assessment Instrument, Laboratory of Community Psychiatry, 1973), providing that the examiner remains aware of important differences in terminology and processes in criminal and delinquency proceedings in many jurisdictions (e.g., although adults are entitled to jury trials, in most proceedings juveniles are not; adults are convicted while juveniles are adjudicated delinquent; adults receive sentences while juveniles receive dispositions).

Conclusion

In the past decade attorneys, judges, and mental health professionals have paid increasing attention to the capacities of juveniles to participate in the justice process as questions have been raised about the purpose and function of the juvenile court and the juvenile justice system. The law has become increasingly clear about what is expected of minors with respect to their participation in legal proceedings, and researchers have begun to describe the abilities and capacities of juveniles to participate in the legal process from the time of their arrest and detention through legal disposition. Juveniles differ from adults in important ways in their understanding of and ability to participate in the legal process. Moreover, the capacities of adolescents change over time and vary both between and within adolescents. Thus, it is important for mental health professionals to consider the psycholegal capacities of juveniles they evaluate in a developmental context.

References

Arizona v. Fulminante, 499 U.S. 279 (1991).

Barnum, R. (2000). Clinical and forensic evaluation of competence to stand trial in juvenile defendants. In T. Grisso & R. G. Schwartz (Eds.), *Youth on trial: A developmental perspective in juvenile justice* (pp. 193–223). Chicago: University of Chicago Press.

Bonnie, R., & Grisso, T. (2000). Adjudicative competence and youthful offenders. In T. Grisso & R. G. Schwartz (Eds.), *Youth on trial: A developmental perspective in juvenile justice* (pp. 73–103). Chicago: University of Chicago Press.

Brown v. Mississippi, 297 U.S. 278 (1936).

Cauffman, E., & Steinberg, L. (2000a). (Im)maturity of judgment in adolescence: Why adolescents may be less culpable than adults. *Behavioral Sciences and the Law, 18,* 1–21.

Cauffman, E., & Steinberg, L. (2000b). Researching adolescents' judgment and culpability. In T. Grisso & R. G. Schwartz (Eds.), *Youth on trial: A developmental perspective in juvenile justice* (pp. 325–343). Chicago: University of Chicago Press.

Colorado v. Connelly, 479 U.S. 157 (1986).

Commonwealth v. King, 17 Mass. App. Ct. 602 (1984).

Commonwealth v. Philip S., 414 Mass. 804 (1993).

Cooper, D. (1997). Juveniles' understanding of trial related information: Are they competent defendants? *Behavioral Sciences and the Law, 15,* 167–180.

Cowden, V., & McKee, G. (1995). Competency to stand trial in juvenile delinquency proceedings: Cognitive maturity and attorney-client relationship. *Journal of Family Law, 33,* 629–660.

Coyote v. United States, 380 F.2d 305 (1967).

Crane v. Kentucky, 106 S. Ct. Rptr. 2142 (1986).

Davis v. United States, U.S. S. Ct. (No. 92-1949) (1994).

Dickerson v. United States, 166 F.3d 667 (2000).

Driver, E. D. (1968). Confessions and the social psychology of coercion. *Harvard Law Review, 82,* 42–61.

Dusky v. United States, 362 U.S. 402 (1960).

Escobedo v. Illinois, 378 U.S. 478 (1964).

Fare v. Michael C., 442 U.S. 707 (1979).

Feld, B. C. (2000). Juveniles' waiver of legal rights: Confessions, *Miranda,* and the right to counsel. In T. Grisso & R. G. Schwartz (Eds.), *Youth on trial: A developmental perspective on juvenile justice* (pp. 105–138). Chicago: University of Chicago Press.

Frumkin, B. (2000). Competence to waive *Miranda* rights: Clinical and legal issues. *Mental and Physical Disability Law Reporter, 24,* 326–331.

Gallagos v. Colorado, 370 U.S. 49 (1962).

G.J.I. v. State, 778 P.2d 485 (Okla. Crim. 1989).

Golding, S. L. Roesch, R., & Schreiber, J. (1984). Assessment and conceptualization of competency to stand trial: Preliminary data on the Interdisciplinary Fitness Interview. *Law and Human Behavior, 8,* 321–334.

Goldstein, A. M. (1994, August). *Competence to confess: Evaluating the validity of Miranda rights waivers and the trustworthiness of confessions.* Workshop presented at the Annual Convention of American Psychological Association, Los Angeles, CA.

Goldstein, A. M. (2003). Overview of forensic psychology. In A. M. Goldstein (Ed.) *Forensic psychology* (pp. 3–20). New York: Wiley.

Goldstein, A. M., & Burd, M. (1990). The role of delusions in trial competency evaluations: Case law and implications for forensic practice. *Forensic Reports, 3,* 361–386.

Goldstein, N. E., Condie, L. O, Kalbeitzer, R., Osman, D., & Geier, J. (2003). Juvenile offenders' Miranda rights comprehension and self-reported likelihood of offering false confessions. *Assessment, 10,* 359–369

Goldstein, N. E., Oberlander, L. B., & Geier, J. (2002, March). *Development and norming of the Miranda rights comprehension instruments-II.* Paper presented at the Biennial Conference of the American Psychology-Law Society, Austin, TX.

Goldstein, N. E., Olubadewo, O., Osman, D., Thomsen, M., Appleton, C., Mesiarik, C., et al. (2001). *Risk factors for false confessions in adolescent offenders.* Paper presented at the European Association of Psychology and Law conference, Lisbon, Portugal.

Graffam Walker, A. (1999). *Handbook on questioning children: A linguistic perspective.* Washington, DC: American Bar Association.

Griffin, P., & Torbet, P. (2002). *Desktop guide to good juvenile probation practice.* Washington, DC: Office of Juvenile Justice and Delinquency Prevention.

Griffin, P., Torbet, P., & Szymanski, L (1998). *Trying juveniles as adults in criminal court: An analysis of state transfer provisions.* Washington, DC: Office of Juvenile Justice and Delinquency Prevention.

Grisso, T. (1981). *Juveniles' waiver of rights: Legal and psychological competence.* New York: Plenum.

Grisso T. (1986). *Evaluating competencies: Forensic assessments and instruments.* New York: Plenum.

Grisso, T. (1996). Society's retributive response to juvenile violence: A developmental perspective. *Law and Human Behavior, 20,* 229–247.

Grisso, T. (1997). The competence of adolescents as trial defendants. *Psychology, Public Policy and Law, 3,* 3–32.

Grisso, T. (1998a). *Assessing understanding and appreciation of Miranda rights: Manual and materials.* Sarasota, FL: Professional Resource Press.

Grisso, T. (1998b). *Forensic evaluation of juveniles.* Sarasota, FL: Professional Resource Press.

Grisso, T. (2000). What we know about youths' capacities as trial defendants. In T. Grisso & R. G. Schwartz (Eds.), *Youth on trial: A developmental perspective on juvenile justice* (pp. 139–170). Chicago: University of Chicago Press.

Grisso, T. (2003a). *Evaluating competencies: Forensic assessments and instruments* (2nd ed.) New York: Kluwer/Plenum.

Grisso, T. (2003b). Forensic evaluation in delinquency cases. In A. M. Goldstein (Ed.), *Forensic psychology* (pp. 315–334). New York: Wiley.

Grisso, T., & Ring, M. (1979). Parents' attitudes toward juveniles' rights in interrogation. *Criminal Justice and Behavior, 6,* 211.

Grisso, T., & Schwartz, R. G. (Eds.). (2000). *Youth on trial: A developmental perspective in juvenile justice.* Chicago: University of Chicago Press.

Grisso, T., Steinberg, L., Woolard, J., Cauffman, E., Scott, E., Graham, S., et al. (in press). Juveniles' competence to stand trial: A comparison of adolescents' and adults' capacities and trial defendants. *Law and Human Behavior.*

Gudjonsson, G. H., Rutter, S., & Clare, I. (1995). The relationship between suggestibility and anxiety among suspects detained at police stations. *Psychological Medicine, 25,* 875–878.

Haley v. Ohio, 332 U.S. 596 (1948).

Hansdottir, I., Thorsteinsson, H., Kristinsdottir, H., & Ragnarsson, R. (1990). The effects of instructions and anxiety on interrogative suggestibility. *Personality and Individual Differences, 11,* 85–87.

Heilbrun, K. (2001). *Principles of forensic mental health assessment.* New York: Kluwer/Plenum.

Heilbrun, K., Marczyk, G. R., & DeMatteo, D. (2002). *Forensic mental health assessment: A casebook.* New York: Oxford University Press.

Heilbrun, K., Warren, J., & Picarello, K. (2003). Third party information in forensic assessment. In A. M. Goldstein (Ed.), *Forensic psychology* (pp. 69–86). New York: Wiley.

In re Causey, 363 So.2d 472 (La. 1978).

In re Gault, 387 U.S. 1 (1967).

In re Morgan, 35 Ill. App. 3d. 10, 341 N.E.2d. 19 (1975).

In the Matter of the Welfare of DDN, 582 N.W.2d 278 (Minn. Ct. App. 1998).

Jackson v. Indiana, 406 U.S. 715 (1972).

Kassin, S. M., & Neumann, K. (1997). On the power of confession evidence: An experimental test of the fundamental difference hypothesis. *Law and Human Behavior, 21,* 469–484.

Kent v. United States, 383 U.S. 541 (1966).

Laboratory of Community Psychiatry. (1973). *Competency to stand trial and mental illness.* New York: Aronson.

Lally, S. J. (2003). What tests are acceptable for use in forensic evaluations? A survey of experts. *Professional Psychology: Research and Practice, 34,* 491–498.

Larson, K. A. (2003). Improving the "kangaroo courts": A proposal for reform in evaluating juveniles' waiver of *Miranda. Villanova Law Review, 18,* 629–666.

Larson, K. A., & Goldstein, N. E. (2003, April). *Reform in the evaluation of juveniles' waiver of Miranda rights.* Paper presented at the Annual Conference of the International Association of Forensic Mental Health Services, Miami, FL.

McCord, J., Spatz-Widom, C., & Crowell, N. A. (Eds.). (2001). *Juvenile crime, juvenile justice.* Washington, DC: National Academy Press.

McGaha, A., McClaren, M., Otto, R. K., & Petrila, J. (2001). Juveniles adjudicated incompetent to proceed: A descriptive study of Florida's competence restoration program. *Journal of the American Academy of Psychiatry and Law, 29,* 427–437.

McKee, G. R., & Shea, S. J. (1999). Competency to stand trial in family court: Characteristics of competent and incompetent juveniles. *Journal of the American Academy of Psychiatry and the Law, 27,* 65–73.

Melton, G. B., Petrila, J., Poythress, N., & Slobogin, C. (1997). *Psychological evaluations for the courts: A handbook for mental health professionals and lawyers.* New York: Guilford Press.

Miranda v. Arizona, 384 U.S. 436 (1966).

Moran v. Burbine, 475 U.S. 412 (1986).

Oberlander, L., Goldstein, N. E., & Ho, C. N. (2001). Preadolescent adjudicative competence: Methodological considerations and recommendations for practice standards. *Behavioral Sciences and the Law, 19,* 545–563.

Oberlander, L. B. (1998). *Miranda* comprehension and confessional competence. *Expert Opinion, 2,* 11–12.

Oberlander, L. B, & Goldstein, N. E. (2001). A review and update on the practice of evaluating *Miranda* comprehension. *Behavioral Sciences and the Law, 19,* 453–471.

Oberlander, L. B., Goldstein, N. E., & Goldstein, A. M. (2003). Competence to confess. In A. M. Goldstein (Ed.), *Forensic psychology* (pp. 335–358). New York: Wiley.

Oberlander, L. B., Goldstein, N. E. S., & Grisso, T. (in preparation). Comprehension of *Miranda* Rights Instruments.

Ohio v. Settles, Ohio App. 3d. LEXIS 4973 (Ohio App. 3d. Sept 30, 1998).

Oregon v. Elstad, 470 U.S. 298 (1985).

Osman, D., Thomson, M., Goldstein, N. E., Weil, J., Oberlander, L. B., & Geier, J.

(2002, March). *Adolescent offenders' demographic characteristics, Miranda rights comprehension, and false confessions.* Paper presented at the Biennial Conference of the American Psychology-Law Society, Austin, TX.

Otto, R. K., & Borum, R. (2004). Juvenile forensic evaluation. In W. O'Donahue & E. Levensky (Eds.), *Forensic psychology* (pp. 873–895). New York: Academic Press.

Otto, R. K., & Heilbrun, K. (2002). The future of forensic psychology: A look toward the future in light of the past. *American Psychologist, 57,* 5–18.

Otto, R. K., Poythress, N. G., Nicholson, R. A., Edens, J. F., Monahan, J., Bonnie, R. J., Hoge, S. K., & Eisenberg, M. (1998). Psychometric properties of the MacArthur Competence Assessment Tool–Criminal Adjudication (MacCAT–CA). *Psychological Assessment, 10,* 435–443.

Peterson-Badali, M., & Abramovitch, R. (1992). Children's knowledge of the legal system: Are they competent to instruct legal counsel? *Canadian Journal of Criminology, 34,* 139–160.

Peterson-Badali, M., & Abramovitch, R., & Duda, C. (1997). Young children's legal knowledge and reasoning ability. *Canadian Journal of Criminology, 39,* 145–170.

People v. Lara, 432 P.2d 202 (1967).

Poythress, N., Bonnie, R., Monahan, J., Otto, R. K., & Hoge, S. (2002). *Adjudicative competence: The MacArthur studies.* New York: Kluwer/Plenum.

Poythress, N., Nicholson, R., Otto, R. K., Edens, J. F., Monahan, J., Bonnie, R., et al. (1999). *Manual for the MacArthur Competence Assessment Tool-Criminal Adjudication.* Odessa, FL: Psychological Assessment Resources.

Redding, R., & Frost, L. (2001). Adjudicative competence in the modern juvenile court. *The Virginia Journal of Social Policy and the Law, 9,* 353–409.

Richardson, G., Gudjonsson, G. H., & Kelly T. P. (1995). Interrogative suggestibility in an adolescent forensic population. *Journal of Adolescence, 18,* 211–216.

Roesch, R., Zapf, P., Golding, S., & Skeem, J. (1999). Defining and assessing competency to stand trial. In A. K. Hess & I. Weiner (Eds.), *The handbook of forensic psychology* (2nd ed., pp. 327–349). New York: Wiley.

Rogers, R., & Bender, S. D. (2003). Evaluation of malingering and deception. In A. M. Goldstein (Ed.), *Forensic psychology* (pp. 109–132). New York: Wiley.

Rogers, R., Salekin, R. T., Sewell, K. W., Goldstein, A. M., & Leonard, K. (1998). A comparison of forensic and non-forensic malingerers: A prototypical analysis of explanatory models. *Law and Human Behavior, 22,* 353–367.

Rogers, R., Sewell, K. W., & Goldstein, A. M. (1994). Explanatory models of malingering: A prototypical analysis. *Law and Human Behavior, 18,* 543–552.

Rhode Island v. Innis, 446 U.S. 291 (1980).

Rosado, L. (Ed.). (2000). *Kids are different: How knowledge of adolescent development theory can aid decision-making in court.* Washington, DC: American Bar Association Juvenile Justice Center.

Savitsky, J., & Karras, D. (1984). Competency to stand trial among adolescents. *Adolescence, 19,* 349–358.

Schmidt, M. G., Reppucci, N. D., & Woolard, J. L (2003). Effectiveness of participation as a defendant: The attorney-juvenile client relationship. *Behavioral Sciences and the Law, 21,* 175–198.

Scott, E. S. (2000). Criminal responsibility in adolescents: Lessons from developmental psychology. In T. Grisso & R. G. Schwartz (Eds.), *Youth on trial: A developmental perspective in juvenile justice* (pp. 291–324). Chicago: University of Chicago Press.

Scott, E. S., Reppucci, N., & Woolard, J. (1995). Evaluating adolescent decision making in legal contexts. *Law and Human Behavior, 19,* 221–244.

Shapiro, D. L. (1991). *Forensic psychological assessment: An integrative approach.* Boston: Allyn & Bacon.

Spano v. New York, 360 U.S. 315 (1959).

Stafford, K. P. (2003). Assessment of competence to stand trial. In A. M. Goldstein (Ed.), *Forensic psychology* (pp. 359–380). New York: Wiley.

State v. Prater, 77 Wash. 2d. 526, 463 P.2d 640 (1970).

Steinberg, L., & Cauffman, E. (1996). Maturity of judgment in adolescence: Psychosocial factors in adolescent decision making. *Law and Human Behavior, 20,* 249–272.

Steinberg, L., & Cauffman, E. (1999, December). A developmental perspective on serious juvenile crime: When should juveniles be treated as adults? *Federal Probation,* 52–57.

Steinberg, L., & Schwartz, R. (2000). Developmental psychology goes to court. In T. Grisso & R. Schwartz (Eds.), *Youth on trial: A developmental perspective on juvenile justice* (pp. 9–31). Chicago: University of Chicago Press.

United States v. Duhon, 104 F.Supp.2d. 663 (W.D. La. 2000).

Warren-Leubecker, A., Tate, C., Hinton, I., & Ozbeck, N. (1989). What do children know about the legal system and when do they know it? In S. Ceci, D. Ross, & M. Toglia (Eds.), *Perspectives on children's testimony* (pp. 158–183). New York: Springer-Verlag.

West v. United States, 399 F.2d 467 (1978).

Wildman, R. W., Batchelor, E. S., Thompson, L., Nelson, F. R., Moore, J. T., & Patterson, M. E. (1978). *The Georgia Court Competency Test: An attempt to develop a rapid, quantitative measure of fitness for trial.* Unpublished manuscript, Milledgeville, GA.

Woolard, J. L., Reppucci, N. D., & Redding, R. E. (1996). Theoretical and methodological issues in studying children's capacities in legal contexts. *Law and Human Behavior, 20,* 219–228.

Wulach, J. S. (1981, Summer). The assessment of competency to waive *Miranda* rights. *Journal of Psychiatry and Law, 8,* 209–220.

Zimring, F. E. (2000). The punitive necessity of waiver. In J. Fagon & F. E. Zimring (Eds.), *The changing borders of juvenile justice: Transfer of adolescents to the criminal court* (pp. 207–226). Chicago: University of Chicago Press.

10

Edward P. Mulvey

Risk Assessment in Juvenile Justice Policy and Practice

The assessment of risk is a central feature of juvenile justice, both for broad policy and for daily practice. At the policy level, a form of risk assessment is implicit in the definitions of the types of adolescents who qualify for particular forms of processing (e.g., as adults or juveniles) or different sanctions or interventions. Defining categories of adolescents for special processing is part of the "wholesale exclusion" strategy for administering juvenile justice (Fagan & Zimring, 2000). In addition, probation officers, judges, and clinicians make risk assessments regarding the adolescents appearing before them every day. These professionals regularly face the tough question of whether having a particular juvenile in the community will significantly endanger others and whether this adolescent has the potential to change positively. Thus, risk assessment is part of the "retail" administration of juvenile justice as well. The challenge is to sort cases, use resources effectively, and reduce risk to the community.

This chapter reviews some of the assumptions about risk assessment that underpin certain juvenile justice policies and practices. It addresses three places where risk assessment plays a central role. First, it provides an overview of policy about transfer to the adult court and how risk assessment notions are built into these statutes. Next, it briefly reviews how risk assessment has been systematized by developing actuarial instruments, highlighting the conditions under which these instruments operate well. Finally, it examines how risk assessment fits into the discretionary judgments made by juvenile court professionals and clinicians on a daily basis. The chapter ends by proposing three points about risk assessment in general that might help to improve policy and practice regarding juveniles specifically.

Transfer Statutes: Risk Assessment in Legal Categories

Juvenile justice policy creates categories of offenders who are treated differently, mainly because they either deserve more retributive punishment or are more likely to benefit from individualized, treatment-oriented interventions. Mandated higher punishments for certain groups of adolescent offenders are justified on several grounds (not all of which are equally sound; see Feld, 2000). Increased and surer punishments are seen as (a) exacting more retribution, thus highlighting societal values; (b) providing a clear deterrent both for that adolescent and others; and (c) achieving some reduction in crime by incapacitating serious offenders, keeping them away from opportunities for crime in the community. Juveniles who are processed with more discretion and access to treatment resources are those who have not had an adequate investment of rehabilitation resources to date or who may be particularly prone to positive change (e.g., less serious, first-time offenders).

Recent changes in transfer statutes (those governing the movement of juvenile offenders into the adult court system) provide perhaps the most dramatic recent example of an effort to integrate risk assessment into juvenile law (Heilbrun, Leheny, Thomas, & Huneycutt, 1997). Over the past decade or so, nearly all states have adopted legislation that allows younger youth who have committed a wider range of offenses to be transferred to the adult system, and many statutes require automatic processing in the adult system. Juvenile court judges have less ability to retain cases in their court, and prosecutors have more discretion in determining which cases get transferred (Griffin, 1998).

As mentioned above, three rationales—retribution, deterrence, and selective incapacitation—have supported the recent expansion of transfer statutes. The appropriateness of retribution as a rationale for increasing juvenile punishments is based largely on values regarding the need for society to exact proportional punishments and the appropriateness of doing this with individuals who are not yet fully adult. The reasonableness of deterrence as a rationale for increasing juvenile punishments rests mainly on beliefs about the susceptibility of adolescents to specific and general deterrence, and there is limited empirical information to guide this determination (e.g., see Paternoster, 1989; Redding, 2000; Schneider & Ervin, 1990). The rationale of selective incapacitation rests mainly on the ability of the statutory guidelines to institute a valid risk assessment strategy.

Selective incapacitation is the idea of identifying repetitive, serious offenders and giving them longer sentences so that these individuals have less opportunity to commit offenses during their most crime-prone years. Simply put, incarcerating the most active and serious criminals should lower the overall crime rate. The most basic requirement of any incapacitation approach is to find those who are "likely to commit more crimes of the same sort or other crimes of other sorts" (Packer, 1968, p. 49).

One obvious limiting factor of this approach is the accuracy of the identification procedure. As the performance of the method for identifying individuals for incarceration deteriorates (i.e., the identified sample has a significantly higher proportion of "false-positive" cases), the efficiency of such an approach to achieve selective incapacitation diminishes. Too many of the wrong people will be locked up.

The seemingly simple calculus of selective incapacitation is not easy to accomplish, however, and many question whether it can ever be an effective approach to reducing crime. One gets very different estimates of the potential impact of selective incapacitation, depending on the assumptions made about rates of offending behaviors, the types of crimes committed by high rate offenders at different points in their criminal careers, and the proportion of high rate offenders in the criminal population (Blumstein, Cohen, Roth, & Visher, 1986). This problem becomes even more difficult when only juvenile criminal careers are considered, since there are often less clear patterns of offending, given the shorter series of events. Nonetheless, the basic idea of finding high rate offenders and keeping them off the street is certainly a lynchpin of the utilitarian case for changes in transfer statutes.

Most automatic transfer statutes make eligibility for transfer contingent upon the age of the adolescent and the type of crime committed. The adolescent must be above a certain minimum age and charged with a sufficiently serious offense. The obvious question is how well these criteria might perform for the straight utilitarian goal of incapacitation—how well they work as a risk assessment instrument.

Based on longitudinal research, age can be expected to perform rather poorly as an initial screening factor when used this way. Age at first arrest is a powerful predictor of continued offending, but the relationship is such that earlier onset of offending indicates markedly increased risk (Piquero, Farrington, & Blumstein, 2003). Limiting the age range to midadolescence (e.g., 14) produces a sample with a confusing mix of "adolescent-limited" and chronic offenders (Broidy et al., 2003). From a strictly utilitarian viewpoint, it seems that younger, repetitive offenders (age 12 or 13) should receive the most stringent sentences (in terms of either incapacitation or intensive supervision), since the likelihood of reoffending is high in this group. Looking at policy more broadly, however, it is clear that such an approach introduces possible iatrogenic effects of intervention and overreaching by the state into family matters. It also has limited general utility because these younger adolescents are a relatively small (but possibly growing; see Snyder, 1998) part of the whole adolescent offender population.

The choice of presenting offense also does little to identify a particularly crime-prone subsample of youth. There is little indication of specialization in juvenile criminal offending, with adolescents who are involved in one type of crime often involved with a variety of other offenses in their early careers (Farrington, Snyder, & Finnegan, 1988; Klein, 1984). There is also limited evidence that severity of presenting offense alone consistently predicts likelihood of future serious offending (Tolan & Gorman-Smith, 1998). There is a demonstrated relationship between frequency of violent and nonviolent offending, and thus adolescents with multiple serious offenses against persons do appear to be at increased risk for continued involvement in this type of behavior (Brame, Mulvey, & Piquero, 2001). The use of a single offense as a criterion for automatic transfer, however, chooses a sample with a sizable proportion of adolescents with a relatively low chance of repeating that crime or a large number of other crimes. The expansion of the category of eligible offenses that has occurred under newer statutes accentuates this problem.

As noted by other commentators (e.g., Redding, 1997, 2000; Scott & Grisso, 1997), the use of age and a broad set of presenting offenses may not be the most effective way of identifying cases most likely to commit future crimes with any regularity. The use of history of offending as a criterion would probably be preferable. Consideration of frequency of offending, age at first arrest, and pattern of offenses could produce a more homogeneous pool of likely repeat offenders. Even more power could probably be obtained from integrating contextual factors related to the adolescent's offending into the case identification process. Knowing an adolescent's neighborhood, the type of family supervision provided, and whether the child has problems in other domains of his/her life (e.g., fights in school) would go a long way toward making a more accurate determination about the likelihood of future offending.

Consideration of these latter contextual factors, however, is probably not reasonable for broad policy purposes. Part of the problem with any strategy used to identify adolescents for transfer or any other selective punishment approach is that the factors considered must not extend beyond those readily ascertainable and related to the offense that brought the juvenile to the attention of the court because such efforts lead easily to discriminatory practices (Feld, 1999). In effect, these cases must be sorted categorically in a "decontextualized" fashion to ensure equal treatment under the law. The consideration of contextual factors such as these in an individualized system relying on the discretion of the judge may be appropriate, but their use as a way to create "classes" of individuals subject to different sanctions would seem questionable.

This example of transfer statutes attempting to operationalize risk assessment illustrates a broader point. Any statutory approach to identifying high-risk groups is inevitably vague and ineffectual for a number of reasons. Such reasons include (a) the legislative process requires language with imprecise interpretation, (b) professionals in human processing organizations accommodate to whatever statutory mandates require, and (c) the link between any socially acceptable method for identifying risk groups and antisocial behavior is bound to be rather weak and indirect. Identification of cases at high risk for antisocial behavior is a delicate enterprise, and the law by its nature is a blunt instrument. As a result, although based on a notion of risk assessment, statutory attempts to identify high-risk groups effectively almost inevitably fall far short of the rhetoric supporting them.

Actuarial Checklists: Risk Assessment in Practice Guidelines

Risk assessment is also built into policy in the form of regulations or guidelines for the placement of juvenile offenders *into* secure facilities or the release of juvenile offenders back into the community *from* secure facilities. Many locales have adopted structured instruments that professionals must use at particular decision points in juvenile justice processing, with scores on these instruments the main determining factor regarding incarceration or release (Guarino-Ghezzi & Loughran, 1997). Although not having the weight of statute, requirements to use actuarial instruments to determine the reasonableness of holding or releasing a juvenile can effectively structure and limit the use of professional discretion. Much of the "business" of courts and social services is done according to guidelines set forth in policy and procedure manuals, with the categories and requirements set out in these documents accepted as the standard for good practice. Actuarial instruments for determining the risk of future offending have become a more commonplace aspect of these regulations and juvenile justice practice (Hoge & Andrews, 1996).

Risk assessment instruments used in juvenile justice are generally straightforward, actuarial checklists that add up points and set a cutoff value for either detaining or releasing a juvenile. These instruments usually collect information about a set of factors related to reoffending (e.g., number of prior arrests, presence of a drug problem) and then calculate a total risk score. The methods for combining information into a score are usually (a) a simple tally of endorsed items or a summation of weighted items indicating overall risk of reoffending or (b) a two-dimensional judgment grid placing a youth in the appropriate category of placement security (LeBlanc, 1998). The logic is rather simple: the more relevant risk factors are present, the more likely the juvenile is to reoffend, and therefore the more justification there is to hold that juvenile. Numerous locales across the United States have devised risk assessment instruments of this sort, based on a combination of local data about rearrest or re-institutionalization and local values regarding the acceptable level of community risk from juvenile crime (Wiebush, Baird, Krisberg, & Onek, 1995).

Despite their growing acceptance, there is only limited research on the accuracy and effectiveness of these instruments (LeBlanc, 1998; Wiebush et al., 1995). Relatively few locales have done successive validation and instrument improvement (for an exception, see Arizona; Krysik & LeCroy, 2002), and while methods for developing these instruments to meet local demands have been developed and applied (e.g., Baird, 1984, 1991), these are oftentimes seen as too costly and involved to implement. As a result, many locales adopt instruments from other jurisdictions without considering whether they are well suited to the risk factors and behaviors seen in their adolescent offenders (Wiebush et al., 1995). Some positive benefits might accrue from this strategy, but it is optimal when a locale uses its own data and a consensus process to develop instruments tailored to its juvenile justice system. There are also several aspects of risk assessment instruments and methods that increase the chances of this approach having a lasting, positive impact.

First, these instruments seem to be most useful when they use information that is readily obtainable, reliable, and interpretable (LeBlanc, 1998). Risk assessment forms are commonly filled out by line staff in institutions or by probation staff, not by highly credentialed professionals conducting an in-depth assessment. As a result, the types of judgments included in the instrument should be straightforward and require minimal inference. An item that asks for the number of prior arrests, for example, is preferable to an item that asks for a scaled judgment about the quality of the adolescent's relationship with his/her parents. The latter judgment would require information that would not be readily available and would be open to idiosyncratic interpretations, both of which would reduce its ability to be collected reliably.

Second, risk assessment instruments are more successful when there is a method for overriding the actuarial determination made from the information supplied (Wiebush et al., 1995). Staff and professionals with an individual adolescent in front of them have to be given some latitude to respond to information not on the form. Actuarial determinations are useful for a variety of situations where categorization must be done consistently, but they can never replace a well-founded clinical conclusion. As noted by Meehl decades ago (Meehl, 1954), no actuarial instrument could possibly come to the conclusion that a person talking about a raven appearing repeatedly in their dreams is concerned about death; no instrument would program in the poetry of Edgar Allan Poe. Similarly, a very dangerous adolescent might not pose an immediate threat if his leg is broken, although it is unlikely that any risk assessment instrument would ask for an inventory of working limbs. When relevant considerations come up, professionals must be able to ignore actuarially based conclusions.

At the same time, allowing clinicians to override actuarial determinations at will defeats the purpose of these instruments. Limits must be set upon the number of times or the conditions that can produce such variations; the Office of Juvenile Justice and Delinquency Prevention (1995) recommends that no more than 15% of the decisions be exceptions. In addition, documentation of the reasons for ignoring the actuarial score should be required so that later reviews of the judgment process can be conducted.

Finally, to work effectively, risk assessment instruments must be tied explicitly to a particular point in the juvenile justice decision-making process. Risk assessment instruments are not generic; their performance may vary considerably when applied at different points in the system. The discriminative power of any actuarial screening device depends heavily on the distribution of the measured characteristics in the sample being assessed and the base rate of the predicted outcomes in that sample (Copas & Tarling, 1986). As a result, an actuarial instrument developed to assess the likelihood of an adolescent reoffending prior to a court appearance (for use at the point of detention) may not function well as a method for assessing risk of crime in the community after adjudication (if used at the point of disposition). The background characteristics of detained youth are different from those of adjudicated youth, the types and frequency of offending prior to court appearance are different from those seen after disposition, and the consequences of the assessment are different (short-term detention vs. longer-term institutional placement). In developing actuarial assessments for juvenile justice, one size does not fit all. To be effective, risk assessment instruments must be developed and validated with the requirements of a particular prediction task clearly in mind.

Several researchers have taken a broader approach to actuarial assessment, going beyond simply a consideration of how likely a juvenile might be to reoffend. These investigators (e.g., see Andrews & Bonta, 1995; Dembo et al., 1996; Hoge & Andrews, 1996; Wiebush et al., 1995) have integrated the assessment of need with that of risk for future offending. Rather than treating risk as a fixed trait, this approach assumes that risk might be lowered by particular interventions or careful monitoring in the community. From this perspective, the task of systematic assessment is to consider not only what aspects of the adolescent's functioning appear to raise the risk of future offending, but also what might be done to reduce the risk of that outcome. The idea here is to acknowledge the malleable nature of adolescents and to identify pivotal aspects of their lives where efforts might be made for positive change. An adolescent with a drug or alcohol problem may be at higher risk for reoffending, but he/she may also be a good candidate for positive community adjustment if that problem can be addressed effectively. The attractive aspect of this risk/need assessment strategy is that it goes beyond the task of sorting adolescents into lower or higher risk groups and instead provides information about how to target interventions to reduce risk. This approach, therefore, raises the chances that an assessment might produce focused intervention rather than just a binary decision about the need for incarceration.

In general, risk assessment instruments for adolescent offenders hold considerable promise for systematizing decision making at several key junctures in the juvenile justice system. The empirical evidence for the value or robustness of these systems, however, is not overwhelming. As we have noted, there is little systematic research on the enduring validity of these instruments for predicting which adolescents might reoffend if left in or released to the community. Much of the value of these approaches, however, may lie in the fact that they are done at all, rather than in the exact specificities or sensitivities of their algorithms.[1]

There are two broad ways that the implementation of actuarial risk assessments can improve decision making in juvenile justice. First, these instruments can simply increase the uniformity of decisions made at certain points in juvenile justice processing. The use of actuarial instruments certainly limits idiosyncratic decision making in a locale, reducing the likelihood of widely disparate outcomes in similarly situated cases. This is a valuable contribution in and of itself, since more consistent application of decision-making rules has been shown to increase overall accuracy even if the model used is less than optimal (Dawes, 1979; Gambrill & Schlonsky, 2000).

---

1. Work is currently being done to refine some potentially promising risk–needs tools. Three that are currently undergoing development or validation are the Youth Level of Service/Case Management Inventory (YLS/CMI; Hoge & Andrews, 2002), the Structured Assessment of Violence Risk in Youth (SAVRY; Borum, Bartel, & Forth, 2002), and the Washington State Juvenile Assessment (WAJA; Barnoski, 2002). The YLS/CMI may be purchased through Multi-Health Systems, 800-456-3003 (U.S.), 800-268-6011 (Canada), or 416-492-2627 (international). E-mail: customerservice @mhs.com. The SAVRY, Version 1, Consultation edition manual may be ordered from Randy Borum, Psy.D., SAVRY Order, Department of Mental Health Law and Policy, Louis de la Parte Florida Mental Health Institute, University of South Florida, 13301 Bruce B. Downs Boulevard, Tampa, FL 33612-3807. E-mail: SAVRYinfo@yahoo.com. The WAJA is not currently available for purchase. Neither the SAVRY nor the WAJA is currently ready for professional use; additional validation research and manual development should be completed on these instruments in the near future.

Second, introduction of these instruments can promote and maintain system improvement. The development of an actuarial decision-making system can often be done as part of a broadly based reformation of the juvenile justice system within a particular locale (see Anne E. Casey Foundation, Juvenile Detention Alternatives Initiative, 2004). The process of having invested stakeholders identify appropriate risk indicators and choose thresholds for particular actions (e.g., detention) can produce increased collaboration and a shared sense of mission among parties involved in the juvenile justice system. In this way, the development of actuarial tools and decision-making guidelines can serve as the content that pushes the positive collaborative process forward, with the ongoing monitoring and adjustment of the guidelines serving to keep these positive contacts alive. In this way, the careful introduction of actuarial risk assessments can be effective in addressing the continuing issue of disproportionate minority confinement (Schirali & Ziedenberg, 2002).

The Application of Professional Discretion: Risk Assessment in Daily Practice

Even though actuarial prediction strategies have and will become more sophisticated, they are not a panacea for assessing risk in adolescent offenders. Actuarial approaches can make the assessment process more routine and focused at particular points in juvenile justice processing, but professionals in this system will still confront the task of judiciously recommending certain interventions or sanctions based on a global assessment of the risk associated with the particular adolescent in front of them. Judges, probation officers, and social service practitioners will still face the task of assessing risk at a variety of decision points, one case at a time and with different amounts and types of information. Whether a case gets processed past intake, whether an adolescent gets referred to a community-based service or sent to a secure facility, or whether certain conditions of probation are imposed are all examples of decisions made by juvenile justice professionals that involve an assessment of the likelihood of future offending or violence.

These assessments may include the administration of a structured risk (or risk/need) instrument like those discussed above. Assessing risk of future offending or violence, however, is generally a more nuanced task than simply the administration of a checklist. Clinicians, social service providers, and court professionals must combine actuarial scores, background information, and impressions about the adolescent's functioning and social context to make specific recommendations regarding the most appropriate action (Grisso, 1998). This requires more than a tally of case characteristics; it instead requires a disciplined weaving together of relevant information about a real person with possibilities for growth and risks for harming other real people.

A professional making a clinical determination regarding risk of harm to others or the likelihood of future offending thus faces a formidable task. Information has to be collected systematically, sifted for validity, weighed carefully, applied thoughtfully, and communicated clearly. The professional stakes for an error are often high, yet the amount of solid guidance for sound practice is rather limited.

The Inherent Difficulties of Assessing Adolescent Behaviors

There are numerous theories at any given time about the most important factors to consider and how to weigh different bits of information in making these assessments. For some time, the triad of bed-wetting, fire setting, and cruelty to animals was thought (mistakenly) to have high predictive value for predicting violence in adolescents (see Mulvey & Lidz, 1984). In current times, the concept of juvenile psychopathy is thought to effectively capture the essential features connected to future violence and reoffending. Whether this construct will stand the test of time as a focus for assessing risk in juvenile offenders seems still to be an open question (Edens, Skeem, Cruise, & Cauffman, 2001). Fads come and go about how to best assess future risk of violence and reoffending, and often the same wine appears in different bottles.

The identification of consistent and enduring indicators of risk for adolescents is an inherently difficult task for several reasons. First, history of behavior is one of our best predictors of future behavior, especially regarding violence and criminal offending, and this information is limited and ambiguous when assessing adolescents. There is simply less of an established pattern of behaviors upon which to base forecasts of future behavior. Furthermore, child and adolescent behavior is more likely to be influenced by context and therefore possibly less indicative of underlying consistencies of character. Children and adolescents have fewer opportunities to choose their everyday settings than do adults, and young people oftentimes display behaviors that indicate the fit between the child and the environment rather than aspects of the child or adolescent that will emerge consistently across settings (Masten & Coatsworth, 1998). A child who is a behavior problem in one school, for instance, may respond favorably to another school, and interpreting disruptive behavior in the first setting as indicative of an established disorder in the child or adolescent could often be a mistaken conclusion.

In addition, adolescents are by definition "works in progress," and making the link between observed behavior and crystallized personality traits is very difficult in this group. It is difficult to make precise determinations about the lines where developmental features stop and personality features begin, especially for the purposes of predicting future criminality (Steinberg & Scott, 2003). Impulsive acts, for example, may be the result of being immature rather than innately impulsive. Making a determination about whether an adolescent is more or less like a "typical" adolescent, therefore, is asking whether an individual can conceivably fit into a category with a wide variability of behaviors; the answer may be affirmative, but it might not tell us much. There is simply less confidence about classification of adolescents, since they are not yet fully formed.

Given this difficulty with achieving reliable characterizations, it is apparent why predicting future behavior becomes difficult. The predictive validity of any classification scheme or dimensional approach is limited when we cannot be sure that we have the right adolescents in the right boxes or that we have them at the right set point on any scale in the first place. Limited reliability measuring risk indicators lowers the achievable predictive validity of any assessment, and we can expect difficulties getting accurate characterizations of adolescents from the outset.

Overcoming these inherent obstacles requires professionals to be especially thoughtful and integrative when assessing adolescents (Grisso, 1998; Melton, Petrila, Poythress, & Slobogin, 1997). It is particularly important, for example, to assess history as a series of incident reports rather than as a reported number of incidents. Prior violent or disruptive incidents indicate how the adolescent functions in certain settings and when confronted with particular challenges. Noting, in and of itself, that an adolescent has a history of aggressive behavior provides very limited information for assessing likelihood of future risk. Considering what precipitated prior aggressive acts, the targets of these acts, and how the child or adolescent responded to them provides much more useful information for considering what actions to take with the youth in the future. Similarly, simply assessing whether an adolescent exhibits seemingly risky behaviors, like a disregard for others or impulsivity, does not address the central question. A more useful tack is to try to make a determination of whether these behaviors are congruent with the level of development seen in the adolescent being assessed, whether these might be expected to change over time or under certain influences, and whether or not these aspects of the adolescent's presentation can be convincingly linked to reoffending or future violence. Answering these more nuanced questions is a much more difficult task, but it seems necessary if the unique aspects of making risk assessments in adolescents are to be taken into account.

Guidance From Longitudinal Studies

Currently, we have a large amount of literature from longitudinal research about the factors related to adolescent criminality and violence (see Loeber & Farrington, 1998; Reppucci, Fried, & Schmidt, 2002; Thornberry & Krohn, 2003), and some of this has applicability to the task of assessing the likelihood of future reoffending or violence. Unfortunately, this literature is voluminous and rather overwhelming. The diversity of methods, the variety of samples, the differences in the case characteristics measured, and the range of possible outcomes all make it difficult to summarize this literature accurately. Identifying particular risk indicators that have emerged across several studies can provide a falsely reassuring sense that science has found the "magic bullets" for easily identifying adolescents with a very high likelihood of future offending or violence. The complexity of the studies in these areas, however, simply makes that impossible; the key to solid risk assessment does not rest with the discovery of some variable or combination of variables that has unsurpassed predictive validity for future outcomes. It instead rests on a systematic consideration of the most relevant broad forces that might increase or decrease the likelihood of future offending or violence.

Taken in this light, a few general findings from this literature can be useful for focusing the assessment process onto domains highlighted by longitudinal studies as valuable to consider (Cottle, Lee, & Heilbrun, 2001).

One basic finding from the longitudinal research is that many adolescents who exhibit serious antisocial behavior do not go on to continued antisocial behavior in adulthood. In fact, estimates are that probably less than half of serious adolescent offenders will continue their adult criminal career into their twenties (see Elliott, 1994; Piquero et al., 2001; Redding, 1997). This is important to consider when assessing risk of future offending or violence with juvenile offenders because it sets the implicit level of expected outcome for the behavior in question. If a professional believes that almost all serious adolescent offenders go on to serious adult crime, then making an assessment that any particular individual is less, rather than more, likely to continue offending requires that individual to be rather distinct from most of the offenders seen. In actuality, it seems that the opposite holds; in a broad sample of adolescent offenders, the presumption to be rebutted is that the adolescent *will* go on to extended criminal involvement.

In addition, the risk indicators identified in longitudinal research are more consistently powerful when predicting the next developmental period rather than long-term outcomes (Cicchetti & Cohen, 1995). As might be expected, risk indicators at one age are most applicable when figuring out what might happen to an adolescent during the next few years. Some indicators of risk, most notably aggression in multiple settings between the ages of 8 and 12 and the presence of a criminal father in males (Loeber, Farrington, Stouthamer-Loeber, Moffitt, & Caspi, 2001), are probably more powerfully related to violent criminality later in life than are other predictors. Nonetheless, the general observation that the power of any risk indicator decreases rather dramatically over time is worth noting because of its relevance to the clinical task of assessing future risk for court or social service actions.

Because risk indicators are generally most valid in the short run, it is important for professionals making risk assessments to be specific about the time frame under consideration and the outcome being predicted. Predictions about long-term outcomes are more likely to be erroneous, whereas focused conclusions about more immediate adjustment have a utility and soundness that can be readily defended. The number of potential intervening influences that can occur in an adolescent's life and the potentially powerful impact of these influences make assertions about long-term outcomes more speculative than scientific. Similarly, a general characterization of an adolescent as a likely repeat offender does little to guide the court's decision making or planning for intervention. Assessments that focus on the likely short-term outcomes of immediate alternatives are likely to be both more scientifically sound and useful.

A second general point emerging from longitudinal studies is that family influences exert a powerful effect on the onset and maintenance of antisocial behavior. Studies of high-risk cohorts (e.g., see Thornberry & Krohn, 2003) consistently identify family functioning as an important risk indicator for young males. The presence of antisocial parents (in particular, the father), poor parent-child relationships, and the presence of abuse/neglect have all been shown to increase risk for future offending in young males (e.g., ages 6–12). In addition, harsh, lax, inconsistent discipline and poor parent-child relationships are relatively useful risk indicators for continued offending in adolescents from ages 12–14 (Satcher, 2001). The effect of family dynamics on offending in older adolescents is less pronounced, as association with antisocial peers becomes more important, but family functioning is still important to consider as something that sets the stage for involvement in a variety of risky behaviors (e.g., lack of parental controls can allow more frequent drug or alcohol use and more involvement in criminal activity). An added indication of the importance of considering family functioning comes from the fact that interventions targeted at stabilizing and clarifying family dynamics (e.g., multisystemic therapy, Henggeler, Schoenwald, Borduin, Rowland, & Cunningham, 1998; functional family therapy, Alexander et al., 1998) have demonstrated records of success at reducing future offending with delinquent adolescents. This would seem to indicate that family functioning is important not only etiologically, but also therapeutically.

A third general conclusion from the longitudinal research is that children who start committing serious offenses at a young age are probably qualitatively different from those adolescents who get in trouble initially at an older age. Age of onset of a criminal career has been shown consistently to be predictive of continued involvement in adult crime (Blumstein et al., 1986; Piquero et al., 2003). In addition, work on the trajectories of offending over adolescence and early adulthood indicate that there may be two oftentimes distinct groups of offenders, i.e., life course persistent and adolescent limited, who follow different patterns of offending over time and who may have different risk factors that precipitate their involvement in offending (Nagin, Farrington, & Moffitt, 1995). It is thought that the life-course-persistent offenders start younger and continue into adult crime because of factors related to their general cognitive and social deficits. Adolescent-limited offenders, on the other hand, engage in criminal activity during adolescence as part of their involvement with social groups that promote such behavior. This group is then presumed to desist from this behavior as their social and developmental demands shift in late adolescence.

A final conclusion that can be gleaned from longitudinal work is the importance of an adolescent's connections to his/her community and social world (Laub & Sampson, 2001). In assessing adolescents for the likelihood of future offending or violence, professionals often look for intrapsychic indicators of future problems. The primary task is often seen as determining how the constellation of traits or personal characteristics observed will dictate the level of future offending or violence. Based on the findings from longitudinal studies, however, considering the social contexts that an adolescent is likely to experience is probably as, or more, useful in assessing risk.

Any individual strengths or problems that an adolescent has operate in a social context, and these contexts interact with individual characteristics to shift the likelihood of a positive or negative outcome significantly. A long history of research has demonstrated the overall impact of neighborhood disorganization and lack of informal social control on aggregate rates of adolescent offending (Sampson, Raudenbush, & Earls, 1997; Shaw, 1929). Recent work has also shown the effects of changes in neighborhood on patterns of offending in individual adolescents' lives, with movement to "better" neighborhoods increasing property offenses for a period, but decreasing violent crime over time (Ludwig, Duncan, & Hirschfield, 2001). In addition, low attachment and commitment to school (Cernkovich & Giordano, 2001), involvement with antisocial peers (Hawkins et al., 1998), and large amounts of unstructured time (Horney, Osgood, & Marshall, 1995) appear to increase the likelihood of continued antisocial activity. Gang involvement in particular has been shown to be a strong indicator of more frequent and more serious offending in adolescence (Thornberry, Krohn, Lizotte, & Chard-Wierschem, 1993).

The broad point is that one of the primary tasks of adolescence is "fitting in" as part of a social group and into a social role. Risk for future reoffending is thus intimately linked to where an adolescent decides to fit in over time and to the opportunities for antisocial activity in the settings encountered (Mulvey et al., 2004). To be complete, a risk assessment has to consider these factors as a major component of figuring out if, how, and why an adolescent might keep reoffending or being violent.

General Principles That Might Help Improve Risk Assessment

So far, I have reviewed three ways that risk assessment is implemented in the juvenile justice system. First, at the broad level of statutes, classes of juvenile offenders are created for differential processing and potentially greater punishments. Second, administrative guidelines regarding incarceration, release, or placement are established, using actuarial formulae based mainly on the presence of indicators related to continued offending. Finally, clinical and court professionals make individualized judgments about risk, combining information about the adolescent's characteristics and history and alternatives available to the court. Each of these activities derives from some implicit and explicit notions about the most appropriate and powerful factors to consider when assessing risk. I have reviewed the validity of some of the general ideas behind these approaches.

Improving these approaches to risk assessment presents new challenges, and it seems that these will require something beyond just a more comprehensive list of empirically validated risk indicators. Indeed, it could be argued that the influences that put an adolescent at higher risk for future offending or violence have been known for some time and that the general contours of what constitutes risk factors for adolescent offenders will change only marginally with increased research. Similar personal, family, peer, and community risk indicators have all been found repeatedly. Depending on what is put into the equation, the relative weights of different indicators shift, but the same factors keep emerging with about the same overall explanatory power in one research project after another. Expanding the content of the list of risk factors or the intricacy of the models about how they relate to each other is not likely to yield much in the way of improved risk assessment.

Broader conceptualizations of the ideas of risk and risk assessment might be needed to improve this practice in juvenile justice. Instead of trying to refine the methods for combining known risk indicators, we may have to think about alternative ways of structuring the basic task. Examining research across other areas of antisocial behavior as well as the broad trends in the research on adolescence can be helpful in this search for alternative models. This section outlines three potentially relevant issues.

Cumulative Risk Versus Specific Risk

Considerable research has shown concurrent associations between different antisocial behaviors in adolescence (Loeber, Farrington, Stouthamer-Loeber, & Van Kammen, 1998). Drinking, school problems, social adjustment problems, and self-reported delinquency regularly occur together. This consistent set of associations among antisocial behaviors has limited the ability of any one type of behavior to serve as a clear precursor of another sort of antisocial behavior. Although there are some general trends about the order of onset of certain antisocial behaviors (e.g., it is likely that an adolescent will shoplift before he/she will commit an armed robbery), antisocial behaviors are more mottled than clearly patterned across adolescence. This observation has prompted some researchers to think that the particular behaviors in question might best be investigated as a "constellation" of behaviors, rather than as distinct entities (Jessor, 1992).

Many antisocial behaviors also have the same types of risk indicators associated with them. The list of conditions or situations that increase risk for mental health problems, self-reported delinquency, or other antisocial behaviors overlap greatly. Living with parents who have a history of antisocial behavior themselves in a bad neighborhood, along with significant cognitive processing difficulties and early disruptive behavior, is one fairly common recipe producing a variety of troubling behaviors in adolescence, including criminal offending. Because of the many ways that risks and individual capacities can play out in an adolescent's life, there is little specificity between particular risk indicators and outcome behaviors. Having a particular risk indicator (or a particular combination of risk indicators) does not invariably produce a particular outcome behavior.

This simple regularity has a straightforward implication for structuring risk assessment and identification strategies. It makes the notion of focusing on children or adolescents with a few particular risk indicators as being at "high risk" for developing a particular later problem seem a bit myopic and inefficient. Since risk seems to play out in many ways in adolescent development, identifying adolescents with only one or two readily identifiable risk indicators will produce a pool of adolescents, some reasonably large proportion of whom will necessarily not be those at the highest likelihood for a negative outcome. Adolescent males without father figures, for example, are not all destined to have tumultuous teen years. The more the definition of risk is limited to a few indicators, the more likely it is to include adolescents who are not at high levels of overall risk.

Thinking about the total risk faced by a child or adolescent (i.e., the cumulative risk), rather than the particular form of that risk, may be most productive for identifying groups for intervention. This approach can still be taken with a set of risk factors that are particularly powerful for some outcome (such as reoffending), but the idea is to avoid worrying about whether an adolescent has one of a small set of risk indicators. It is instead to determine how many of a given set of indicators an individual adolescent faces. Identifying those with the most overall risk is a generally sounder way to proceed than picking those who might fit a popularized stereotype of those adolescents destined to continue in criminal offending (e.g., adolescents who have school difficulties and problems at home).

Risk Markers Versus Risk Factors

The old adage that "correlation is not causation" is often forgotten in risk research with juvenile offenders and other populations. The co-occurrence of two events (say X and Y) can be the result of one event "causing" the other or the product of other processes affecting the likelihood of these events occurring together (either in time or in the same types of cases). It may be that (a) X causes Y, (b) Y causes X, and we just have not taken sufficiently fine-grained observations to establish the causal order of these events, (c) there is a reciprocal relationship between the two where an increase in either X or Y corresponds to an increase in the other, or (d) the relationship between the two is spurious and simply indicative of some other underlying process that raises the likelihood of both events occurring simultaneously. The implication of this logic is that the mere presence of associated events or conditions does not mean that a powerful risk indicator has been identified.

This point was highlighted in an article by Helena Kraemer and her colleagues (Kraemer et al., 1997), which introduced the useful distinction between *risk markers* and *risk factors*. The basic argument is that researchers and practitioners should be more careful about whether something seems to have a causal relationship with a negative outcome or whether it simply seems to occur in close temporal proximity to that outcome. This distinction is important because it implies different strategies for assessing risk and undertaking interventions designed to reduce the occurrence or intensity of antisocial behavior.

If a risk indicator is a *risk marker*, its occurrence is associated with and may even precede offending. In short, it co-occurs regularly with the antisocial behavior of interest and may be promoted by some of the same influences that promote that antisocial behavior. If it is a *risk factor*, there is a causal link between the identified risk indicator and the antisocial behavior, with a reduction in the occurrence of the risk indicator reducing the likelihood of the antisocial behavior. A risk indicator is a risk factor for antisocial behavior if its occurrence temporally precedes the antisocial behavior and the occurrence of the risk indicator can be shown to increase the likelihood of the antisocial behavior occurring.

Risk markers are obviously very valuable for the identification of high risk groups. Focusing prevention efforts on groups likely to develop later problems makes good sense. Deciding how to intervene, however, rests largely on the identification of risk factors. Those responsible for interventions (and the assessments that set the stage for them) need to decide what aspects of functioning to focus on with this high-risk group. Interventions obviously should be focused on causal and changeable risk factors to maximize impact.

Unfortunately, identifying risk factors is not a straightforward task. Making a claim that a risk indicator is indeed a risk factor, rather than a risk marker, requires a substantial body of information beyond the demonstration of an association. It is necessary to have empirical results indicating that reduction in the risk indicator produces substantial reduction in the antisocial behavior. At this point in the development of risk research on adolescent offending and violence, though, we are still short of demonstrating that we have found a large number of powerful risk factors for antisocial behavior. We have considerable convergence on the associations between certain risk indicators (e.g., parental supervision, age of onset of problem behavior) and serious antisocial behavior, but there is limited information about whether these risk indicators are pivotal points for intervention whose reduction substantially reduces the likelihood of later antisocial behavior. Such evidence requires careful longitudinal work examining interventions as well as carefully conceptualized tests of specific types of possible interventions. The amount of work that meets these criteria is relatively small (Satcher, 2001).

For the purposes of risk assessment per se, the identification and assessment of risk markers is probably adequate. Those adolescents with the presence of risk markers that regularly precede reoffending or violence are at more "risk" for these subsequent behaviors. If, however, one is pursuing risk assessment with an eye toward recommendations for intervention, this distinction between risk markers and risk factors becomes crucial. Assessment of needs should focus on those risk indicators that, if changed, can reduce the likelihood of the negative outcome. Unfortunately, there is often little attempt to sort out risk markers from risk factors, and interventions are assumed to be useful if they are directed toward any risk indicator with a demonstrated association with the negative outcome.

Risk Status, Risk State, and Risk Management

Finally, it is worth noting that risk is not static; it has a dynamic quality. People are not at the same level of risk at all points in their lives or under every set of conditions that they might encounter. Antisocial activity is not the sole product of an internal propensity manifesting itself in a set of behaviors. Like other behaviors, it is some combination of individual proclivity and "environmental press" (Murray, 1938).

It is reasonable to assume, therefore, that risk for involvement in particular behaviors shifts over time, even for people who are at higher overall risk than others for involvement in antisocial behavior. Individuals may be in a high *risk status* group (i.e., the likelihood of involvement in antisocial activity is higher for people like them than it is for the rest of the reference group), but their likelihood of involvement in antisocial activities may still shift considerably over time, depending on the situations that confront them. This fluctuation in the likelihood of engaging in antisocial behavior over time has been referred to as change in *risk state* (Mulvey & Lidz, 1995, 1998), and the importance of considering these changes in managing risk for violence has been emphasized (Heilbrun, 1997).

This general point is particularly relevant when considering risk assessment in juvenile offenders, since change is a fundamental aspect of adolescence. Whether criminally active or not, individuals undergo marked physiological, psychosocial, and cognitive developmental changes during middle and late adolescence that can have an effect on their antisocial behavior (Mulvey et al., 2004). Some of these changes during this period are rather predictable and positive, often increasing the capacity for making sound judgments (e.g., a reduction in impulsivity). In addition, individuals may attain skills and competencies during middle and late adolescence that prepare them for the challenge of entering the workforce or living independently. Other changes, unfortunately, may mark the beginning of enduring limitations for that individual (e.g., the onset of a serious mental disorder during late adolescence). Finally, adolescents often change their social contexts, confronting and mastering new dimensions of identity. Moving out of the house, establishing more stable romantic relationships, and reconstructing peer networks are all changes that occur with considerable frequency for adolescents and have a high likelihood of affecting involvement in antisocial activity.

One obvious corollary of this simple observation is that evaluating risk, whether for purposes of policy or practice, requires a consideration of the developmental stage and social context of the adolescent at issue. Indicators of risk change over the course of childhood and adolescence because (a) the same behaviors do not mean the same things when done by individuals of different ages and (b) key developmental challenges change with age. As a result of developmental changes, the normative quality of certain troublesome behaviors at particular ages has to be considered in assessing that behavior as a risk indicator. Drinking at age 12, for instance, is a much more powerful indicator of risk than drinking at age 17 (Satcher, 2001). Along the same lines, having certain skills and capacities to address the next developmental challenge is a critical consideration. For example, having appropriate job-related behaviors is more important for success at age 18 than it is at age 14.

Despite this apparent truism, a large number of policies or programs conceptualize risk as invariant with age. Certainly there are characteristics of an adolescent that might increase risk rather robustly across different ages (e.g., the presence of a serious learning disorder). However, there are also *age-specific risks*—situations in which the behavior or condition might contribute very differently to risk, depending on the age of the child (Cicchetti & Cohen, 1995). Aggressiveness with peers, while a rather consistent indicator of trouble, appears to be a much stronger marker for continued aggression when it happens in boys 9–11 years of age than when it emerges later in adolescence, while disorganized neighborhoods are more influential with older rather than younger adolescents (Thornberry & Krohn, 2003). In thinking about identifying groups of adolescents at highest risk for reoffending or in assessing individual adolescents regarding their level of likely risk for reoffending, it is important to choose indicators of risk that are particularly relevant for different age groups. Like shirts, what fits a 13-year-old doesn't necessarily fit a 16-year-old.

The implications of this simple observation are rather far reaching. If one were to take seriously the idea that risk changes substantially with age and with context, then risk/need assessment for juvenile offenders would necessarily be much more differentiated than it is currently. At the policy level, this would argue for blended sentences that reassess the most serious adolescent offenders when they are likely to be punished in the adult system (Redding & Howell, 2000). Regarding actuarial risk assessments and professional discretion, there would be different domains of factors considered for particular age groups. This would also seem to argue that risk should be reassessed periodically for youth who have long-term involvement with the juvenile justice system.

Conclusion

The idea of risk assessment is a consistent undercurrent in juvenile justice policy and practice. As long as the juvenile justice system has the responsibility for ensuring public safety as one of its main missions, policy-makers and practitioners in this area cannot escape their responsibilities to sort adolescent offenders by their likelihood of doing continued community harm. Doing this more effectively requires both consideration of whether we are currently doing it well and a search for some leads from other areas about how to improve.

As we have seen above, building risk assessment into statutory schemes is inherently limited. Classifications that are acceptable for legal purposes are necessarily rather poor at identifying a homogeneous group of high-risk adolescents. At the same time, there has been considerable progress in the development of actuarial instruments for assessing risk and needs. These instruments need to be tested, revised, and implemented with an eye toward making them work well given the conditions in local juvenile justice systems. Better clinical strategies for assessing risk will require the integration of a developmental perspective to produce thoughtful assessment approaches.

In the larger picture, two types of information would be particularly useful for improving the risk assessment of juvenile offenders. First, it would be useful to have more information about the patterns of desistance in serious adolescent offenders. Knowing if there are distinct, identifiable pathways out of involvement with juvenile crime rather than just likelihoods of involvement in future crime or violence would refine our current state of knowledge. Ideally, identifying the characteristics of the adolescents who progress along each of these pathways could eventually reframe the risk assessment enterprise.

Identifying distinguishable pathways out of the juvenile justice system would contribute to risk assessment by allowing justice professionals and clinicians to think in terms of the factors related to different classes of offenders (e.g., a high-frequency, continuing offender or a likely desister by age 20), rather than just the likelihood of future crime or violence. Currently, assessing risk in serious adolescent offenders is generally a matter of gauging whether the severity of the present offense and the history of prior treatment warrants institutional placement, and professionals and locales vary widely in their sophistication regarding this task. Having more knowledge about the types of factors that might differentiate among serious offenders, once initially identified, could focus practice and planning in this area.

Second, it would be useful to know the impacts of the strategies used most commonly with these high-risk offenders. Comparisons of different types of interventions (e.g., secure confinement vs. community supervision) or sanctions (e.g., longer-term vs. shorter-term confinement) would be valuable for guiding court dispositional practices. Judges and probation officers are often faced with decisions about allocating scarce court resources with little empirical guidance about when these particular interventions or sanctions will be most effective for reducing risk. Empirical information about the optimal payoff for investment with particular types of offenders could provide a rational structure for these decisions.

The types of information described above are potentially useful both for policy purposes and for improving the individualized assessments of serious adolescent offenders. Such data would provide policy audiences with evidence about the utility of different sanctioning and processing options, a topic that is hotly debated in the midst of today's trend toward a more retributive juvenile justice process. For practitioners, this information should provide a richer base of information to consider in risk assessments, as well as what signs to monitor or assess on an ongoing basis with serious adolescent offenders.

No research can provide a dispositive answer to the question of how much risk to take with serious offenders or what "should be done with" them. This is a complex sociopolitical issue beyond the scope of any empirical test. Future work can, however, enrich the field's understanding of how sanctions and developmental events exert influences and interact in the lives of these adolescents. A more refined picture of this sort would be a large step forward toward debate and practice based more on reason than rhetoric.

References

Alexander, J. F., Barton, C., Gordon, D., Grotpeter, J., Hansson, K., Harrison, R., et al. (1998). *Blueprints for violence prevention, book three: Functional family therapy.* Boulder: University of Colorado, Center for the Study and Prevention of Violence.

Andrews, D. A., & Bonta, J. (1995). *Level of service inventory–revised.* Toronto: Multi-Health Systems.

Anne E. Casey Foundation, Juvenile Detention Alternatives Initiative. (2004). Retrieved February 24, 2004, from www.aecf.org

Baird, S. C. (1984). *Classification of juveniles in corrections: A model systems approach.* Madison, WI: National Council on Crime and Delinquency.

Baird, S. C. (1991). *Validating risk assessment instruments used in community corrections.* Madison, WI: National Council on Crime and Delinquency.

Barnoski, R. (2002). Monitoring vital signs: Integrating a standardized assessment into Washington state's juvenile justice system. In R. Corrado, R. Roesch, S. Hart, &

J. Gierowski (Eds.), *Multi-problem violent youth: A foundation for comparative research on needs, interventions, and outcomes* (pp. 219–231). Washington, DC: IOS Press.

Blumstein, A., Cohen, J., Roth, J., & Visher, C. (Eds.) (1986). *Criminal careers and "career criminals."* Washington, DC: National Academy Press.

Borum, R., Bartel, P., & Forth, A. (2002). *Manual for the Structured Assessment of Violence Risk in Youth (SAVRY)*. Tampa, FL: University of South Florida.

Brame, R., Mulvey, E. P., & Piquero, A. (2001). On the development of different kinds of criminal activity. *Sociological Methods and Research, 29*, 319–341.

Broidy, L. M., Nagin, D., S., Tremblay, R. E., Bates, J. E., Brame, R., Kenneth, A., et al. (2003). Developmental trajectories of childhood disruptive behaviors and adolescent delinquency: A six-site, cross-national study. *Developmental Psychology, 39*, 222–245.

Cernkovich, S. A., & Giordano, P. C. (2001). Stability and change in antisocial behavior: The transition from adolescence to early adulthood. *Criminology, 39*, 371–410.

Cicchetti, D., & Cohen, D. (Eds.). (1995). *Developmental psychopathology, Vol. 1: Theory and methods*. London: Wiley.

Copas, J. B., & Tarling, R. (1986). Accuracy of prediction models. In A. Blumstein, J. Cohen, J. A. Roth, & C. A. Visher (Eds.), *Criminal careers and "career criminals"* (Vol. II, pp. 291–313). Washington, DC: National Academy Press.

Cottle, C. C., Lee, R. J., & Heilbrun, K. (2001). The prediction of criminal recidivism in juveniles: A meta-analysis. *Criminal Justice and Behavior, 28*, 367–394.

Dawes, R. M. (1979). The robust beauty of improper linear models in decision making. *American Psychologist, 3*, 571–582.

Dembo, R., Turner, G., Schmeidler, J., Sue, C. C., Borden, P., & Manning, D. (1996). Development and evaluation of a classification of high risk youths entering a juvenile assessment center. *Substance Use and Misuse, 31*, 303–322.

Edens, J. F, Skeem, J. L, Cruise, K. R, & Cauffman, E. (2001). Assessment of "juvenile psychopathy" and its association with violence: A critical review. *Behavioral Sciences and the Law, 19*, 53–80.

Elliott, D. S. (1994). Serious violent offenders: Onset, developmental course, and termination. The American Society of Criminology 1993 presidential address. *Criminology, 32*, 1–21.

Fagan, J., & Zimring, F. (Eds.) (2000). *The changing borders of juvenile justice*. Chicago: University of Chicago Press.

Farrington, D., Snyder, H., & Finnegan, T. (1988). Specialization in juvenile court careers. *Criminology, 26*, 461–487.

Feld, B. (1999). *Bad kids: Race and the transformation of juvenile court*. New York: Oxford University Press.

Feld, B. (2000). Legislative exclusion of offenses from juvenile court jurisdiction: A history and critique. In J. Fagan & F. Zimring, *The changing borders of juvenile justice* (pp. 83–144). Chicago: University of Chicago Press.

Gambrill, E., & Schlonsky, A. (2000). Risk assessment in context. *Children and Youth Services Review, 22*, 813–837.

Griffin, P. (1998). Trying juveniles as adults in criminal court: An analysis of state transfer provisions. Washington, DC: U.S. Department of Justice, Office of Justice Programs, Office of Juvenile Justice and Delinquency Prevention.

Grisso, T. (1998). *Forensic assessment of juveniles*. Sarasota, FL: Professional Resource Press.

Guarino-Ghezzi, S., & Loughran, E. (1997). *Balancing juvenile justice*. New Brunswick, NJ: Transaction.

Hawkins, J. D., Herrenkohl, T., Farrington, D. P., Brewer, D., Catalano, R. F., & Harachi, T. W. (1998). A review of predictors of youth violence. In R. Loeber & D. P. Farrington (Eds.), *Serious and violent juvenile offenders: Risk factors and successful interventions* (pp. 106–146). Thousand Oaks, CA: Sage.

Heilbrun, K. (1997). Prediction versus management models relevant to risk assessment: The importance of legal decision-making context. *Law and Human Behavior, 21,* 347–359.

Heilbrun, K., Leheny, C., Thomas, L., & Huneycutt, D. (1997). A national survey of U.S. statutes on juvenile transfer: Implications for policy and practice. *Behavioral Sciences and the Law, 15,* 125–149.

Henggeler, S. W., Schoenwald, S. K., Borduin, C. M., Rowland, M. D., & Cunningham, P. B. (1998). *Multisystemic treatment of antisocial behavior in children and adolescents.* New York: Guilford Press.

Hoge, R., & Andrews, D. A. (1996). *Assessing the youthful offender: Issues and techniques.* New York: Plenum.

Hoge, R., & Andrews, D. A. (2002). *The Youth Level of Service/Case Management Inventory (YLS/CMI) user's manual.* North Tonawanda, NY: Multi-Health Systems.

Horney, J., Osgood, D. W., & Marshall, I. H. (1995). Criminal careers in the short-term: Intra-individual variability in crime and its relation to local life circumstances. *American Sociological Review, 60,* 655–673.

Jessor, R. (1992). Risk behavior in adolescence: A psychosocial framework for understanding and action. *Developmental Review, 12,* 374–390.

Klein, M. (1984). Offence specialization and versatility among juveniles. *British Journal of Criminology, 24,* 185–194.

Kraemer, H., Kazdin, A., Offord, D., Kessler, R., Jensen, P., & Kupfer, D. (1997). Coming to terms with the terms of risk. *Archives of General Psychiatry, 54,* 337–343.

Krysik, J., & LeCroy, C. W. (2002). The empirical validation of an instrument to predict risk of recidivism among juvenile offenders. *Research on Social Work Practice, 12,* 71–81.

Laub, J., & Sampson, R. (2001). Understanding desistance from crime. In M. Tonry (Ed.), *Crime and justice: A review of research* (Vol. 28, pp. 1–69). Chicago: University of Chicago Press.

LeBlanc, M. (1998). Screening of serious and violent juvenile offenders. In R. Loeber & D. P. Farrington (Eds.), *Serious and violent offenders: Risk factors and successful interventions* (pp. 167–193). Thousand Oaks, CA: Sage.

Loeber, R., & Farrington, D. (Eds.). (1998). *Serious and violent juvenile offenders: Risk factors and successful interventions.* Thousand Oaks, CA: Sage.

Loeber, R., Farrington, D. P., Stouthamer-Loeber, M., Moffitt, T. E., & Caspi, A. (2001). The development of male offending: Key findings from the first decade of the Pittsburgh Youth Study. In R. Bull (Ed.), *Children and the law: The essential readings. Essential readings in developmental psychology* (pp. 336–378). Malden, MA: Blackwell.

Loeber, R., Farrington, D. P., Stouthamer-Loeber, M., & Van Kammen, W. B. (1998). Multiple risk factors for multiproblem boys: Co-occurrence of delinquency, substance use, attention deficit, conduct problems, physical aggression, covert behavior, depressed mood, and shy/withdrawn behavior. In R. Jessor (Ed.), *New perspectives on adolescent risk behavior* (pp. 90–149). Cambridge: Cambridge University Press.

Ludwig, J., Duncan, G. J., & Hirschfield, P. (2001). Urban poverty and juvenile crime: Evidence from a randomized housing-mobility experiment. *Quarterly Journal of Economics, 116,* 665–679.

Masten, A., & Coatsworth, J. (1998). The development of competence in favorable and unfavorable environments: Lessons from research on successful children. *American Psychologist*, 53, 205–220.

Meehl, P. (1954). *Clinical vs. statistical prediction: A theoretical analysis and a review of the evidence*. Minneapolis: University of Minnesota Press.

Melton, G., Petrila, J., Poythress, N., & Slobogin, C. (1997). *Psychological evaluations for the courts: A handbook for mental health professionals and lawyers* (2nd ed.). New York: Guilford Press.

Mulvey, E., & Lidz, C. (1984). Clinical considerations in the prediction of dangerousness in mental patients. *Clinical Psychology Review*, 4, 379–401.

Mulvey, E., & Lidz, C. (1995). Conditional prediction: A model for research on dangerousness to others in a new era. *International Journal of Law and Psychiatry*, 18, 117–143.

Mulvey, E., & Lidz, C. (1998). The clinical prediction of violence as a conditional judgment. *Social Psychiatry and Psychiatric Epidemiology*, 33, 107–113.

Mulvey, E., Steinberg, L., Fagan, J., Cauffman, E., Piquero, A., Chassin, L., et al. (2004). Theory and research on desistance from antisocial activity among serious juvenile offenders. *Youth Violence and Juvenile Justice: An Interdisciplinary Journal*, 2, 213–236.

Murray, H. A. (1938). *Explorations in personality*. New York: Oxford University Press.

Nagin, D., Farrington, D., & Moffitt, T. (1995). Life course trajectories of different types of offenders. *Criminology*, 33, 111–139.

Office of Juvenile Justice and Delinquency Prevention. (1995). *Guide for implementing the comprehensive strategy for serious, violent, and chronic juvenile offenders*. Washington, DC: Department of Justice, Office of Juvenile Justice and Delinquency Prevention.

Packer, H. (1968). *The limits of the criminal sanction*. Stanford, CA: Stanford University Press.

Pasternoster, R. (1989). Absolute and restrictive deterrence in a panel of youth: Explaining the onset, persistence/desistance, and frequency of offending. *Social Problems*, 36, 289–309.

Piquero, A., Blumstein, A., Brame, R., Haapanen, R., Mulvey, E., & Nagin, D. (2001). Assessing the impact of exposure time and incapacitation on longitudinal trajectories of criminal offending. *Journal of Adolescent Research*, 16, 54–74.

Piquero, A., Farrington, D., & Blumstein, A. (2003). The criminal career paradigm. In M. Tonry (Ed.), *Crime and Justice: A review of research*, 30. Chicago: University of Chicago Press.

Redding, R. (1997). Juveniles transferred to criminal court: Legal reform proposals based on social science research. *Utah Law Review*, 3, 709–763.

Redding, R. (2000). Deterrence effects of transfer laws. *Juvenile justice fact sheet*. Charlottesville, VA: University of Virginia, Institute of Law, Psychiatry, and Public Policy.

Redding, R., & Howell, J. (2000). Blended sentencing in American juvenile courts. In J. Fagan & F. Zimring (Eds.), *The changing borders of juvenile justice* (pp. 145–180). Chicago: University of Chicago Press.

Reppucci, N. D., Fried, C. S, & Schmidt, M. G. (2002). Youth violence: Risk and protective factors. In R. Corrado, R. Roesch, S. Hart, & J. Gierowski (Eds.), *Multi-problem violent youth: A foundation for comparative research on needs, interventions and outcomes* (pp. 3–22). Amsterdam: IOS Press.

Sampson, R., Raudenbush, S., & Earls, F. (1997). Neighborhoods and violent crime: A multilevel study of collective efficacy. *Science*, 277, 918–924.

Satcher, D. (2001). *Youth violence: A report of the Surgeon General*. Washington, DC: Office of the Surgeon General. Retrieved February 20, 2004, from http://www. surgeongeneral.gov/library/youthviolence/

Schirali, V., & Ziedenberg, J. (2002). *Reducing disproportionate minority confinement: The Multnomah County Oregon success story and its implications*. San Francisco: Center on Juvenile and Criminal Justice.

Schneider, A. L., & Ervin, L. (1990). Specific deterrence, rational choice, and decision heuristics: Applications in juvenile justice. *Social Science Quarterly, 71*, 585–601.

Scott, E., & Grisso, T. (1997). The evolution of adolescence: A developmental perspective on juvenile justice reform. *Journal of Criminal Law and Criminology, 88*, 137–189.

Shaw, C. (1929). *Delinquency areas*. Chicago: University of Chicago Press.

Snyder, H. (1998). Serious, violent and chronic juvenile offenders—an assessment of the extent of and trends in officially recognized serious criminal behavior in a delinquent population. In R. Loeber & D. Farrington (Eds.), *Serious and violent juvenile offenders: Risk factors and successful interventions* (pp. 428–444). Thousand Oaks, CA: Sage.

Steinberg, L., & Scott, E. (2003). Less guilty by reason of adolescence: Developmental immaturity, diminished responsibility, and the juvenile death penalty. *American Psychologist, 58*, 1009–1018.

Thornberry, T., & Krohn, M. (2003). *Taking stock of delinquency: An overview of findings from contemporary longitudinal studies*. New York: Kluwer.

Thornberry, T. P., Krohn, M. D., Lizotte, A. J., & Chard-Wierschem, D. (1993). The role of juvenile gangs in facilitating delinquent behavior. *Journal of Research in Crime and Delinquency, 30*, 55–87.

Tolan, P., & Gorman-Smith, D. (1998). Development of serious and violent offending careers. In R. Loeber & D. Farrington (Eds.), *Serious and violent juvenile offenders: Risk factors and successful interventions* (pp. 68–85). Thousand Oaks, CA: Sage.

Wiebush, R. G., Baird, C., Krisberg, B., & Onek, D. (1995). Risk assessment and classification for serious, violent, and chronic juvenile offenders. In J. C. Howell, B. Krisberg, J. Hawkins, & J. Wilson (Eds.), *Sourcebook on serious, violent, and chronic offenders* (pp. 171–212). Thousand Oaks, CA: Sage.

11

RICHARD E. REDDING AND BARBARA MROZOSKI

Adjudicatory and Dispositional Decision Making in Juvenile Justice

Juvenile court judges and others working in the juvenile justice system have a wide variety of dispositional and sentencing options available for the juvenile offenders under their jurisdiction. For serious, violent, or chronic offenders, these options increasingly involve transferring juveniles from juvenile court for trial and sentencing in the criminal court or blended juvenile and adult sentences. This chapter provides an overview of the adjudicatory and dispositional options available for handling juvenile offenders in the juvenile and criminal justice systems. The limited research on adjudicatory and dispositional decision making is also reviewed, and directions for future law and policy development are proposed.

Juvenile Court Adjudications and Dispositions

A juvenile may be brought to the juvenile court by parents, other adults, or police (who handle about 25% of cases informally simply by warning and releasing the juvenile; Federal Bureau of Investigations, 1997). When a juvenile is brought to the juvenile court, court intake workers (also called juvenile probation officers) conduct an initial intake screening to determine, usually in consultation with the local prosecutor, whether to file a petition against the juvenile in juvenile court, resulting in an adjudicatory hearing before the judge. State statutes define the types of cases in which juvenile court intake workers have such discretion. Typically, they are required to file a petition (provided there is sufficient evidence) when the alleged offense is a serious one. In some states, however, intake workers have no such discretion and must refer all criminal offenses to the local prosecutor, who then decides whether to file charges (Binder, Geis, & Bruce, 2001). Juvenile court intake units and prosecutors differ on how they make their charging decisions. Some largely comply with the wishes of the victim, while others conduct a needs assessment to determine the level of risk and the juvenile's need for services (Rubin, 2003). Theft, assault, and drug violations are the most common offenses resulting in court referral (Stahl, 1999). National data indicate that a court petition is filed in about 57% of cases, while 43% are handled through informal probation (in which the juvenile agrees to probation in lieu of court adjudication), case dismissal, or diversion (Puzzanchera, 2000).

Roughly 60% of cases referred to the juvenile court for adjudication result in a finding of delinquency by the judge (Stahl, 1999), thus giving the court jurisdiction to intervene and make dispositional decisions (Elrod & Ryder, 1999). The juvenile then moves to the sentencing phase, called the dispositional hearing. Dispositional hearings can be complex, as they are designed to promote an individualized disposition best suited to the child's needs while considering available resources and programs and the need to ensure community protection. "[I]t is an adversarial proceedings with a mixture of recommendations by probation and social workers; reports of social and academic histories; and interactions within the court among the legal participants, the offender and his or her family, probation staff, and, perhaps, psychologists and social workers" (Binder et al., 2001, p. 286). Dispositional plans are often tailored to the individual. This usually includes consideration of a detailed social history report prepared by the court intake staff. There is little research on the role that these social histories play in dispositional decision making, although they appear to substantially influence judges' decisions.

Elrod and Ryder (1999) list the 10 dispositional alternatives commonly available to juvenile courts: (a) probation in the juvenile's own home; (b) probation with placement in the home of a relative or a foster home; (c) probation with restitution to victims and/or the community; (d) house arrest or other intensive probation; (e) detention followed by probation; (f) placement in a private institution; (g) placement in a boot camp for about 30 to 300 days; see Zaehringer, 1998; (h) placement in a state facility under commitment laws; (i) placement in a private correctional facility; and (j) some combination of these alternatives. Probation, which is the disposition in 54% of juvenile cases, is the most common sanction (Snyder & Sickmund, 1999). But residential placements (e.g., juvenile correctional facility, boot camp, drug treatment facility, group home) are becoming more common, increasing 51% between 1987 and 1996. The cases most likely to result in residential placement are those involving serious person offenses, such as homicide, rape, robbery, or aggravated assault (Snyder & Sickmund, 1999).

Diversion programs (see Chapin & Griffin, ch. 8 in this volume) that promote alternatives to court referral for juvenile offenders are another popular alternative. Diversion has a variety of forms, such as informal case handling by law enforcement or court referral to outside programs. Diversionary programs have been developed all over the country, though they are not found in all jurisdictions, often due to lack of resources. Many offer specialized treatment and rehabilitation services for specific populations, such as family crisis intervention programs, individual and family counseling programs combined with educational, employment, and recreational services, and programs involving restitution and community service.

Research on the efficacy of diversion programs has been decidedly mixed (see Chapin & Griffin, ch. 8). Reviewing a number of diversion studies, Elrod and Ryder (1999) concluded that "although some evaluation studies indicate that diversion programs can reduce recidivism or are at least as effective as formal processing at reducing recidivism, other studies have found that some diversion programs are associated with higher levels of subsequent offending" (p. 173). Ironically, some diversion programs may have a net-widening effect, since they target youth that otherwise may have been "left alone" entirely by the justice and social services systems (Elrod & Ryder, 1999).

Judges have wide discretion when determining the disposition and are not bound by recommendations made by caseworkers, probation officers, or social workers (Senna & Siegel, 1992). Research shows that the severity of offense, prior record, and age of the offender are among the strongest factors influencing the severity of the disposition imposed (Campbell & Schmidt, 2000; Elrod & Ryder, 1999; Hoge, Andrews, & Leschied, 1995). Other important factors considered by court probation officers and judges include whether the parents will supervise the juvenile and participate in his rehabilitation, the level of family dysfunction, and whether the juvenile is attending school (Campbell & Schmidt, 2000; Horwitz & Wasserman, 1980; Sanborn, 1996). Several studies have found substantial agreement rates between probation or social worker recommendations and judges' dispositions (see Campbell & Schmidt, 2000), although the very limited available research on this point suggests caution in accepting it. In addition, judges' dispositional decision making is likely influenced by judicial philosophies toward juvenile offenders and the availability of local resources. This is illustrated by Mulvey and Reppucci's (1988) study, which found that mental health and juvenile court workers' judgments about juvenile offenders' amenability to treatment and the likely effectiveness of those treatments varied according to the level of resources locally available. Indeed, financial resources and program availabilities often affect judges' dispositional decisions. A juvenile may be more likely to avoid incarceration if there is facility overcrowding, for example (Brummer, 2002).

African American youth are overrepresented throughout all stages of the juvenile justice process and comprise a disproportionately high percentage of the juvenile offenders (about 40%) arrested each year (Redding & Arrigo, in press). Race (or factors correlating with race, such as socioeconomic status) may play a significant role in choice of disposition. Research findings are conflicting on whether juveniles' race influences decision making in the juvenile justice system (Bortner, Zatz, & Hawkins, 2000; Redding & Arrigo, in press), but the scholarly consensus is that there may be small effects of race throughout the process that have a cumulative impact on adjudicatory and dispositional outcomes, with the greatest effects likely occurring at the early states of justice system processing (arrest, juvenile court intake, and detention) (Redding & Arrigo, in press). There also appears to be emerging a scholarly consensus that the over-representation of minority youth in the juvenile justice system is so substantial (compared to any possible discriminatory effects) that it must in part reflect a real difference in offending patterns and rates for violent offenses among White versus African American youth (Redding & Arrigo, in press; Rutter, Giller, & Hagell, 1998). In turn, these differences in offending rates are linked to socioeconomic disadvantage and a constellation of interrelated family, peer, and neighborhood risk factors for delinquency more commonly found in African American communities (Redding & Arrigo, in press).

Moreover, prosecutorial and judicial decision making may exacerbate racial disparities through practices that focus on such risk factors as a way of identifying those youth who are less amenable to treatment. A Florida study, for example, found that harsher punishments were given to juveniles who came from single-parent homes lacking the support for parents to be actively involved in the child's court proceedings and rehabilitation (Bishop & Frazier, 1996). White and upper-class youth may be underrepresented in the juvenile justice system (relative to their rates of offending) because of their greater access to private mental health services and placements that divert them away from the justice system or correctional placements (Redding & Arrigo, in press). Minority youth are also more likely to be placed in secure detention facilities, while White youth tend to be housed in private facilities or diverted away from the juvenile justice system entirely (Snyder & Sickmund, 1999).

Graduated Sanctions

Juvenile justice systems have begun adopting integrated and standardized policies for determining dispositions, including largely age- and offense-based determinate and mandatory sentencing guidelines (Feld, 2003). Another important development is the U.S. Justice Department's Office of Juvenile Justice and Delinquency Prevention's (OJJDP) Comprehensive Strategy for Serious, Violent, and Chronic Juvenile Offenders (Wilson & Howell, 1995), which proposes a continuum of sanctions and services based on a juvenile's offense severity and offending history (see Wilson & Howell, 1995). The comprehensive strategy promotes the use of multiple interventions to address the multiple risk factors present across settings for a given youth. A needs assessment determines the presence and severity of problems in a particular juvenile's life. Risk and placement assessments are used to identify public safety and rehabilitation considerations. Consideration is always given to the important areas of substance abuse, family relationships, mental health needs, school problems, and peer relationships (Howell, 1997). The integrated assessment of these problem areas is necessary to ensure the proper treatment and level of restrictiveness tailored for the specific offender.

The goal of the comprehensive strategy is to improve the "juvenile justice response to delinquent offenders through a system of graduated sanctions and a continuum of treatment alternatives that includes immediate intervention, intermediate sanctions, and community-based corrections sanctions, incorporating restitution and community service when appropriate" (Wilson & Howell, 1995, p. 37). The program targets serious, violent, and chronic juvenile offenders, so that as offenses become more severe or repetitive, treatment and accountability sanctions become more progressively structured and intensive (Howell, 1997).

However, the comprehensive strategy also emphasizes early intervention for first-time offenders. First-time and nonserious repeat offenders receive immediate sanctions such as diversion, restitution, informal probation, or community service. But if the youth's first offense is serious or violent, intermediate sanctions may be warranted, including intensive supervision, substance abuse treatment, electronic monitoring, day treatment, community-based residential treatment, and brief stays in confinement. Implicitly, the strategy focuses on controlling the 4% of juvenile offenders who are the serious, violent, and chronic offenders, the 15% who are chronic offenders committing most of the serious juvenile offenses (Snyder, 1998), and those most likely to continue their offending in adulthood (see Moffitt, 1993). These offenders are often placed in secure confinement, although some community-based facilities may provide the intensive services needed.

In addition to providing continuum of service plans for individual offenders, the comprehensive strategy calls on communities to conduct a detailed assessment of the juvenile crime risk and protective factors present in their community, in order to determine needed prevention and intervention strategies. In 1996, OJJDP developed three pilot sites (Lee and Duval counties, FL; San Diego, CA) to implement and evaluate the comprehensive strategy (Coolbaugh & Hansel, 2000). The results demonstrated that implementation "enhanced community-wide understanding of prevention services and sanction options" and "expanded networking capacity and (resulted in) better coordination among agencies and service providers" (Coolbaugh & Hansel, 2000). The early success of these pilot programs has initiated additional studies in other states. A jurisdiction using this strategy will "examine its capacity to address the identified community risks and ensure that the right resources are available to each youth (and family) at the right time" (Coolbaugh & Hansel, 2000).

Transfer to Criminal Court: Adjudicating and Sentencing Juveniles as Adults

Statutes known as "transfer laws" (also called "waiver" or "certification" laws), which transfer juveniles from the juvenile court for trial and sentencing in adult criminal court, are found in every state and the District of Columbia (Heilbrun, Leheny, Thomas, & Huneycutt, 1997). The age at which juveniles can be transferred to the adult system varies across states, though most states will transfer those aged 14 and older (Beresford, 2000), and four states (Florida, Nevada, New York, and Pennsylvania) automatically transfer juveniles of any age who commit certain (usually violent) offenses. State laws usually fall into four broad categories of offenses for which juveniles of a certain age may be transferred: (a) any crime, (b) capital crimes and murder, (c) certain violent felonies, and (d) certain crimes committed by juveniles with prior records (Snyder & Sickmund, 1999). (For recent comprehensive lists of states' recent transfer statutes, listing statutory requirements, see Feld, 2000; Snyder & Sickmund, 1999; Steiner & Hemmens, 2003.)

There are three types of transfer laws: legislative transfer ("automatic transfer"), judicial-discretionary ("judicial transfer"), and prosecutorial-discretionary ("prosecutorial transfer"). Most states have two or three coexisting types of transfer laws. For example, 40 states and the District of Columbia have judicial as well as prosecutorial transfer statutes (with the prosecutorial statutes often applicable only to older and/or more serious offenders) (Sanborn, 2003).

Each type of transfer law defines the kind of juvenile offender eligible for transfer under the statute, specifying certain offenses and often minimum age criteria. Legislative transfer laws (currently in 31 states, see Steiner & Hemmens, 2003) require automatic transfer of a juvenile if statutory requirements are met. Generally, violent felonies such as murder, rape, kidnapping, and crimes committed with a firearm are automatically transferred to criminal court. The offender's age and previous offenses are also often determinative (Beresford, 2000). Judicial transfer laws vest discretion in juvenile court judges to decide, after the prosecution files a transfer motion, whether a juvenile should be transferred. Prosecutors file transfer motions in fewer than 5–10% of eligible cases (Dawson, 2000; Feld, 2000), and perhaps because of this selectivity, prosecutor's motions for transfer often are successful (Dawson, 2000). Prosecutorial transfer laws (currently available in 14 states and the District of Columbia; see Steiner & Hemmens, 2003) vest the discretion with prosecutors, allowing them to decide whether to file charges in juvenile or criminal court. Often, the same prosecutor who decides which charges to file also decides the court in which to file (DeFrances & Strom, 1997), and the prosecutor's decision is generally not subject to judicial review (Beresford, 2000).

Finally, some states also have a "reverse waiver," which can ameliorate overinclusive juvenile transfer laws. In a reverse waiver jurisdiction, the judge overseeing the case in criminal court, upon a motion of the defendant and after a hearing, has the discretion to issue an order to transfer the defendant back to the juvenile court (or to juvenile status for sentencing purposes) (Kole, 2001). The defendant, however, bears the burden of persuasion that the case should be transferred to juvenile court (Dawson, 2000).

As Sanborn (2003) points out, there is an inherent discretionary element in all transfer statutes, even "automatic" transfer statutes, since the prosecutor has the initial charging discretion as to whether to charge a greater or less serious offense (or not to charge at all). But considerably greater discretion, of course, is to be found in the judicial and prosecutorial transfer laws. In the 1966 case of *Kent v. United States*, the U.S. Supreme Court listed the eight discretionary criteria present in the District of Columbia's judicial transfer statute.[1] These criteria

---

1. The criteria were:

(a) The seriousness of the alleged offense to the community and whether the protection of the community requires waiver
(b) Whether the alleged offense was committed in an aggressive, violent, premeditated, or willful manner
(c) Whether the alleged offense was against persons or against property, greater weight being given to offenses against persons, especially if personal injury resulted

have subsequently been adopted and modified by many states in their discretionary transfer statutes, particularly in judicial transfer statutes (Redding, 1997). Judicial transfer statutes often require the judge to consider the (a) offender's treatment needs and amenability, (b) risk assessment of the likelihood of future offending, (c) offender's sophistication-maturity, (d) presence of mental retardation or mental illness, and (e) offense characteristics (Heilbrun et al., 1997). States vary on the extent to which they articulate such factors, but all states require consideration of the seriousness of the offense (and thus the need to protect the community); most consider the child's characteristics and the system's rehabilitative capacities as well. The juveniles' sophistication-maturity and amenability to treatment are not always required nowadays. Some statutes allow judges to consider such factors as they see fit, while others require that greater weight be given to certain factors. Many statutes include rebuttable presumptions of transfer for certain offense/juvenile age combinations that guide and constrain judicial discretion (Dawson, 2000).

In response to public and legislator demands to "get tough" on juvenile crime (see Heilbrun, Sevin Goldstein, & Redding, ch. 1 in this volume), states have revised their transfer laws or passed new laws that have reduced the minimum age for transfer, expanded the number of offenses for which a juvenile can be transferred, expanded prosecutorial power, and reduced or eliminated judicial discretion (see Redding, 1997; Steiner & Hemmens, 2003). In 1979, only 14 states had automatic transfer statutes, but by 1995 twenty-one states had such statutes, with 31 states having these laws by 2003 (Steiner & Hemmens, 2003). In addition to transfer statutes, 13 states have lowered the age at which juvenile court jurisdiction ends, to age 15 or 16 (Sanborn, 2003). In these states, everyone aged 15–16 or above is an adult for purposes of criminal prosecution.

Trying a juvenile in criminal court carries serious implications. In *State v. RGD* (1987), the Supreme Court of New Jersey observed, "Waiver to the adult court is the single most serious act the juvenile court can perform . . . . the child loses all protective and rehabilitative possibilities available" (p. 835). Al-

(d) The prosecutive merit of the complaint, i.e., whether there is evidence upon which a Grand Jury may be expected to return an indictment . . .

(e) The desirability of trial and disposition of the entire offense in one court when the juvenile's associate's in the alleged offense are adults who will be charged with a crime . . .

(f) The sophistication and maturity of the juvenile as determined by a consideration of his home, environmental situation, emotional attitude, and pattern of living

(g) The record and previous history of the juvenile, including previous contacts with the Youth Aid Division, other law enforcement agencies, juvenile courts, and other jurisdictions, prior periods of probation to this Court, or prior commitments to juvenile institutions

(h) The prospects for adequate protection of the public and the likelihood of reasonable rehabilitation of the juvenile (if he is found to have committed the alleged offense) by the use of procedures, services, and facilities currently available to the Juvenile Court

though in some states criminal courts can impose juvenile sentences, transferred juveniles are at risk of receiving criminal convictions and sentences, including lengthy incarceration in adult prisons. A felony conviction usually results in the loss of a number of civil rights and privileges (see Redding, 2003). Moreover, in 30 states, once convicted in criminal court, a juvenile will automatically be tried as an adult for any subsequent offenses (Sanborn, 2003). Due to the potentially onerous consequences for the juvenile, it is not surprising that transfer hearings often are time-consuming and hard fought (Dawson, 2000).

Studies have consistently found that the juvenile's age, the seriousness of the offense, the prior record, and the number of prior property offenses are the most significant predictors of transfer (Dawson, 1992; Fagan, Forst, & Vivona, 1987; Poulos & Orchowsky, 1994). Other common factors influencing transfer decision making include the treatment and rehabilitation prognoses, the facilities available for rehabilitation, and the community's attitude toward the offense (Strasburger, 1988). While some other studies have found substantial racial effects in the transfer process, even when controlling for prior record and offense seriousness, others have failed to find such racial effects (Bortner et al., 2000).

Fewer studies have examined decision making by the personnel who make transfer recommendations, such as prosecutors, probation officers, and mental health professionals. Some research indicates that juvenile court workers perceive the juvenile's family functioning, criminal record, current offense, school record, and prior case dispositions as the most significant factors that should be, and often are, considered when sentencing juveniles. Other factors include the juvenile's character, capacity for rehabilitation, mental health issues and treatment needs, and prior drug abuse (Sanborn, 1996). Grisso, Tomkins, and Casey (1988) presented 1,423 prosecutors, defense attorneys, mental health professionals, and juvenile court probation officers with hypothetical cases to examine the factors influencing their transfer recommendations. Juveniles' psychosocial makeup and family functioning were related to the recommendations made, but the seriousness of the offense and person variables such as age, gender, and race were not. The child's willingness to accept intervention, behavioral compliance, prior juvenile justice system contacts, and academic or work functioning were the strongest predictors.

Effects of Transfer Laws

Many feel that the juvenile system, created with the goal of rehabilitation, has failed. In turn, they support transferring juveniles to the adult system with the belief that harsher sentences and lower recidivism will follow (see Taylor, 2002). Yet research strongly suggests that transfer laws have little or no deterrent effect on juvenile crime and that transferring juveniles to criminal court exacerbates recidivism.

According to two well-designed studies, automatic transfer laws have no deterrent effect on juvenile crime. Jensen and Metsger's (1994) time-series analysis found a 13% increase in arrest rates for violent juvenile crime in Idaho after the State implemented its automatic transfer law. In a similar analysis, Singer and

McDowall (1988) found that a state law that automatically sent violent juvenile offenders to criminal court (by lowering the age for criminal court jurisdiction) had no deterrent effect, even though the law was widely used and publicized.

On the other hand, the results of a recent multistate analysis do suggest some deterrent effects for juvenile offenders (Levitt, 1998). In this study, an age-associated decrease (when states lowered the jurisdictional age for criminal court from 18 to 17) in juvenile crime rates was found of 25% for violent crime and 10–15% for property crime across states. The greatest decreases were found in those states with a greater disparity in the severity of punishment between its criminal and juvenile courts, suggesting the deterrent effect of transfer laws. Anecdotal reports and data collected in some communities also suggest that transfer laws have deterrent effects. In Jacksonville, Florida, for example, the juvenile arrest rate decreased 30% and the juvenile violent crime rate decreased 44% in just 1 year (between 1993 and 1994) after the local prosecutor instituted aggressive policies to prosecute and incarcerate serious juvenile offenders as if they were adults (Bennett, DiIulio, & Walters, 1996). According to Glassner, Ksander, Berg, and Johnson (1983), some juvenile offenders decided to stop or reduce their offending when they reached age 16 because they knew they could be tried as if they were adults on reaching that age.

It is difficult to reconcile previous studies showing that transfer laws have no deterrent effect with Levitt's (1998) study and with anecdotal reports that transfer laws deter crime. Some have argued that the recent decline in the crime rate is attributable to get tough policies (see Bennett et al., 1996; Scheidegger & Rushford, 1999) and that zero tolerance policies have worked in some juvenile justice contexts (see Kennedy, 1997). Recent reviews of the research on deterrence (Nagin, 1998; Von Hirsch, Bottoms, Burney, & Wikstrom, 1999) conclude that criminal sanctions are effective deterrents, at least for adult offenders. The research on adult deterrence, however, does not necessarily translate to youth, who may not weigh the severity or swiftness of punishment in the same way as adults. The psychosocial immaturity of youth (see Scott, Reppucci, & Woolard, 1995) could make rational choice models of deterrence, which assume that perceived consequences influence decisions about committing crime, less applicable (see Schneider & Ervin, 1990).

In addition to the questionable deterrent effects of transfer laws, recent large-scale studies indicate that youth tried in criminal court have greater recidivism rates after release than those tried in juvenile court, particularly youth convicted of person offenses. Fagan (1996) examined the recidivism rates of 800 randomly selected juvenile offenders aged 15 and 16 who were charged with robbery or burglary. Controlling for eight variables (prior offenses, offense severity, race, gender, age at first offense, case length, sentence length, and court), this natural experiment compared offenders charged in New Jersey's juvenile courts with offenders charged in New York's criminal courts under the state's automatic transfer law. Both geographical areas shared similar demographic, socioeconomic, sociolegal, and crime indictor characteristics. Thus, the study allows comparison of recidivism rates as a function of whether cases are processed in juvenile or criminal court, without as many of the sample selection problems inherent in studies comparing cases within a single jurisdiction wherein prosecutors or judges decide which cases to transfer. Youth who had committed robbery and were sentenced in criminal court had a higher postrelease recidivism rate than those who were tried in juvenile court, but the recidivism rates for burglary offenders tried in criminal and juvenile courts were similar. The findings on robbery offenders suggest that criminal court processing, irrespective of whether youth are incarcerated in juvenile or adult facilities, produces a higher recidivism rate. In addition, youth sentenced to probation in criminal court had a substantially higher recidivism rate than those receiving a term of incarceration in the juvenile justice system.

Bishop, Frazier, Lanza-Kaduce, and Winner (1996) compared the 1-year recidivism rate of 2,738 juvenile offenders transferred to criminal court in Florida with a matched sample of 2,738 juvenile offenders who had not been transferred. The study, which controlled for seven variables (race, gender, age, most serious prior offense, number of referrals to juvenile court, number of charges, and most serious charge), revealed that the rearrest rates were higher (30 vs. 19%) and the period before reoffending was shorter (135 vs. 227 days) for the transferred youth across seven offense types (ranging from violent felonies to minor misdemeanors). Following the same Florida offenders 6 years after the initial study, Winner, Lanza-Kaduce, Bishop, and Frazier (1997) found higher recidivism rates among those transferred to criminal courts, with the exception of property felons. Florida relies almost exclusively on transfer by prosecutors, who typically make their transfer decisions very soon after arrest, before gaining access to information about the youth's background. Therefore it is less likely that the youth who were not transferred had lower recidivism rates due to selection factors (Bishop, 2000).

A similar study (Myers, 2001), controlling for offense-related and demographic variables (e.g., age of onset of offending, prior offenses, use of a firearm), examined the recidivism rates of 557 violent juvenile offenders in Pennsylvania. Youth who were judicially transferred to criminal court were rearrested more quickly upon their return to the community than youth who were retained in juvenile justice system during the same period. Moreover, transferred youth who were incarcerated for longer periods had a lower recidivism rate upon release than those incarcerated for shorter periods. Finally, Podkopacz and Feld (1996) compared transferred with nontransferred juvenile offenders in Minnesota and found higher recidivism rates among those transferred.

These five studies involving all three types of transfer laws (automatic, judicial, prosecutorial) used fairly large sample sizes (557 to 5,476), different methodologies (natural experiment, matched groups) and were conducted in different jurisdictions (Florida, New Jersey, New York, Minnesota, Pennsylvania). But they each had significant methodological limitations, primarily in not being able to control completely for possible differential selection effects (vis-à- vis juveniles' amenability to treatment, for example) between those cases retained in the juvenile court versus those that were transferred.

However, armed with two very recent large-scale studies that better control for possible selection effects, the research now permits us to conclude with a fair degree of confidence that transfer generally does increase recidivism, though remaining methodological limitations do not allow for definitive conclusions. Fagan, Kupchik, and Liberman's (2003) recent finding of greater recidivism for transferred juveniles (charged with robbery, burglary, or assault) replicates Fagan's (1996) previous study but with a larger data set (2,400 juveniles) and methodology that better controls for important variables relating to possible selection effects. As in the previous study, by controlling for sentence lengths, the study showed that criminal court processing per se (rather than differential sentences between the juvenile and criminal courts) increased recidivism. Similarly, Lanza-Kaduce, Frazier, Lane, and Bishop's (2000) recent follow-up study to the Bishop et al. (1996) Florida recidivism study also replicated their previous findings of higher recidivism rates for transferred juveniles as a function of criminal court processing per se (rather than differential sentences), using better matching techniques to control for possible selection effects, more extensive recidivism data, and data drawn from six Florida judicial circuits in rural and urban jurisdictions.

Several factors may contribute to the generally higher recidivism rates for youth tried in criminal court. These factors include the rehabilitative services provided by the juvenile justice system versus the counter-rehabilitative effects of processing and incarceration in the criminal justice system. In particular, the negative effects of labeling juveniles as convicted adult felons, the decreased focus on family support in the adult system, the stigmatization that often results, and the learning of criminal mores and behavior from adults have been singled out as possible reasons for the increase in recidivism rates among this population (see Bazemore & Umbreit, 1995; Hirschi, 1969; Thomas & Bishop, 1984).

Significantly, Forst, Fagan, and Vivona (1989) found a relative lack of programming and services for youth in adult facilities. Staffs in juvenile facilities were more likely to be in, and rewarded for, helping and counseling residents and counseling in juvenile facilities was provided by line staff as part of their regular duties. In addition, youth in juvenile facilities gave higher marks than youth in adult facilities to the available treatment and case management services, which youth in detention described as helpful in providing counseling, obtaining needed services, encouraging participation in programs, teaching the consequences of rule breaking, and deepening their understanding of their problems.

A recent study captures well the differences between juvenile and criminal courts and detention facilities and correctional institutions. Bishop and Frazier (2000) conducted interviews with serious and chronic juvenile offenders in Florida who were transferred to the criminal justice system and incarcerated in correctional facilities. Many of these offenders had experience with the juvenile justice system, which they perceived positively. In comparison, the transferred youth perceived the criminal court quite negatively; they saw the lawyers and judges as having little interest in them and the court procedures as too adversarial. They also were angry and resentful at what they viewed to be unfair sentences. Despite the punitive rhetoric of juvenile justice in Florida, Bishop and Frazier (2000, p. 255) found that the juvenile institutions "were clearly treatment oriented," and juvenile offenders felt that staff members cared about them and taught them appropriate behaviors. These findings contrasted with the clearly custodial nature of Florida prisons, where youth spent much of their time learning criminal behavior from adult inmates, to whom they had to prove their toughness through aggression and defiance of authority. According to Bishop and Frazier (2000, p. 265), "Compared to the criminal justice system, the juvenile system seems to be more reintegrative in practice and effect."

Blended Sentencing: The Convergence of Juvenile and Criminal Sentencing

Many states have turned to "blended sentencing," which increases the sentencing options available in the juvenile court through a limited blending of juvenile and adult sentences. Blended sentencing has become an appealing option for many states, because it allows them to retain serious and violent juvenile offenders under juvenile court jurisdiction, while demanding greater accountability through the possibility of a criminal sentence. The possible consequence of an adult sentence if the juvenile commits a new offense, violates probation, or fails to respond to rehabilitation is designed to hold juveniles accountable (Torbet et al., 1996). It offers offenders a "last chance" at rehabilitation within the juvenile system and an incentive to respond to treatment in order to avoid the consequences of an adult sentence (Clarke, 1996).

Roughly half of the states have adopted one of three blended sentencing options for their juvenile courts, allowing the court to (a) impose either a juvenile or an adult sentence, (b) impose both a juvenile and an adult sentence, or (c) impose a sentence exceeding the normal time limit of juvenile court jurisdiction and conduct a hearing when the juvenile reaches age 17 to 21 (depending on the jurisdiction) to determine if an adult sentence should then be imposed. But blended sentencing in juvenile court does not always mean a more lenient sentence than if the case were transferred to criminal court. In Massachusetts, Rhode Island, and Texas, for example, the juvenile court may impose the maximum adult sentence, with the option to suspend the balance of that sentence once juvenile jurisdiction ends. In other states, the blended sentencing option is exercised not in the juvenile court, but in the criminal court, allowing the criminal court to impose a juvenile sentence or both a juvenile and (typically suspended) adult sentence. (Only a few states have blended sentencing available in *both* juvenile and criminal courts. This comes closest to bridging the gap between the juvenile and criminal courts, by allowing juvenile courts to impose adult sentences or extend their jurisdiction and by also allowing criminal courts to impose juvenile sentences.)

Most blended sentencing statutes target juveniles who otherwise meet the criteria for transfer to criminal court under the state transfer law. Rhode Island, for example, requires the court first to find that the juvenile is eligible for transfer before blended sentencing may be considered. Statutes usually require the prosecution to prove that blended sentencing (as opposed to regular juvenile court jurisdiction) is warranted in the instant case. While the standard of proof for determining whether a case is eligible for blended sentencing varies across states, most adhere to the intermediate standard of clear and convincing evidence. (The standard of proof for ultimate adjudication, however, still requires proof beyond a reasonable doubt.) There usually is not a right to a jury trial in juvenile court delinquency proceedings, since they can only result in a juvenile disposition. But under blended sentencing jurisdiction, all states but Connecticut provide the right to a jury trial, since a criminal conviction and sentence is a possible eventual outcome (Redding & Howell, 2000).

Once the prosecution files a petition requesting blended sentencing, the juvenile court judge uses her discretion in determining whether to proceed under this authority, guided by the statutory criteria. The statutory factors are very similar to those found in discretionary transfer statutes and include (a) the seriousness of the offense, (b) the amount of violence involved, (c) whether the alleged offense was against a person, (d) the sophistication and maturity of the juvenile as determined by considering his home, environmental situation, emotional attitude, and pattern of living, (e) the previous criminal record of the juvenile, and (f) the likelihood of rehabilitation (Redding & Howell, 2000).

Some states also have transfer/adult sentencing hearings that review similar criteria shortly before a juvenile, previously sentenced under blended sentencing, "ages out" of the juvenile justice system (at age 17.5 to 21, depending on the state). The purpose of this later hearing is to determine whether the adult sentence that was stayed until the completion of the juvenile disposition should be imposed or if the juvenile should be released from court jurisdiction. If the juvenile violates the terms of the juvenile disposition or commits another offense, the judge will often impose the adult sentence at this second hearing or at the time of the violation (Brummer, 2002).

Effects of Blended Sentencing: Net Narrowing or Net Widening?

It is unclear whether blended sentencing keeps more juveniles from entering the criminal system (net narrowing) or whether it only subject more juveniles to adult sentences (net widening). Initial data from three states (New Mexico, Minnesota, and Texas) that have enacted blended sentencing laws suggest that both net narrowing and net widening may be occurring.

Indeed, in Texas, the blended sentencing law was intended to have both net-narrowing and net-widening effects. The purpose of Texas's blended sentencing law (Texas Family Code, 1999) was twofold: (a) to serve as an alternative to the transfer of 15- and 16-year-old juveniles, for whom the length of confinement available in the juvenile system was insufficient, and (b) to respond to violent offenses committed by adolescents as young as 10 years old, who were below the state's minimum transfer age of 15. The law enables juvenile courts to impose sentences of up to 40 years in prison on children as young as 10 years of age who commit violent offenses. Dawson (1990) found that 47% of the Texas blended sentencing cases were *not* transfer-eligible, thus enabling the juvenile court to impose adult sentences that would otherwise not have been available. In addition, 60% of the juveniles that prosecutors referred for blended sentencing had no prior offenses, thus subjecting many first-time offenders to the possibility of criminal sanctions. But 53% of the cases *were* transfer-eligible, and the blended sentencing option may have kept those juveniles out of the adult system.

Prior to 1995, Minnesota had a typical judicial transfer law that authorized a juvenile court judge to transfer jurisdiction based on the juvenile's suitability for treatment and public safety concerns (Podkopacz & Feld, 2001). The 1995 legislative changes focused the transfer criteria primarily on public safely and gave "extended juvenile jurisdiction" authority to juvenile courts, allowing them to impose a juvenile sentence along with a suspended adult sentence. A study of the dispositions of youth before and after the legislative changes was conducted to determine the effects of the blended sentencing legislation (Podkopacz & Feld, 2001). Under the new blended sentencing and transfer law, prosecutors more than doubled the average number of transfer ("certification") motions made per year, from 47 to 108, and filed motions for blended sentencing jurisdiction against 36% of all eligible juvenile offenders (Podkopacz & Feld, 2001). Many juveniles sentenced under blended sentencing subsequently had their juvenile probation revoked and an adult sentence imposed, demonstrating the reality of the net-widening effect in Minnesota. Judges revoked probation in 35% of these cases, most of the time (76%) for probation violations rather than the commission of a new offense, sending 49% of these juveniles to prison and 51% to the workhouse. In addition, the juveniles under blended sentencing authority typically were younger and had less extensive prior records than the transferred youth. Their technical probation violations, which often resulted in the automatic imposition of the stayed adult sentence, were not offenses that would have resulted in transfer in the first place (Podkopacz & Feld, 2001).

Thus, blended sentencing in Minnesota "apparently had widened-the-net and created a 'back door' to prison for youth who likely would never have been [transferred] . . . It appears that the blended sentencing law which the legislature hoped would give juveniles 'one last chance' for treatment has instead become their 'first and last chance' for treatment, widened the net of criminal social control, and moved larger numbers of younger and less serious or chronic youth into the adult correctional system indirectly through the 'back door' of probation revocation proceedings rather than through [transfer] hearings" (Podkopacz & Feld, 2001, pp. 1062, 1070).

New Mexico's new blended sentencing law (which resulted in the state's abolishing transfer except in homicide cases) apparently has produced a change in prosecutorial charging or case selection practices. Previously, only 63% of transfer-referred juveniles were charged with a violent felony. But with the new blended sentencing law emphasizing public safety, 83% of transfer-referred juveniles are now charged with crimes against persons (Podkopacz & Feld, 2001). Prosecutors also now charge 67% of these youth with use of a weapon compared to only 48% previously, a significant change that suggests prosecutors are tailoring their blended sentencing motions to focus on youth committing violent offenses (Podkopacz & Feld, 2001). Although the number of transfer motions by prosecutors has more than doubled (27 vs. 108 per year) under the blended sentencing law, judges have responded by transferring less than one third of the eligible juveniles compared to two thirds previously under the old law.

Adjudicating and Sentencing Juvenile Offenders: Future Directions for Law and Policy

The newest legal development in sentencing law for juvenile offenders—blended sentencing—offers a compromise between rehabilitative and get tough ideals that retains juvenile court authority over serious offenders while increasing and extending the accountability sanctions available. Blended sentencing laws have been increasing nationwide, becoming a standard option for juvenile court systems. Importantly, they provide an alternative to transfer for juveniles whose serious offenses require periods of incarceration or court supervision exceeding the traditional age jurisdiction of the juvenile court. Some blended sentencing regimes, however, widen the net of adult sanctions over juveniles by including less serious or younger offenders who otherwise would not be subject to adult sanctions. Moreover, adult sanctions often are imposed under blended sentencing for minor probation violations, and blended sentencing may only "supplement rather than supplant" transfer laws when prosecutors file transfer motions and then plea-bargain down to blended sentencing (Tanenhaus & Drizin, 2002, p. 696.) Blended sentencing will not be an effective alternative to transfer unless it is not linked to the availability of evidence-based juvenile offender rehabilitation programs in the juvenile justice system. At the end of the day, "whether or not blended sentences give juvenile offenders a real chance at earning their way out of adult sanctions depends on the quality of programming the juvenile system offers" (Tanenhaus & Drizin, 2002, p. 697).

But the extant research, conducted in only a few states, is far from conclusive on the effects of blended sentencing, particularly given the apparent variability in prosecutorial practices. (Dawson [1990] noted, for example, that the practices of local prosecutors varied widely across the state of Texas, referring anywhere from 0 to 87% of the eligible cases for blended sentencing.) Substantial research is needed to determine the cases prosecutors and judges select for blended sentencing and the factors relevant in their decision making, how blended sentencing narrows or widens the net of adult sanctions over juvenile offenders, the nature and quality of judicial decision making on the revocation of juvenile sentences and the imposition of adult sentences, case outcomes under various blended sentencing regimes, and the general and specific deterrence effects of blended sentencing (Redding & Howell, 2000). Similarly, a jurisprudence of blended sentencing must be developed and implementation issues addressed. For example, what kinds of cases are ideal for blended sentencing and how should these cases differ from those targeted for transfer, how will blended jurisdiction affect juvenile court resources, and are juvenile courts equipped for jury trials (Brummer, 2002)?

Prosecutors often use the threat of transfer to criminal court as plea bargaining leverage against juveniles to persuade them to plead guilty and/or agree to a particular sentence under blended sentencing authority (Dawson, 1990; Podkopacz & Feld, 2001). Juveniles' competence to enter into such agreements is questionable, particularly because lawyers' tendency to encourage defendants to plead guilty or accept a plea agreement may compromise a juvenile's rights (Mears, 1998). When juveniles face the possibility of an adult sentence (through either transfer or blended sentencing), a competency hearing should be conducted to determine whether the juvenile is competent to stand trial (Bonnie & Grisso, 2000). But while adult adjudicative competency standards are well defined, it is unclear, in both law and practice, the extent to which maturity factors ought to be evaluated and considered in determining a juvenile's competence (see Redding & Frost, 2002). Additionally, juvenile plea agreements should be examined closely for evidence of coercion (see *People v. Simpson*, 2001). Some have argued that enhanced protections should be afforded to ensure that juvenile waivers are fully voluntary, knowing, and intelligent (Redding, 1997).

Under blended sentencing, the constitutionality and ethics of imposing lengthy criminal sentences on juvenile offenders, particularly life sentences without the possibility of parole, is also a serious concern. With most states currently permitting life sentences for juveniles, and only a few expressly limiting the option to those 16 years and older (Logan, 1998), some youth waived from the juvenile system will remain incarcerated for of a life term "without a chance of meaningful appellate review of their sentences," unlike similarly situated peers retained in the juvenile system (Logan, 1998, p. 709). Very long sentences or sentences of life without parole may be disproportionate sentences for juveniles, as a matter of prudence, morality, or penal philosophy.

In older decisions, the Kentucky and Nevada State Supreme Courts struck down sentences of life without parole for young juvenile offenders on Eighth Amendment (cruel and unusual punishment grounds). In *Naovarath v. Nevada* (1989), the Nevada Supreme Court struck a life without parole sentence for a 13-year-old convicted of murder, stating, "When a child reaches twelve or thirteen, it may not be universally agreed that a life sentence without parole should never be imposed, but surely all agree that such a severe and hopeless sentence should be imposed on prepubescent children, if at all, only in the most exceptional of circumstances. Children are and should be judged by different standards from those imposed upon mature adults" (pp. 946–947).

Despite these court decisions, however, the current trend has been to allow harsh sentences for juveniles. If these sentencing options are here to stay, then efforts should be made to ensure that the criminal court judiciary is sensitive to the juvenile's maturity level, social and mental health history, and culpability (Logan, 1998).

While blended sentencing is a new development in the landscape of juvenile justice, transfer laws have long existed. But their reach over juveniles has expanded considerably in recent years as states have revised their transfer laws to lower the minimum age for transfer, expand the number of transfer-eligible offenses, and reduce or eliminate judicial discretion by vesting discretion in prosecutors or making transfer automatic for certain crimes. Whether the appropriate locus for discretion lies with prosecutors or judges is highly debatable (see Feld, 2000; Sanborn, 2003). But among the legal and social science scholars of transfer, there is a strong consensus that the expansion of automatic transfer laws is unwise (e.g., Feld, 2000; Redding, 1997; Zimring & Fagan, 2000).

Automatic transfer laws are overinclusive, failing to take into account the wide variability among juvenile offenders in cognitive and emotional maturity (and thus culpability) and rehabilitative potential (Steinberg & Cauffman, 2000). Their overinclusiveness is particularly troubling when considering the counterdeterrent effects of transfer. Minimizing the number of juvenile cases transferred to criminal court, especially first-time offenders, is an important policy goal suggested by the extant research showing higher recidivism rates for transferred youth (Redding, 1997). Yet minimizing the number of youth transferred to criminal court does not mean that transfer should be abolished. Transfer serves as a necessary safety valve vis-à-vis those serious juvenile offenders who cannot or should not be retained in the juvenile justice system. In some cases, rehabilitative options have been exhausted, the seriousness or heinousness of the offense demands "the punitive necessity of waiver" (Zimring, 2000b), or retention in the juvenile system will put other juveniles at risk. "It is interesting how those who fear placing chronic/violent juvenile offenders with adults voice no corresponding concern for he plight of less violent and criminal juveniles who are forced to cohabitate with youth who arguably should have been excluded from juvenile court" (Sanborn, 2002, p. 204). Although a solution to this problem is to offer separate programs for chronic or violent offenders, this often is not done in practice.

A related policy implication of recent research is that incarceration in adult facilities be reserved for only the most serious and chronic offenders (Redding, 2002). The use of graduated sanctions, determined by the juvenile's offending history and offense seriousness, is one way to preserve long-term incarceration as a last resort for offenders who have not responded well to previous interventions. Recognizing and treating juveniles' needs early in their offending careers may also aid in reducing the recidivism rates of juvenile offenders. Graduated sanctions programs have produced positive results: reduced costs, enhanced responsiveness to the treatment needs of juveniles, and increased accountability for juveniles as well as communities (Krisberg & Howell, 1998).

The result of transfer and blended sentencing is that some—perhaps many—juveniles lacking adult maturity and competence are being tried and sentenced as mature adults. Research has shown that compared to juvenile nonoffenders, juvenile delinquents have lower IQs (see Redding & Arrigo, in press), a higher prevalence of learning disabilities (Tulman, 2003) and mental illness, often have poor social problem-solving skills (Dodge & Frame, 1982), and may not fully understand their legal rights (Grisso & Schwartz, 2003). Indeed, a separate juvenile justice system was created out of the belief that children, because of their immaturity, do not bear the same culpability as adults for their crimes (Redding, 1997). Courts may accept diminished capacity claims by adults who can prove impaired cognitive functioning. Unfortunately, juveniles are not afforded a similar "diminished capacity" status as a means for avoiding transfer to the adult system.

Older juveniles often are transferred to the adult system so that incarceration can continue after the child reaches the age of majority (Bishop & Frazier, 1991), and for this reason, the child's age is a key if not determining factor considered by judges when making discretionary transfer decisions (Redding, 1997). As the Alaska Court of Appeals stated, "even if a child's best chance for rehabilitation would be in a juvenile institution, waiver must be ordered when the evidence shows a likelihood that the child cannot be rehabilitated before reaching twenty years of age" (*DEP v. State*, 1986). Thus, transfer laws often target first-time serious offenders, who research has shown are less likely to recidivate than those having prior contacts with the system. The number of contacts with the juvenile justice system has been found to be a better predictor of recidivism than the seriousness of the first offense (Feld, 1987), and many first-time offenders do not commit other violent acts (Redding, 1997). Replacing automatic transfer laws with statutory schemes that guide judicial discretion may more accurately identify those juveniles who will be best served in each system.

However, transfer laws often lack concrete guidelines, resulting in considerable variability in outcomes across similarly situated cases (Redding, 1997). The discretionary decisions of prosecutors, court personnel, and judges often lack uniformity (Redding, 1997) and in some cases may reflect biases based on offender race or socioeconomic status or misconceptions about juvenile offenders. A recent empirical study of judicial transfer concluded that judges decided the cases of similarly situated offenders significantly differently (Podkapacz & Feld, 1996, p. 492). Thus, more explicit statutory guidance and decision-making criteria are needed for judges to make more informed and uniform transfer decisions (Redding, 1997). Research has consistently found that actuarial (i.e., statistically based) predictions are equal, and usually superior, to those based on clinical judgment. To improve decision-making accuracy and uniformity, transfer criteria should be predicated, in part, on actuarial models of the likelihood of recidivism as a function of various offender, offense, and offense history characteristics (Redding, 1997). Moreover, requiring prosecutors to issue written opinions detailing their reasons for a transfer decision may minimize the risk that juveniles who are amenable to rehabilitation will be transferred, because prosecutors will have to articulate compelling reasons justifying a transfer decision (Arteaga, 2002). It is also likely to reduce "the disparate treatment of similarly situated juveniles" by allowing the public to compare transfer decisions in different cases (Arteaga, 2002).

While the extant research on transfer permits the above policy recommendations, many of the effects of trying and sentencing juveniles as adults remain unclear. In particular, research is needed on the general deterrent effects of such laws, whether transfer laws offer a sufficiently certain threat of punishment, and the extent to which juveniles are aware of these laws and the deterrent effects of such awareness (Redding, 2003). Redding and Fuller's (2004) interviews with serious juvenile offenders indicate that many are not aware of such laws, do not think they will be applied to them, and do not believe they will face serious punishment. With increasing numbers of juveniles being incarcerated in adult facilities, research is urgently needed on the comparative effects of adult and juvenile facilities on juveniles' psychological and behavioral functioning (Redding, 2003). Perhaps the most important challenge for future research is to determine what features of criminal court processing increase recidivism, an important question for policy-making. For example, are there changes that could be made in the criminal court processing of juveniles to make it less detrimental? In what ways should the juvenile justice system be on guard against those features of the criminal justice system that serve to increase recidivism? How can blended sentencing systems incorporate the best features of both systems while avoiding the iatrogenic features of the criminal justice system?

Finally, effective legal advocacy is one of the most practical ways to improve the quality of justice and programming afforded to youth in the juvenile court. The quality of legal representation afforded juveniles in juvenile court adjudicatory and dispositional hearings, as well as in transfer and blended sentencing hearings, is abysmal (Redding, 2002). The poor quality of representation has been noted by numerous commentators and found in many studies of the juvenile court since the U.S. Supreme Court's landmark *In re Gault* (1967) decision extending full due process rights to juvenile delinquency proceedings. A recent American Bar Association study concluded that "many young people in juvenile court are significantly compromised, and that many children are literally left defenseless" (American Bar Association, 1995, p. 7). Professor Ainsworth noted, after observing a number of juvenile trials, that "one gets the overall impression that defense counsel prepared minimally or not at all" (Ainsworth, 1991, p. 1128). Lack of attorney expertise and training is a key factor making it difficult for public defenders and court-appointed counsel to provide effective representation (American Bar Association, 1995).

Lawyers and juvenile justice professionals must be trained on the relevant juvenile mental health, forensic, and rehabilitative programming issues (see Rosado, ch. 14 in this volume). Meaningful representation is often completely lacking at the dispositional hearing, when lawyers frequently defer to the probation officer's recommendation or argue nothing more than that the recommendation is too punitive, without proffering any alternatives to the court. As Roche (1987) points out, lawyers must be equipped to provide the court with specific and detailed recommendations for dispositional alternatives, either because probation officers often will fail to make well-informed recommendations or because their recommendations may be too punitive. Roche recommends imposing on juvenile court attorneys an ethical and legal duty of effective representation at dispositional hearings and creating rules of court that require counsel to file with the court a statement of dispositional recommendations. Juvenile court dispositional and transfer recommendations will be influenced by the decision-maker's knowledge about the effectiveness and availability of treatment options (see Mulvey & Reppucci, 1988). The best emphasis for advocates should be whether the juvenile is amenable to rehabilitation, not whether and how the juvenile is amenable given locally available resources. "A finding of amenability places some pressure on the courts to provide adequate treatment to youth who are amenable to treatment" (Salekin, 2002, p. 67).

Additionally, there is evidence that programs aimed at educating judges and other juvenile justice professionals can have substantial positive effects in reducing the number of juveniles receiving adult sanctions. The Miami–Dade County Public Defender's Office developed the Juvenile Sentencing Advocacy Project (JSAP), a highly effective program that has produced a 350% increase the number of transferred cases receiving a juvenile (rather than an adult) sanction (Mason, 2000). A key component of JSAP was the development of training programs for judges and attorneys on adolescent development, effective treatment and rehabilitation programs for juvenile offenders, and sentencing options, along with the development of greater linkages to community resources.

Conclusion

The juvenile court system was created over 100 years ago "to save kids from the savagery of the criminal courts and prisons" by removing juveniles from the criminogenic influences of the criminal justice system while providing rehabilitative interventions (Zimring, 2000a, p. 2480). Significantly, "the protective impact of a diversionary juvenile court on sanctions for youth crime is largest when punitive policies are at their most dominant in criminal courts . . . in ages like the American present," as shown by the fact that the discrepancy between the proportional number of young adults versus juveniles incarcerated is greater than ever in our history (Zimring, 1998, p. 2491). This explains the reason for the continued public and legislative pressure on the juvenile justice system to "get tough" despite declines in the rates of violent juvenile crime — "the political forces that had produced extraordinary expansion through the rest of the penal system had been stymied in juvenile courts" (Zimring, 1998, p. 2494).

In part, these forces have turned to transfer and blended sentencing as ways to increase the availability of adult sanctions for juvenile offenders. At the same time, however, research is mounting on the counter-rehabilitative effects on juveniles of adult sanctions while the effectiveness of evidence-based rehabilitative programs is clearly shown in rigorous recent studies (see Sheidow & Henggeler, ch. 12 in this volume). It remains to be seen whether the juvenile justice system will continue to resist the penal pressures of the adult criminal justice system.

References

Ainsworth, J. E. (1991). Re-imagining childhood and reconstructing the legal order: The case for abolishing the juvenile court. *North Carolina Law Review, 69*, 1083–1133.

American Bar Association. (1995). *A call for justice: An assessment of access to counsel and quality of representation in delinquency proceedings.* Washington, DC: Author.

Arteaga, J. A. (2002). Juvenile injustice: Congressional attempts to abrogate the procedural rights of juvenile defendants. *Columbia Law Review, 102*, 1051–1085.

Bazemore, G., & Umbreit, M. (1995). Rethinking the sanctioning function in juvenile court: Retributive or restorative responses to youth crime. *Crime and Delinquency, 41*, 296–316.

Bennett, W. J., Dilulio, J. J., & Walters, J. P. (1996). *Body count: Moral poverty and how to win America's war against crime and drugs.* New York: Simon & Schuster.

Beresford, L. S. (2000). Is lowering the age at which juveniles can be transferred to adult criminal court the answer to juvenile crime? A state-by-state assessment. *San Diego Law Review, 37,* 783–848.

Binder, A., Geis, G., & Bruce, D. D. (2001). *Juvenile delinquency: Historical, cultural and legal perspectives* (3rd ed.). Cincinnati, OH: Anderson.

Bishop, D. M. (2000). Justice offenders in the adult criminal justice system. In M. Tonry (Ed.), *Crime and justice: A review of research* (Vol. 26, pp. 81–167). Chicago: University of Chicago Press.

Bishop, D. M., & Frazier, C. E. (1991). Transfer of juveniles to criminal court: A case study and analysis of prosecutorial waiver. *Notre Dame Journal of Legal Ethics and Public Policy, 5,* 281–302.

Bishop, D. M., & Frazier, C. E. (1996). Race effects in juvenile justice decision making: Findings from a statewide analysis. *Journal of Criminology & Criminal Law, 86,* 392–414.

Bishop, D. M., & Frazier, C. E. (2000). Consequences of transfer. In J. Fagan & F. E. Zimring (Eds.), *The changing borders of juvenile justice: Transfer of adolescents to the criminal court.* Chicago: University of Chicago Press.

Bishop, D. M., Frazier, C. E., Lanza-Kaduce, L., & Winner, L. (1996). The transfer of juveniles to criminal court: Does it make a difference? *Crime and Delinquency, 42,* 171–191.

Bonnie, R., J., & Grisso, T. (2000). Adjudicative competence and youthful offenders. In T. Grisso & R. Schwartz (Eds.), *Youth on trial: A developmental perspective on juvenile justice* (pp. 73–103). Chicago: University of Chicago Press.

Bortner, M. A., Zatz, M. S., & Hawkins, D. F. (2000). Race and transfer: Empirical research and social context. In J. Fagan & F. E. Zimring (Eds.), *The changing borders of juvenile justice: Transfer of adolescents to the criminal court* (pp. 277–320). Chicago: University of Chicago Press.

Brummer, C. E. (2002). Extended juvenile jurisdiction: The best of both worlds? *Arkansas Law Review, 54,* 777–822.

Campbell, M. A., & Schmidt, F. (2000). Comparison of mental health and legal factors in the disposition outcome of young offenders. *Criminal Justice and Behavior, 27,* 688–715.

Clarke, E. E. (1996). A case for reinventing juvenile transfer: The record of transfer of juvenile offenders to criminal court in Cook County, Illinois. *Juvenile and Family Court Journal, 47,* 3–21.

Coolbaugh, K., & Hansel, C. J. (2000). The comprehensive strategy: Lessons learned from the pilot sites. In *Juvenile justice bulletin.* Washington, DC: U.S. Department of Justice, Office of Juvenile Justice and Delinquency Prevention.

Dawson, R. O. (1990). The violent offender: An empirical study of juvenile determinate sentencing proceedings as an alternative to criminal prosecution. *Texas Tech Law Review, 21,* 1897–1939.

Dawson, R. O. (1992). An empirical study of Kent style juvenile transfers to criminal court. *St. Mary's Law Journal, 23,* 975–1055.

Dawson, R. O. (2000). Judicial waiver in theory and practice. In J. Fagan & F. E. Zimring (Eds.), *The changing borders of juvenile justice: Transfer of adolescents to the criminal court* (pp. 45–81). Chicago: University of Chicago Press.

DeFrances, C. J., & Strom, K. J. (1997). *National survey of prosecutors, 1994: Juveniles prosecuted in state criminal courts.* Washington, DC: United States Department of Justice, Bureau of Justice Statistics.

DEP v. State, 727 P.2d 800 (Alaska Ct. App. 1986).

Dodge, K. A., & Frame, C. L. (1982). Social cognitive biases and deficits in aggressive boys. *Child Development, 55*, 163–173.

Elrod, P., & Ryder, R. S. (1999). *Juvenile justice: A social, historical, and legal perspective.* Gaithersburg, MD: Aspen.

Fagan, J., Forst, M., & Vivona, S. (1987). Racial determinants of the judicial transfer decision: Prosecuting violent youth in criminal court. *Crime and Delinquency, 33*, 259–286.

Fagan, J., Kupchik, A., & Liberman, A. (2003). *Be careful what you wish for: The comparative impacts of juvenile versus criminal court sanctions on recidivism among adolescent felony offenders* (Pub. Law Research Paper No. 03-61). New York: Columbia University Law School.

Fagan, J. A. (1996). The comparative advantage of juvenile versus criminal court sanctions on recidivism among adolescent felony offenders. *Law and Policy, 18*, 77–113.

Federal Bureau of Investigation. (1997). *Uniform crime reports.* Washington, DC: Author.

Feld, B. C. (1987). The juvenile court meets the principle of the offense: Legislative changes in juvenile waiver statutes. *Journal of Criminal Law & Criminology, 78*, 471–533.

Feld, B. C. (2003). Legislative exclusion of offenses from juvenile court jurisdiction: A history and critique. In J. Fagan & F. E. Zimring (Eds.), *The changing borders of juvenile justice: Transfer of adolescents to the criminal court.* Chicago: University of Chicago Press.

Forst, M., Fagan, J., & Vivona, S. T. (1989). Youth in prisons and training schools: Perceptions and consequences of the treatment-custody dichotomy. *Juvenile and Family Court Journal, 40*, 1–14.

Glassner, B., Ksander, M., Berg, B., & Johnson, B. D. (1983). A note on the deterrent effect of juvenile versus adult jurisdiction. *Social Problems, 31*, 219–221.

Grisso, T., & Schwartz, R. G. (2003). *Youth on trial: A developmental perspective on juvenile justice.* Chicago: University of Chicago Press.

Grisso, T., Tomkins, A., & Casey, P. (1988). Psychosocial concepts in juvenile law. *Law and Human Behavior, 12*, 403–437.

Heilbrun, K., Leheny, C., Thomas, L., & Huneycutt, D. (1997). A national survey of U.S. statutes on juvenile transfer: Implications for policy and practice. *Behavioral Sciences and the Law, 15*, 125–149.

Hirschi, T. (1969). *Causes of delinquency.* Berkeley: University of California Press.

Hoge, R. D., Andrews, D. A., & Leschied, A. (1995). Investigation of variables associated with probation & custody dispositions in a sample of juveniles. *Journal of Clinical Child Psychology, 24*, 279–286.

Horwitz, A., & Wasserman, M. (1980). Formal rationality, substantive justice, and discrimination. *Law and Human Behavior, 4*, 103–115.

Howell, J. C. (1997). *Juvenile justice and youth violence.* Thousand Oaks, CA: Sage.

In re Gault, 387 U.S. 1 (1967).

Jensen, E. L., & Metsger, L. K. (1994). A test of the deterrent effect of legislative waiver on violent juvenile crime. *Crime and Delinquency, 40*, 96–104.

Kennedy, D. M. (1997). *Juvenile gun violence and gun markets in Boston.* Washington, DC: U.S. Department of Justice, Office of Justice Programs, National Institute of Justice.

Kent v. United States, 383 U.S. 541 (1966).

Kole, T. (2001). Juvenile offenders. *Harvard Journal on Legislation, 38,* 231–247.

Krisberg, B., & Howell, J. C. (1998). The impact of the juvenile justice system and prospects for graduated sanctions in a comprehensive strategy. In R. Loeber & D. P. Farrington (Ed.), *Serious and violent juvenile offenders: Risk factors and successful interventions* (pp. 346–366). Thousand Oaks, CA: Sage.

Lanza-Kaduce, L., Frazier, C. E., Lane, J., & Bishop, D. M. (2000). *Juvenile transfer to criminal court study: Final report.* Tallahassee, FL: Florida Department of Juvenile Justice.

Levitt, S. D (1998). Juvenile crime and punishment. *Journal of Political Economy, 106,* 1156–1185.

Logan, W. A. (1998). Proportionality and punishment: Imposing life without parole on juveniles. *Wake Forest Law Review, 33,* 681–725.

Mason, C. A. (2000). *Juvenile sentencing advocacy project: Evaluation report.* Miami, FL: Miami–Dade County Public Defender's Office.

Mears, D. P. (1998). *Theorizing and predicting juvenile justice sanctioning.* Presented at the annual meeting of the American Society of Criminology, Washington, DC.

Moffitt, T. E. (1993). Adolescence-limited and life-course-persistent antisocial behavior: A developmental taxonomy. *Psychological Review, 100,* 674–701.

Mulvey, E. P., & Reppucci, N. D. (1988). The context of clinical judgment: The effect of resource availability on judgments of amenability to treatment in juvenile offenders. *American Journal of Community Psychology, 16,* 525–545.

Myers, D. L. (2001). *Excluding violent youths from juvenile court: The effectiveness of legislative waiver.* New York: LFB Scholarly.

Myers, D. L. (2003). Adult crime, adult time: Punishing violent youth in the adult criminal justice system. *Youth Violence and Juvenile Justice, 1,* 173–197.

Nagin, D. S. (1998). Criminal deterrence research at the outset of the twenty-first century. *Crime and Justice: A Review of Research, 23,* 5–91.

Naovarath v. Nevada, 779 P.2d 944 (Nev.1989).

People v. Simpson, 51 P.3d 1022 (Cob. App. 2001).

Podkopacz, M., & Feld, B. (2001). The back-door to prison: Waiver reform, blended sentencing, and the law of unintended consequences. *Journal of Criminal Law & Criminology, 91,* 997–1071.

Podkopacz, M. R., & Feld, B. C. (1996). The end of the line: An empirical study of judicial waiver. *Journal of Criminal Law & Criminology, 86,* 449–492.

Poulos, T. M., & Orchowsky, S. (1994). Serious juvenile offenders: Predicting the possibility of transfer to criminal court. *Crime and Delinquency, 40,* 3–17.

Puzzanchera, C. (2000). *Juvenile court statistics, 1997.* Washington, DC: U.S. Department of Justice, Office of Juvenile Justice and Delinquency Prevention.

Redding, R. E. (1997). Juveniles transferred to criminal court: Legal reform proposals based on social science research. *Utah Law Review, 1997,* 709–763.

Redding, R. E. (2002). Using juvenile adjudications for sentence enhancement under the federal sentencing guidelines: Is it sound policy? *Virginia Journal of Social Policy and the Law, 10,* 231–260.

Redding, R. E. (2003). The effects of adjudicating and sentencing juveniles as adults: Research and policy implications. *Youth Violence and Juvenile Justice, 1,* 128–155.

Redding, R. E, & Arrigo, B. (in press). Multicultural perspectives on juvenile delinquency: Etiology and intervention. In C. Frisby & C. Reynolds (Eds.), *Handbook of multicultural school psychology.* New York: Wiley.

Redding, R. E., & Frost, L. E. (2002). Adjudicative competence in the modern juvenile court. *Virginia Journal of Social Policy and the Law, 9,* 353–410.

Redding, R. E., & Fuller, E. (2004, Summer). What do juvenile offenders know about being tried as adults? Implications for deterrence. *Juvenile and Family Court Journal*, 35–45.

Redding, R. E., & Howell, J. C. (2000). Blended sentencing in American juvenile courts. In J. Fagan & F. E. Zimring (Eds.), *The changing borders of juvenile justice: Transfer of adolescents to the criminal court* (pp. 145–180). Chicago: University of Chicago Press.

Roche, J. L. (1987). Juvenile court dispositional alternatives: Imposing a duty on the defense. *Santa Clara Law Review*, 27, 279–297.

Rubin, H. T. (2003, April/May). Juvenile court intake: Developments in practice. *Juvenile Justice Update*, 3–4, 16.

Rutter, M., Giller, H., & Hagell, A. (1998). *Antisocial behaviors by young people*. Cambridge: Cambridge University Press.

Salekin, R. T. (2002). Clinical evaluation of youth considered for transfer to adult criminal court: Refining practice and directions for science. *Journal of Forensic Psychology Practice*, 2, 55–72.

Sanborn, J. B. (1996). Factors perceived to affect delinquent dispositions in juvenile court: Putting the sentencing decision into context. *Crime and Delinquency*, 42, 99–113.

Sanborn, J. B. (2003). Hard choices or obvious ones: Developing policy for excluding youth from adult court. *Youth Violence and Juvenile Justice*, 1, 198–214.

Scheidegger, K., & Rushford, M. (1999). The social benefits of confining habitual criminals. *Stanford Law and Policy Review*, 11, 59–64.

Schneider, A. L., & Ervin, L. (1990). Specific deterrence, rational choice, and decision heuristics: Applications in juvenile justice. *Social Science Quarterly*, 71, 585–601.

Scott, E. S., Reppucci, N. D., & Woolard, J. L. (1995). Evaluating adolescent decision making in legal contexts. *Law and Human Behavior*, 19, 221–244.

Senna, J., & Siegel, L. J. (1992). *Juvenile law: Cases and comments*. St. Paul, MN: West.

Singer, S. I., & McDowall, D. (1988). Criminalizing delinquency: The deterrent effects of the New York juvenile offender law. *Law and Society Review*, 22, 521–535.

Snyder, H. N. (1998). Serious, violent, and chronic juvenile offenders—An assessment of the extent of and trends in officially recognized serious criminal behavior in a delinquent population. In R. Loeber & D. P. Farrington (Eds.), *Serious and violent juvenile offenders: Risk factors and successful intervention* (pp. 428–444). Thousand Oaks, CA: Sage.

Snyder, H. N., & Sickmund, M. (1999). *Juvenile offenders and victims: 1999 national report*. Washington, DC: U.S. Department of Justice, Office of Juvenile Justice and Delinquency Prevention.

Stahl, A. L. (1999). Offenders in juvenile court, 1996. In *OJJDP bulletin*. Washington, DC: U.S. Department of Justice, Office of Juvenile Justice and Delinquency Prevention.

State v. RGD, 527 A.2d 834 (N.J. 1987).

Steinberg, L., & Cauffman, E. (2000). A developmental perspective on jurisdictional boundary. In J. Fagan & F. E. Zimring (Eds.), *The changing borders of juvenile justice: Transfer of adolescents to the criminal court*. Chicago: University of Chicago Press.

Steiner, B., & Hemmens, C. (2003, Spring). Juvenile waiver 2003: Where are we now? *Juvenile and Family Court Journal*, 1–24.

Strasburger, L. H. (1988). The juvenile transfer hearing & the forensic psychiatrist. In R. Rosner (Ed.), *Critical issues in American psychiatry and the law* (Vol. 4). New York: Plenum.

Tanenhaus, D. S., & Drizin, S. A. (2002). "Owing to the extreme youth of the accused": The changing legal response to juvenile homicide. *Journal of Criminal Law &Criminology*, 92, 641–705.

Taylor, J. (2002). California's proposition 21: A case of juvenile injustice. *Southern California Law Review*, 75, 983–1019.

Texas Family Code Ann. 53.045, 54.04, 54.11 West 1996 & Supp. (1999).

Thomas, C. W., & Bishop, D. M. (1984). The impact of legal sanctions on delinquency: A longitudinal comparison of labeling and deterrence theories. *Journal of Criminal Law and Criminology*, 75, 1222–1245.

Torbet, P., Gable, R., Hurst, H., Montgomery, I., Szymanski, L., & Thomas, D. (1996). *State responses to serious and violent juvenile crime*. Washington, DC: U.S. Department of Justice, Office of Juvenile Justice and Delinquency Prevention.

Tulman, J. B. (2003). Disability and delinquency: How failures to identify, accommodate, and serve youth with education-related disabilities leads to their disproportionate representation in the delinquency system. *Whittier Journal of Child and Family Advocacy*, 3(1), 3–76.

Von Hirsch, A., Bottoms, A. E., Burney, E., & Wikstrom, P. O. (1999). *Criminal deterrence and sentence severity: An analysis of recent research*. Oxford, U.K.: Hart.

Webb, J. A., & Willems, E. P. (1987). Certifying juveniles for adult court: An attribution analysis. *Journal of Applied Social Psychology*, 17, 896–910.

Wilson, J. J., & Howell, J. C. (1995). Comprehensive strategy for serious, violent, and chronic juvenile offenders. In J. C. Howell, B. Krisberg, J. D. Hawkins, & J. J. Wilson (Eds.), *Sourcebook on serious, violent, and chronic juvenile offenders* (pp. 35–46). Thousand Oaks, CA: Sage.

Winner, L., Lanza-Kaduce, L., Bishop, D. M., & Frazier, C. E. (1997). The transfer of juveniles to criminal court: Reexamining recidivism over the long term. *Crime and Delinquency*, 43, 548–563.

Zaehringer, B. (1998). Juvenile boot camps: Cost and effectiveness versus residential facilities. *Cotch Crime Institute*, 4.

Zimring, F. E. (1998). The youth violence epidemic: Myth or reality. *Wake Forest Law Review*, 33, 727–744.

Zimring, F. E. (2000a). The common thread: Diversion in juvenile justice. *California Law Review*, 88, 2477–2495.

Zimring, F. E. (2000b). The punitive necessity of waiver. In J. Fagan & F. E. Zimring (Eds.), *The changing borders of juvenile justice: Transfer of adolescents to the criminal court* (pp. 207–226). Chicago: University of Chicago Press.

Zimring, F. E., & Fagan, J. (2000). Transfer policy and law reform. In J. Fagan & F. E. Zimring (Eds.), *The changing borders of juvenile justice: Transfer of adolescents to the criminal court* (pp. 407–424). Chicago: University of Chicago Press.

12

ASHLI J. SHEIDOW AND SCOTT W. HENGGELER

Community-Based Treatments

Recent syntheses of intervention research have concluded that treatments for juvenile delinquency produce quite divergent results, but that community-based treatments are showing greater promise than most other approaches. For example, Lipsey and Wilson's 1998 meta-analysis of intervention studies for serious juvenile offenders found an overall average effect size of .12 for recidivism, indicating a difference between treatment and control groups of only about one tenth of a standard deviation unit. However, effect sizes ranged from as high as .52 (i.e., one half of a standard deviation unit) to as low as −.17 (i.e., the treatment group fared worse than the control group). Likewise, other recent reviews have supported the view that community-based interventions are the most promising treatments available for juvenile offenders. For example, of the more than 500 programs reviewed in the Office of Juvenile Justice and Delinquency Prevention's (OJJDP) Blueprints for Violence Prevention Initiative (Mihalic, Irwin, Elliott, Fagan, & Hansen, 2001), the model programs identified as effective for treating juvenile offenders were all family- and community-based.

This chapter examines the community-based treatment models for juvenile offending that have established effectiveness or are promising. Specifically, brief summaries of their clinical procedures, findings from clinical trials, and cost-related outcomes are provided. In addition, parallels among these community-based models and corresponding implications for clinical practice and future research are discussed.

How Can We Tell What Works?

The Lipsey and Wilson (1998) meta-analysis identified 200 experimental or quasi-experimental studies that included treatment of juvenile offenders. Some community-based treatments, in particular, have received increased research attention compared to other treatments for juvenile delinquency. However, the confidence one can have in the conclusions generated by research differs depending on the type and quality of research. Further, a research base cannot be the sole justification for identifying a treatment as a model program when other issues, such as ease of implementation and cost, determine which treatments get disseminated.

Extending work by Chambless and Hollon (1998) for identifying empirically supported psychotherapies,[1] Kazdin and Weisz (1998) proposed standards for ascertaining efficacy among child and adolescent treatments:

1. *Multiple randomized control trials*—A randomized controlled trial (RCT) is a study where interventions are compared using random allocation of individuals into treatment and control groups. Well-implemented RCTs are considered the "gold standard" for determining the effectiveness of interventions. However, such trials are costly and time-consuming, so relatively few treatments have been subjected to them. Furthermore, randomized designs can be challenging to implement within the juvenile justice system because community-based treatment of serious juvenile delinquents is often perceived as an increased risk to public safety when serving as an alternative to restrictive placement. Nevertheless, well-implemented randomized trials are the best way to evaluate the effectiveness of interventions.

2. *Well-described, replicable treatment procedures*—For treatments to be conducted by service providers in the "real world" (i.e., by clinicians not affiliated with the treatment developer), clinical procedures must be clearly specified. Defining clinical procedures for community-based interventions is especially difficult given the complexity of such interventions; it is a time-consuming process and, thus, is often overlooked during treatment development.

3. *Uniform therapist training and monitoring of treatment fidelity*—Developing a training protocol and a protocol to ensure adherence can be accomplished only after the treatment model is well-specified. Like standardizing treatment protocols, this step is time-consuming and is further challenging due to the complexity of community-based treatment models. However, accurate replication cannot be accomplished without both training protocols and quality assurance protocols.

4. *Use of clinical samples*—Rather than using a nonclinical sample,

---

1. With input from various American Psychological Association Task Forces, Chambless and Hollon (1998) proposed criteria for empirically supported psychological therapies, including therapies showing statistically significantly better outcomes than no treatment, alternative treatment, or placebo within multiple studies that are replicable (were conducted using a treatment manual, defined inclusion criteria, reliable assessment tools, and appropriate data analysis).

treatment research should use a referred sample. For juvenile delinquency, a clinical sample would include only youth who were offenders (vs. at-risk youth or youth with general conduct problems). Without using clinical samples, one cannot be certain that the treatment model will generalize to the target population.

5. *Broad-based assessment of outcomes (e.g., evidence of clinical significance and of "real world" functioning)* — Treatment research should include multimethod, multisource assessments and should focus on clinically significant changes rather than relying solely on statistical significance. In addition, such research should include evaluation of clinically meaningful data, such as symptom level, as well as functional outcomes, such as school performance and maintenance in less restrictive placements. Such comprehensive evaluations substantially increase the expense of conducting treatment research and are often sacrificed in lieu of service costs.

6. *Evidence of long-term outcomes* — In addition to immediate success, the optimal treatment model would have positive long-term effects, but would, at a minimum, sustain the gains made during treatment. Without continued tracking of outcomes, one cannot determine if treatment progress holds, if youth improve even further, or if treated individuals fare worse than individuals in the control group over time. Like other recommended processes, tracking long-term outcomes is quite expensive and greatly extends the time it takes to evaluate a treatment model.

As discussed by Kazdin and Weisz, studies meeting these criteria are currently our best method for evaluating effectiveness across treatment models and are usually achieved through a systematic program of clinical research informed by clients, researchers, clinicians, and others involved in the provision and utilization of services.

Similarly, reports by the U.S. Surgeon General (U.S. Public Health Service, 1999, 2001) and a National Institute of Mental Health task force (National Advisory Mental Health Council Workgroup on Child and Adolescent Mental Health Intervention Development and Deployment, 2001; U.S. Public Health Service, 1999, 2001) provide recommendations for adolescent treatment development and evaluation. They suggest that model treatments should:

1. Use the science base of known risk factors for the development and maintenance of conduct problems
2. Provide an effective alternative to costly and largely ineffective restrictive placements for youth offenders
3. Use respectable scientific methods (e.g., matched comparison or randomized clinical trials) to evaluate effectiveness

The extensive review of interventions in OJJDP's Blueprints for Violence Prevention (Mihalic et al., 2001) endorsed similar criteria. Thus, federal stakeholders have identified high-quality research as a cornerstone for evaluating interventions, but also have highlighted the need for interventions to accomplish effectiveness at a substantial cost savings.

A blend of the more stringent criteria proposed by Kazdin and Weisz (1998) and the more pragmatic criteria proposed by federal entities (National Advisory Mental Health Council Workgroup on Child and Adolescent Mental Health Intervention Development and Deployment, 2001; U.S. Public Health Service, 1999, 2001) provides useful evaluation criteria for community service providers. While strong research methods and evidence of meaningful treatment effects for the target population are paramount to showing efficacy, the issues of treatment specification, training and quality assurance, and cost savings are clearly important for service providers and funders of mental health interventions for juvenile offenders. Thus, this chapter presents both exemplary and promising community-based interventions. However, priority is given to those treatment approaches that have empirical support for lowering recidivism (i.e., between-group comparisons presented in peer-reviewed publications) among juvenile offenders (i.e., clinical population). Further priority is given to those treatment models that have well-described treatment procedures, defined therapist training protocols, monitoring procedures for treatment fidelity, evidence of long-term outcomes, and/or documented cost benefit.

Exemplary Community-Based Interventions

Specific community-based treatment models that meet the blended criteria detailed above are presented in this section. A brief introduction to the models and their clinical procedures is provided; more detailed information can be obtained through the respective treatment manuals or references. The level of treatment specification is described, as well as the degree of specification for training and for quality assurance. In addition to introducing the treatment models, the controlled outcome for juvenile offending and available cost analyses are presented for each model.

Multisystemic Therapy (MST)

Guided by ecological and systems theory, the MST assessment process and intervention protocols focus on the individual, family, peer, school, and social network variables that are linked with identified problems, as well as on the interface of these systems. With five randomized controlled trials demonstrating success in treating juvenile offenders, MST is the most frequently cited community-based intervention for juvenile delinquency. MST clinical procedures are clearly specified for adolescent antisocial behavior in a clinical volume (Henggeler, Schoenwald, Borduin, Rowland, & Cunningham, 1998), and procedures for supervision are specified in a separate volume (Henggeler & Schoenwald, 1998). In addition, a recent volume describes MST adaptations to treat youth with serious emotional disturbance and their families (Henggeler, Schoenwald, Rowland, & Cunningham, 2002b). Therapist and supervisory training also have been standardized, as has an extensive quality assurance protocol (Henggeler & Schoenwald, 1999).

TREATMENT PROVISION

MST employs a home-based (e.g., home, school, community) model of service delivery that aims to decrease barriers to service access and increase engagement in treatment (e.g., Henggeler, Pickrel, Brondino, & Crouch, 1996). MST is provided by full-time master's level therapists who carry caseloads of four to six families. Three to four therapists work within a team, supervised by an advanced master's level or doctoral level supervisor, to provide 24-hour/7-day-a-week availability so that therapists can react quickly to crises that may threaten goal attainment (i.e., prevent out-of-home placement). Services are time limited, entailing an average of 60 hours of direct service over 3 to 6 months. The model of service delivery utilized by MST is particularly effective at engaging and retaining families in treatment. For example, in two recent trials of MST (Henggeler et al., 1996, 1999b), 98% of the youth and families randomly assigned to the MST conditions completed treatment.

CLINICAL PROCEDURES

The fundamental goal of MST is to empower families to effectively resolve and manage the serious clinical problems presented by their youth, as well as the potential problems that are likely to occur during the youth's adolescence. Thus, therapists aim to help youth and their families develop the capacity to cope with problems that have a multisystemic set of causal and sustaining factors, utilizing resources within the families' ecologies to develop this capacity. Rather than providing a rigid manualized plan for treatment, the MST manual provides a framework in which treatment occurs. Specifically, MST therapists and supervisors follow a set of nine core principles that guide all assessment practices and the integration of evidence-based interventions within the MST framework (Henggeler et al., 1998). These nine principles[2] are used to identify targets for intervention and to design interventions to meet the goals of treatment.

2. (a) The primary purpose of assessment is to understand the "fit" between the identified problems and their broader systemic context. (b) Therapeutic contacts emphasize the positive and use systemic strengths as levers for change. (c) Interventions are designed to promote responsible behavior and decrease irresponsible behavior among family members. (d) Interventions are present-focused and action-oriented, targeting specific and well-defined problems. (e) Interventions target sequences of behavior within or between multiple systems that maintain the identified problems. (f) Interventions are developmentally appropriate and fit the developmental needs of the youth. (g) Interventions are designed to require daily or weekly effort by family members. (h) Intervention effectiveness is evaluated continuously from multiple perspectives, with providers assuming accountability for overcoming barriers to successful outcomes. (i) Interventions are designed to promote treatment generalization and long-term maintenance of therapeutic change by empowering caregivers to address family members' needs across multiple systemic contexts.

The MST team designs particular intervention strategies by adapting empirically based interventions from pragmatic, problem-focused treatments that have at least some empirical support. These may include strategic family therapy (Haley, 1987), structural family therapy (Minuchin, 1974), behavioral parent training (Munger, 1993), and cognitive behavior (Kendall & Braswell, 1993) therapies. In addition, if evidence of biological contributors to identified problems is found, psychopharmacological treatment is integrated with psychosocial treatment. Specific goals for treatment may be at the individual, family, peer, school, and social network levels. However, the MST model views the caregivers as key to achieving desired outcomes, and interventions typically focus on empowering the family to interface with key systems.

QUALITY ASSURANCE

As research trials of MST began to expand to multiple sites and as the MST treatment protocol was disseminated to community provider organizations across the country, specification of quality assurance mechanisms became necessary to maintain the internal validity of the treatment model. Further, several empirical studies have supported linkages between adherence to MST treatment principles and clinical outcomes (Henggeler, Melton, Brondino, Scherer, & Hanley, 1997; Henggeler, Pickrel, & Brondino, 1999a; Huey, Henggeler, Brondino, & Pickrel, 2000; Schoenwald, Henggeler, Brondino, & Rowland, 2000; Schoenwald, Sheidow, & Letourneau, 2003; Schoenwald, Sheidow, Letourneau, & Liao, 2003). Thus, the MST model includes a comprehensive quality assurance system with an overriding purpose of helping therapists and supervisors achieve desired clinical outcomes for youth and families by supporting treatment fidelity.

The treatment developers initially provided all program development and ongoing support to new and distal MST sites, but in 1996 a new organization, MST Services, was formed with the mission of supporting the effective transport and dissemination of MST programs for serious juvenile offenders. Hence, MST programs, operating in more than 30 states and eight nations as of early 2003, include multiple layers of clinical and programmatic support. Specifically, provider organizations receive extensive organizational consultation to assure the provision of necessary resources (e.g., funding, small caseloads, and interagency collaboration) prior to and following the development of MST programs. The assessment, intervention, supervision, and consultation processes are all manualized and focus on the nine guiding principles of MST. Treatment integrity is sustained through initial didactic and experiential training, followed by regular booster sessions by MST experts, weekly supervision within the MST treatment team (consisting of therapists and MST supervisor), and weekly consultation with a MST expert. Supervision and consultation include feedback from measures of treatment integrity, including monthly caregiver-reported ratings of therapist adherence (Henggeler & Borduin, 1992). Thus, therapist adherence to the treatment model is monitored continuously.

CONTROLLED OUTCOME RESEARCH

MST is widely regarded as one of the best validated juvenile delinquency inter-ventions in the field, with federal entities such as the Surgeon General (U.S. Public Health Service, 1999, 2001), National Institute on Drug Abuse (1999), and Center for Substance Abuse Prevention (2001), as well as leading reviewers (e.g., Burns, Hoagwood, & Mrazek, 1999; Elliott, 1998; Farrington & Welsh, 1999; Kazdin & Weisz, 1998; Mihalic et al., 2001; Stanton & Shadish, 1997), identifying MST as a model program for treating youths' criminal behavior. These conclusions are based on the findings from six published outcome studies (five randomized, one quasi-experimental) with juvenile offenders and their families.

In the first MST outcome study, Henggeler et al. (1986) used a quasi-experi-mental design (i.e., MST youth were matched with control youth on key charac-teristics) to evaluate the short-term effectiveness of MST with juvenile offenders ($N = 57$). MST was more effective than usual diversion services at improving both self-reported and observed family relations, as well as decreasing youth behavior problems and youth association with deviant peers. These favorable findings led to three randomized trials of MST with chronic and violent juvenile offenders that were published in the 1990s. Henggeler, Melton, and Smith (1992) evaluated the capacity of MST to serve as an effective community-based alternative to incarceration for a sample ($N = 84$) of serious juvenile offenders. MST services were delivered by real world clinicians (not graduate students) working in a community mental health center. In addition to being more effec-tive than usual juvenile justice services at improving family and peer relations, MST reduced recidivism by 43% and out-of-home placement by 64% at 59-week follow-up. Moreover, a 2.4-year follow-up (Henggeler, Melton, Smith, Schoen-wald, & Hanley, 1993) showed that MST doubled the survival rate (i.e., the percentage of youth not rearrested) of these serious offenders. Similarly, in a ran-domized trial that included 176 chronic juvenile offenders, Borduin and col-leagues (1995) demonstrated improved family functioning and decreased psychi-atric symptomatology at posttreatment, as well as a 69% decrease in recidivism at a 4-year follow-up compared to individual counseling. Finally, in a randomized trial of MST with 155 violent and chronic juvenile offenders conducted at two community sites, Henggeler et al. (1997) found that MST was more effective than usual juvenile justice services at decreasing youth psychiatric sympto-matology at posttreatment and produced a 50% reduction in incarceration at a 1.7-year follow-up. Although recidivism was reduced by only 26%, analyses showed significant associations between therapist adherence to MST treatment principles, which was allowed to vary considerably by design, and long-term out-comes.

A randomized trial of MST versus usual community services in the treat-ment of 118 juvenile offenders meeting diagnostic criteria for substance abuse or dependence (Henggeler et al., 1999a) showed decreased drug use at posttreat-ment for youth receiving MST, as well as a 50% reduction in days in out-of-home placement and a 26% reduction in recidivism (statistically nonsignificant) at 1-year follow-up. In addition, MST increased attendance in regular school settings at 6-month follow-up (Brown, Henggeler, Schoenwald, Brondino, & Pickrel, 1999), and 4-year follow-up data (Henggeler, Clingempeel, Brondino, & Pickrel, 2002a) showed that MST significantly reduced violent criminal activity and increased drug use abstinence.

To date, the only published randomized trial in the field of juvenile sexual offender treatment was a MST study directed by Borduin, Henggeler, Blaske, and Stein (1990). Although the sample was small ($N = 16$), MST demonstrated significantly lower recidivism for both sexual offending and criminal offending in comparison with individual counseling.

In sum, reductions in rates of recidivism have ranged between 26 and 69% across studies for youth treated with MST compared to treated control groups, and group differences have been observed as much as 4 years posttreatment. Together, findings from these studies have demonstrated the capacity of MST to change key determinants of antisocial behavior (e.g., family relations, peer relations) and to produce significant reductions in rearrest and out-of-home placement for juvenile offenders.

COST ANALYSES

Identifying the importance of cost-effectiveness, Schoenwald and colleagues (Schoenwald, Ward, Henggeler, Pickrel, & Patel, 1996) evaluated the costs of MST compared to usual services for the sample of substance abusing and dependent delinquents studied by Henggeler et al. (1999a). The incremental cost of MST was offset by the reduced placement of youth in the MST condition at 1-year postrecruitment (Schoenwald et al., 1996). Specific monetary costs for the victim and the system-level costs for treating juvenile offenders were recently evaluated by researchers unaffiliated with a specific treatment approach (Aos, Phipps, Barnoski, & Lieb, 2001). This initiative, conducted by the Washington State Institute for Public Policy, evaluated available empirical research on treatments for juvenile offenders and estimated total cost savings (i.e., victim costs, victim quality of life costs, and system costs) for numerous intervention models. To evaluate the ability to generalize findings about a treatment to real world settings, Aos and colleagues (2001) also assessed whether studies had been performed by the treatment developer or by researchers other than the developer and whether studies had been conducted in community settings or in university settings. The report placed the highest level of confidence in the findings of MST studies (i.e., produced a rating of 5 on a 5-point scale of confidence in study findings), noting that some studies had been carried out by researchers other than the developers and were conducted in real world community settings. According to the report, MST cost an average of $4,743 per family and had an average effect size of $-.31$, producing $31,661 in reduced placement and juvenile justice system costs. Further savings from costs to victims increased this figure to $131,918 per participant.

Oregon Treatment Foster Care (OTFC)

Like MST, OTFC was developed as an alternative to incarceration for serious juvenile offenders. Based on principles of social learning theory, developers began specifying and evaluating OTFC in the early 1980s. They have conducted one quasi-experimental investigation and one randomized controlled trial to establish the efficacy of the intervention for juvenile offenders. OTFC is specified in a treatment manual (Chamberlain & Mihalic, 1998) entitled *Multidimensional Treatment Foster Care* and published as part of the OJJDP Blueprints for Violence Prevention series (Mihalic et al., 2001) and in a recently published volume (Chamberlain, 2003). The developers have established training and supervision procedures, which they use to support treatment fidelity, but they have not yet developed or tested measures of quality assurance.

TREATMENT PROVISION

Youth receiving OTFC are placed with trained foster parents in lieu of restrictive residential placement, with an ultimate goal of the youth transitioning home to the biological or adoptive family. Typically, only one youth is placed with each foster family at a time. Treatment is provided by a team, consisting of trained foster parents, a full-time case manager, individual and family therapists, and other resource staff. Treatment is intensive, with each team responsible for 10 active cases and the case manager providing 24-hour/7-day-a-week availability over a 6- to 12-month period. Foster parents are contacted daily by the case manager to review the youth's behavior and modify the treatment plan. Treatment teams also meet weekly, and family therapy is provided to prepare the biological/adoptive family for the youth's return.

CLINICAL PROCEDURES

The main objectives of OTFC are to provide (a) close supervision, (b) fair and consistent limits, (c) predictable consequences for rule breaking, (d) a supportive relationship with a mentoring adult(s), and (e) reduced exposure to delinquent peers while encouraging prosocial youth relationships. Thus, specific interventions occur in a variety of environmental contexts. As in the case of MST, a range of treatment modalities is integrated to achieve change in youth with severe behavior problems.

For instance, behavioral parent training is employed for teaching both foster parents and biological parents to manage the youth's behavior in a consistent and noncoercive manner. Here, an individualized behavioral program is tailored for each youth through collaboration of the OTFC treatment team. This program includes a comprehensive point system that rewards normative behaviors each day (e.g., school attendance, completion of chores, completing activities on time, having a cooperative attitude). The youth's compliance with the behavioral program is linked with a three-level system of privileges, where each level relates to an expansion of available privileges. A loss of points results in loss of privileges, demotion to a lower level, or addition of chores (prespecified in behavioral plan). Other family-level interventions include intensive supervision of the youth's activities and monitoring of his or her interactions with peers. Family therapy sessions with the biological family (or other aftercare resource) are also conducted throughout placement in foster care. These sessions emphasize the development of caregiver skills in supervision, encouragement, discipline, and problem solving. Youth have home visits that begin with short (e.g., 1- to 2-hour) stays, increasing to overnight visits as treatment progresses.

OTFC also incorporates school-based behavioral interventions and academic supports. For instance, the individualized behavioral program includes daily tracking of school behavior, with teachers signing off on attendance, completion of work, and attitude. The OTFC treatment team offers full collaboration with school counselors and teachers, including provision of support if the youth becomes disruptive while in school. In addition, OTFC includes individual therapy for the youth that is integrated into treatment. This may include psychiatric consultation and medication management that is coordinated by the case manager. In particular, individual therapy includes skills training for youth to develop skills for having positive relationships with adults and for generating relationships with prosocial peers. Such treatment is behaviorally oriented and may include development of problem-solving skills, social perspective taking, and nonaggressive methods of self-expression.

QUALITY ASSURANCE

OTFC maintains quality assurance through standardized training and close supervision of treatment providers (Chamberlain & Mihalic, 1998). Foster care parents are trained during a 20-hour didactic and experiential program. Upon successful completion of this program, which includes screening of the foster home and parents, daily contact between case managers and OTFC parents and weekly supervision meetings of OTFC teams provide further instruction that maintains treatment integrity. The daily contact between case managers and foster parents is also used to review the youth's progress on the behavioral treatment plan and to coordinate other services (e.g., psychiatric consultation, school supports). This daily contact is structured, with data collected on the Parent Daily Report Checklist (see Chamberlain & Mihalic, 1998), and the daily point cards are collected at weekly supervision meetings. These data are reviewed periodically by the program director, who is responsible for treatment integrity and provides weekly supervision to the OTFC case managers and therapists. Other than the Parent Daily Report Checklist, there currently are no quantifiable measures of adherence to the OTFC model for ongoing treatment programs. However, as part of a research investigation of OTFC, staff in the comparison conditions (group homes) and OTFC foster parents have been interviewed to assess treatment integrity (Chamberlain, Ray, & Moore, 1996). Significant differences were observed for types of additional services, adult mentoring, peer involvement, and perceived mechanisms of change.

CONTROLLED OUTCOME RESEARCH

Federal entities such as the U.S. Surgeon General (U.S. Public Health Service, 1999) and OJJDP's Blueprints for Violence Prevention initiative (Mihalic et al., 2001) have identified OTFC as a model treatment program. Two empirical studies have been conducted in real world settings to test the effectiveness of OTFC for treating juvenile offenders (Chamberlain, 1990; Chamberlain & Reid, 1998). As OTFC is intended to treat youth that have exhausted less restrictive methods of treatment, youth in these two trials were severe and chronic offenders. The initial investigation of OTFC treated sixteen 13- to 18-year-olds, matched by age, sex, and date of commitment to sixteen youth in other community residential treatment settings. Youth receiving OTFC were less likely to run away from the treatment setting, more likely to complete treatment, and experienced fewer days of incarceration during the 2 years posttreatment.

The second investigation was a randomized trial of 79 male 12- to 17-year-olds receiving either OTFC or standard group care (Chamberlain & Reid, 1998). Youth treated with OTFC were again less likely to run away and more likely to complete treatment. Notably, during the year after commitment to OTFC or group care, youth in the OTFC condition spent an average of 59 days residing with biological parents or relatives, in contrast to 31 days for youth in the group care condition. Youth in OTFC spent an average of 53 days in detention facilities, compared to an average of 129 days for youth in group care. Further, youth who received OTFC engaged in fewer offenses at 1 year posttreatment, as measured by both official arrests and self-reports of criminal offenses. These two trials, both using clinical samples and respectable scientific methods, demonstrate the capacity of OTFC to produce significant reductions in incarceration and criminal behavior among juvenile offenders.

COST ANALYSES

The Washington State Institute for Public Policy cost analysis (Aos et al., 2001) included the two studies described above, with a cost estimate of approximately $2,052 per youth, in addition to the cost of the foster placement. With reasonable confidence in conclusions about treatment differences, Aos and colleagues concluded that OTFC had an average effect size of −.37 for basic recidivism, generating $21,836 in reduced placement and juvenile justice costs compared to placement in group homes. Adding costs to victims produced savings of $87,622 per participant.

Functional Family Therapy (FFT)

FFT has been used for nearly 30 years in the treatment of youth conduct problems. One randomized controlled trial with juvenile status offenders and two quasi-experimental investigations with serious juvenile offenders have established the efficacy of the intervention. The treatment is described in an earlier clinical volume (Alexander & Parsons, 1982) and a recent treatment manual

(Alexander et al., 1998) published as part of the Blueprints for Violence Prevention series. Like OTFC, the developers of FFT have established training and supervision procedures, which they use to support treatment fidelity, but they have not yet developed or tested measures of quality assurance.

TREATMENT PROVISION

FFT treatment is provided by a single part-time or full-time therapist (FFT therapists have been student trainees, paraprofessionals, and professionals), and therapists are responsible for 12 to 16 active cases. FFT averages 12 sessions over 3 months, with more difficult cases requiring 26 to 30 hours of direct service, and treatment often occurs in the home.

CLINICAL PROCEDURES

FFT includes three sequential phases of treatment, with different intervention techniques used to achieve the goals of each phase (Alexander et al., 1998; Alexander & Sexton, 2002; Sexton & Alexander, 2002).

PHASE 1. ENGAGEMENT AND MOTIVATION. One goal of this phase is to enhance the family members' perceptions of therapist responsivity and credibility. Therapists accomplish this goal by behaving responsively and respectfully toward the family and making family members feel as comfortable as possible through dress, attitude, affect, and availability. A second goal is to create a therapist–family context that is conducive to desired change. For example, FFT emphasizes the importance of creating a balanced alliance with each family member. To achieve this goal, the practitioner works to reduce anger, blaming, hopelessness, and other negative behaviors and emotions among family members using techniques such as reframing.

PHASE 2. BEHAVIOR CHANGE. This stage focuses primarily on changing family interactions through building interpersonal and problem-solving skills. As Alexander et al. (1998) noted, FFT change techniques fall into two categories: parent training and communication training. Parent training is usually emphasized with families of younger children and follows relatively well-specified protocols developed in the behavioral parent training literature. Communication skills training is also based primarily on the behavioral literature and emphasizes elements such as brevity, directness, and active listening. During this phase, relationship skills remain important, but therapist interactions primarily focus on restructuring family relations in ways that will facilitate desired behavior change (Alexander & Sexton, 2002).

PHASE 3. GENERALIZATION. The goal of this final phase is to extend positive intrafamily change by incorporating relations with community systems, such as mental health and juvenile justice authorities. Here, the therapist acts largely as a case manager or collaborates with a case manager in attempting to anchor the family in a supportive community context. To accomplish this goal, therapists must possess extensive knowledge of community resources and have positive relations with community social service agencies.

QUALITY ASSURANCE

The FFT model maintains quality assurance through standardized training of therapists and supervisors, therapist reports from each session, supervision of therapists, and consultation with FFT experts (Alexander et al., 1998). Specifically, quality assurance includes (a) an initial 2- to 3-day training workshop by the treatment developers; (b) an on-site consultation visit each year, including group and individual meetings; (c) individual telephone consultations with each intervention staff member once or more per year; (d) a process summary measure completed by the therapist following each client session; (e) a counseling process questionnaire completed by family members after every other treatment session; and (f) weekly supervision by a FFT supervisor with at least a master's degree, including review of process measures and occasional review of audio-taped client sessions. Importantly, an innovative Internet-based system for tracking therapist performance and clinical progress from multiple perspectives (i.e., client, therapist, supervisor) across FFT dissemination sites has recently become operational. Such systems have the clear potential to promote program fidelity and corresponding youth and family outcomes.

CONTROLLED OUTCOME RESEARCH

Like MST and OTFC, federal entities such as the U.S. Surgeon General (U.S. Public Health Service, 1999) and OJJDP's Blueprints for Violence Prevention initiative (Mihalic et al., 2001) have identified FFT as a model treatment program. The initial study of FFT (Alexander & Parsons, 1973) was a randomized trial of male and female offenders, aged 13 to 16 years, who were referred by the Salt Lake County Juvenile Court for primarily status offenses. Forty-six families received FFT through the University of Utah, while 40 comparison families received client-centered family group therapy, psychodynamic family therapy, or no treatment. The recidivism rate for status offenses of those youth receiving FFT was less than those of the three other groups by 50% or more.

In a replication (Gordon, Arbuthnot, Gustafson, & McGreen, 1988) with 54 rural Ohio youth who were more disadvantaged and had committed more serious offenses than youth in the initial trial, FFT was conducted in-home (vs. the clinic-based treatment previously utilized) and averaged 16 sessions. Youth referred for FFT as a condition of probation were matched to control youth randomly selected from those not referred for family treatment based on schools attended. FFT resulted in a recidivism rate of 11% compared to 67% for the no-treatment controls, a reduction in recidivism of over 80%. In addition, Barton, Alexander, Waldron, Turner, and Warburton (1985) reported three quasi-experimental evaluations of FFT ($N = 74$) that included therapists with different levels of training (e.g., undergraduates, probation officers) treating youth presenting different levels of problem severity (e.g., status offenders, youth returning from placement) and their families. Results were generally favorable, though few methodological details were provided for these studies.

The most recent investigation of FFT, yet to be submitted for peer review, was an urban, community-based trial for the treatment of violent, drug abusing youth (Sexton, Ostrom, Bonomo, & Alexander, 2000, as reported in Sexton & Alexander, 2002). Results of this matched trial indicate a reoffense rate for youth receiving FFT of 20% versus 36% for the matched controls receiving usual services. Furthermore, youth receiving FFT committed fewer crimes and engaged in less severe criminal acts. Overall, FFT research has found a significant reduction in recidivism compared to treated and untreated controls (Alexander et al., 1998), and outcomes have been stable for as long as 5 years (Gordon et al., 1988) posttreatment.

COST ANALYSES

The Washington State Institute for Public Policy report (Aos et al., 2001) indicated that studies of FFT, some of which had been carried out by researchers independent of the treatment developers, were reasonably strong in their research design (i.e., produced a rating of 3 to 4 on a 5-point scale of confidence in study findings). After controlling for confidence ratings of research designs, FFT had an effect size of $-.25$ for basic recidivism (proportion of offenders to nonoffenders). At an average cost of $2,161 per participant, FFT produced an average of $14,149 in placement and juvenile justice savings for each treated youth compared to the standard juvenile justice program. When crime victim costs were included in the formula, the savings reached $59,067 per participant.

Promising Community-Based Interventions

While the treatments described above can be considered efficacious, other community-based interventions have shown promise for treating juvenile delinquency. These models may lack the degree of specification needed to replicate them in the field and/or the research base needed to adequately determine effectiveness for treating juvenile delinquency. Some of these promising treatment models are described here.

Wraparound

The Wraparound model (see Burchard, Bruns, & Burchard, 2002; Burns & Goldman, 1999) was developed primarily from grassroots movements across the country to coordinate already available services in the community when treating child problems. The Wraparound approach has been employed in a wide array of service sectors (e.g., mental health, education, child welfare, and juvenile justice) and aims to be child and family centered, focused on child and family strengths, community-based, culturally relevant, flexible, and coordinated across agencies (Burchard et al., 2002).

Wraparound has experienced enormous proliferation with support from the federal Center for Mental Health Services as communities look to improve services for youth in a cost-efficient manner. However, this rapid dissemination has resulted in a wide assortment of approaches being called "wraparound," even though they may have little resemblance to what the developers proposed. In an effort to develop standards for Wraparound providers and to understand the effectiveness of the model, the intervention's definitions, values, essential elements, and requirements for practice have been more clearly specified (Burns & Goldman, 1999). Training procedures are also becoming more standardized (Meyers, Kaufman, & Goldman, 1999), and a quality improvement protocol is under development. Emerging research is supporting the relation of outcomes to a measure of fidelity to Wraparound principles (Bruns, Suter, Burchard, Force, & Dakan, 2003), suggesting the value of a quality assurance protocol. Although outcome research of Wraparound for juvenile offenders has not been conducted, an investigation is beginning to evaluate Wraparound for youth diverted from detention in Baltimore, Maryland (E. J. Bruns, personal communication, February 2003). Cost analyses specifically for the Wraparound model have not been conducted.

Parent Management Training (PMT)

PMT (see Kazdin, 1996, 1997; Mabe, Turner, & Josephson, 2001) is based on social learning theory and teaches parents to modify parent-child interactions and to use operant conditioning procedures to reduce problem youth behaviors and develop prosocial youth behaviors. PMT was developed over 30 years ago and, through its strong research track record, has become recognized as an effective evidence-based treatment for young children with behavioral problems (Kazdin & Weisz, 1998). Although much research has been conducted on using PMT to treat young children or youth with less acute problems, only one controlled trial has focused specifically on youth offenders. Bank, Marlowe, Reid, Patterson, and Weinrott (1991) evaluated 55 chronic offenders randomized to either PMT or usual juvenile justice services and conducted yearly follow-up assessments for 3 years. Although both PMT and usual services significantly reduced recidivism, reductions occurred more quickly in the PMT condition. Youth receiving PMT also spent less time incarcerated than youth receiving usual services. PMT treatment procedures are specified, although training and quality assurance protocols are not standardized. Cost comparisons for PMT have not been conducted.

Juvenile Counseling and Assessment Program (JCAP)

Researchers and professionals at the University of Georgia (UGA), the Georgia Department of Juvenile Justice, and the Athens–Clarke County Juvenile Court developed and evaluated the JCAP for adjudicated youth (Kadish, Glaser, Calhoun, & Risler, 1999). Master's students provided services, supervised by doctoral students and doctoral-level UGA faculty members. Based on social learning theory, JCAP includes individual counseling, group counseling, psychological assessments, and family consultations, with counseling focused on problem-solving skills, social skills, anger management, and education. In a quasi-experimental trial using JCAP to treat delinquent youth, significant group differences emerged within the 6 months following treatment (Kadish et al., 1999). Of the 55 youth receiving JCAP, 14 youth reoffended in the 6 months posttreatment (6 had 1 reoffense, 8 had 2+ reoffenses), while 35 of the 55 matched control youth reoffended (12 had 1 reoffense, 23 had 2+ reoffenses). Although JCAP is not well specified at this time, these preliminary data suggest the promise of the community-based intervention model.

Treatment Commonalties

Community-based interventions have been identified as model approaches to youth treatment in reviews by the U.S. Surgeon General (U.S. Public Health Service, 1999, 2001) and the National Advisory Mental Health Council Workgroup on Child and Adolescent Mental Health Intervention Development and Deployment (2001), and researchers continue to highlight such treatments of serious antisocial behavior in adolescents as "best practice" and exemplary treatments (Kazdin & Weisz, 1998). Although each of the community-based interventions described in this chapter was developed independently, many of them share several commonalties in their conceptualization, delivery, and procedures. As these approaches are disseminated into community settings, the bases of their success and the parallels among the approaches become of heightened interest.

Evidence-Based Development and Integration in Community-Based Treatment

Whereas the typical services (e.g., residential, probation) for juvenile offenders primarily focus on the individual youth, community-based treatment models aim to alter the aspects of the environment that developed and sustained deviant youth behavior. Thus, treatment may occur in multiple systems within the youth's environment (e.g., family, peers, school, neighborhood), and treatment foci may include emphases on improving family interactions and caregiver functioning, developing the family's social support system, increasing the youth's prosocial peer relationships, minimizing youth contact with antisocial peers, or enhancing school supports and interactions.

Such a model makes sense in light of the literature on the causes and correlates of antisocial behavior in adolescents. This literature has provided clear evidence for a multidetermined, ecological conceptualization of juvenile delinquency. As summarized in several recent reviews (Hann & Borek, 2001; Hawkins et al., 1998; Lipsey & Derzon, 1998), associations between deviant behavior and individual, family, peer, school, and community constructs have been identified across numerous longitudinal and cross-sectional samples. For instance, individual factors that have been linked to antisocial behavior include biological processes (e.g., adrenal hormones, serotonin levels, teratogenic effects) and cognitive functioning (e.g., social information processing, problem solving, and verbal ability). Family factors include caregiver characteristics (e.g., drug use, maternal age, caregiver psychopathology) and family-level characteristics (e.g., conflict management, monitoring, and supervision). Peer influences include association with deviant peers, lack of association with prosocial peers, and poor socialization skills. School-related predictors of conduct problems include low academic achievement, dropout, low commitment to education, and poor structure within the school. Finally, community constructs, such as violence exposure, neighborhood criminal activity, neighborhood supports, and mobility, have been predictive of antisocial behavior. As evidence for a multisystemic set of causes and correlates for antisocial behavior in youth has become available, community-based intervention approaches have garnered increasing support among reviewers and policy-makers.

In general, the approaches described in this chapter use the existing knowledge base in child psychopathology and treatment in the conceptualization, design, and implementation of interventions. Treatment planning is informed by evidence of known risk factors across the youth and family's social ecology (Atkins & McKay, 2001). For instance, MST, OTFC, and FFT recognize involvement with antisocial peers as a vital contributor to antisocial behavior, and specific interventions are aimed at reducing this negative influence. Family structure and monitoring of youth are also identified as critical areas of intervention across the models. In addition, the evidence base on psychotherapy research is incorporated into many of these treatment models. For example, behavioral techniques are used across the approaches to provide structure within home and school settings.

Demand and Dissemination

The success of the exemplary community-based models, in combination with significant national need for effective services for youth with serious antisocial behavior, has created considerable demand for such treatment approaches. In response to this demand, the exemplary models presented in this chapter (i.e., MST, OTFC, and FFT) are all highly specified treatments whose developers have defined a comprehensive dissemination protocol. These protocols include clearly defined treatment procedures, as well as standardized training procedures and quality assurance systems. Promising programs such as Wraparound also are moving toward this paradigm. As evidenced by great variation in implementation across the country for promising programs like Wraparound, clarifying the various protocols prior to promulgation is essential for evaluation and successful implementation of a treatment model. Indeed, the importance of specification and quality assurance for promoting favorable treatment outcomes for youth was highlighted by the U.S. Surgeon General (U.S. Public Health Service, 2001).

Development of specified procedures is the initial step in accurate replication and supports the development of measurable fidelity. Given that recent empirical studies of MST have demonstrated linkages between therapist adherence to MST treatment principles and short- and long-term clinical outcomes (Henggeler et al., 1997, 1999a; Huey et al., 2000; Schoenwald et al., 2000) and that evidence from Wraparound developers suggests that adherence to the Wraparound model is related to youth outcomes (Bruns et al., 2003), this step is fundamental to the successful dissemination of community-based treatments. Although some of the treatments presented here monitor fidelity through different mechanisms (e.g., OTFC and FFT monitor adherence through structured supervision; MST tracks fidelity through supervisory and expert consultation protocols and through adherence measures), functional adherence procedures are becoming a recognized issue for successful dissemination.

Transport of a complex community-based practice to field settings requires a different set of skills than those needed in the development and evaluation of these models. The exemplary treatments presented here are utilizing very different methods than the "workshop" model of dissemination that historically has dominated the treatment field. For instance, the developers of MST and, more recently, OTFC have pursued strategies that emphasize the creation of new organizations that are explicitly committed to effective transport and dissemination. The emphases of these organizations on ongoing fidelity monitoring and quality assurance by teams of experts is somewhat unique in the services sector. It remains to be seen, however, which dissemination strategies are more effective at promoting youth and family outcomes.

Commitment to Rigorous Evaluation

The efficacious treatments, as well as the promising treatments, presented in this chapter have evidenced a commitment to developing a strong evidence base. MST, OTFC, and FFT have each generated empirical support through multiple clinical trials that aimed to systematically evaluate treatment effectiveness. Matched group and randomized trials of FFT have evaluated a wide array of clinical outcomes. Randomized control trials, the "gold standard" for clinical research, have frequently been used to test the effectiveness of MST. The effectiveness of OTFC has been examined using both matched and randomized trials. In addition, promising interventions like Wraparound and JCAP are in the process of developing a research base. Most important to establishing effectiveness in this multiproblem population, outcome studies of these treatment models have typically included "real-world" youth in community settings. That is, treatment was provided in a manner consistent with what could be provided by a community agency, rather than within a university setting. Further, youth research participants have been clinically impaired and accurately represent the population of youth with conduct problems.

Treatment Process

As noted previously, intervention guidelines have been specified in manuals and texts for most of the community-based interventions presented here. For many of the interventions, these guidelines focus on similar sets of issues. For example, strategies to promote treatment engagement and reduce barriers to service access are emphasized. MST and OTFC provide clinician availability 24 hours a day, 7 days a week. MST clinicians provide all services within the youth's ecology, and FFT devotes the initial phase of treatment to obtaining adequate engagement. These procedures have resulted in extraordinarily high rates of treatment engagement and completion. Youth treated with OTFC completed treatment programs at a rate of 73% compared to 36% for the control group. FFT research reports a treatment completion rate of 80%, while recent MST studies have achieved 97 and 98% treatment completion rates.

Similarly, the community-based models typically maintain a focus on generalization of treatment progress. Although the treatments may be time limited (except in the case of Wraparound), substantial portions of time are devoted to establishing supports and resources that will help to maintain changes made during treatment. For instance, FFT devotes an entire phase of treatment to this focus, while OTFC continues to provide individual and family therapy as the youth transitions back to the home. MST focuses on generalization throughout treatment, utilizing and enhancing resources and supports already present within the youth's surroundings to maintain treatment change. The clear ecological concentration on generalization that these evidence-based models maintain is instrumental in producing long-term change and makes them very unusual among treatments for adolescent behavior problems.

Clinical and Research Implications

While MST, OTFC, and FFT have developed an evidence base to support denotation as efficacious for treating juvenile delinquency, the promising treatments presented are generally making progress toward developing such an evidence base (e.g., specifying protocols, conducting randomized trials, and the like). Regardless, the development, validation, and dissemination activities of the community-based models presented here have important, and possibly unsettling, implications for typical modes of clinical practice. In general, these treatment models (and a wealth of services research—see Weisz & Jensen, 1999) suggest that current practice methods are probably not effective. Importantly, they suggest several directions in the establishment of more effective practice.

Address Known Risk Factors

Many approaches to treating juvenile delinquency have not necessarily focused on known risk factors, yet a wealth of knowledge has emerged during the past several decades regarding the determinants of delinquency in adolescents. Most of the community-based models presented here are clear in their focus on these factors. As someone recovering from a heart attack should address known risk factors (e.g., exercise, smoking, drug use, hypertension, cholesterol, obesity) if he or she desires to reduce the probability of a second attack, it makes sense for therapists to focus on known risk factors when treating adolescents with antisocial behavior.

Follow Treatment Protocols

The efficacious approaches presented here, MST, OTFC, and FFT, are operationalized with flexible, yet structured, protocols. Therapists are provided guidelines in which certain types of interventions are appropriate for certain types of situations, and other types of interventions are proscribed. For example, each of these treatments integrates behavioral interventions within ecological conceptual frameworks. Similarly, some of the models proscribe certain interventions (e.g., group treatment) that are used widely in community practice.

Embrace Quality Assurance Systems

Serious antisocial behavior in adolescents can be extremely difficult to treat, and such youth are often embedded in families with many other challenging problems (e.g., caregiver mental illness and drug abuse, poverty, high stress, low social support). To expect a lone clinician to treat this array of problems effectively on a consistent basis is unrealistic. Clinicians should be surrounded with strong clinical support from peers, supervisors, and possibly even other experts in the field. This support should endeavor to optimize clinical outcomes by helping therapists adhere to validated treatment protocols and to develop and implement strategies for overcoming barriers to desired clinical outcomes.

Reward Accountability and Effectiveness

As indicated in the cost-effectiveness analyses, effective clinicians can save service systems considerable costs, most immediately and directly by preventing expensive out-of-home services. It seems only fair that a proportion of those savings should be passed on to the treatment program and effective clinician. Such extrinsic rewards for clinical success are rare, however, and require structures in which outcomes are tracked and accountability is high. Almost everyone can win in an effective accountability system (e.g., performance contracts) — youth and family functioning are improved, clinicians and their program benefit from their success, funders save money from reduced placements, and fewer community members are victimized.

Conclusion

This chapter identified several exemplary and promising community-based interventions for treating juvenile offenders, as well as similar features among the interventions that most likely account for their success. Future treatment developers should consider these features in the design and specification of new treatment models. In addition, the validation and initial transport of MST, OTFC, and FFT to community agencies across the nation have opened up new lines of research that are on the cutting edge of the National Institutes of Health agenda—research examining the transport of evidence-based practices to community settings. Such research, as well as studies to further develop the promising models presented here, holds the potential to significantly improve the nation's outcomes for youth with serious clinical problems and their families.

References

Alexander, J., Barton, C., Gordon, D., Grotpeter, J., Hansson, K., Harrison, R., et al. (1998). *Blueprints for violence prevention: Book Three. Functional Family Therapy.* Boulder, CO: Center for the Study and Prevention of Violence.

Alexander, J. F., & Parsons, B. V. (1973). Short-term behavioral intervention with delinquent families: Impact on family process and recidivism. *Journal of Abnormal Psychology, 81,* 219–225.

Alexander, J. F., & Parsons, B. V. (1982). Functional family therapy: Principles and procedures. Carmel, CA: Brooks/Cole.

Alexander, J. F., & Sexton, T. L. (2002). Functional family therapy (FFT) as an integrative, mature clinical model for treating high risk, acting out youth. In J. Lebow (Ed.), *Comprehensive handbook of psychotherapy: Vol. IV. Integrative/eclectic* (pp. 111–132). New York: Wiley.

Aos, S., Phipps, P., Barnoski, R., & Lieb, R. (2001). *The comparative costs and benefits of programs to reduce crime* (Document 01-05-1201). Olympia: Washington State Institute for Public Policy.

Atkins, M. S., & McKay, M. M. (2001). Conduct disorder. In M. Hersen & V. B. Van Hasselt (Eds.), *Advanced abnormal psychology* (2nd ed., pp. 209–222). New York: Kluwer Academic/Plenum.

Bank, L., Marlowe, J. H., Reid, J. B., Patterson, G. R., & Weinrott, M. R. (1991). A comparative evaluation of parent-training interventions for families of chronic delinquents. *Journal of Abnormal Child Psychology, 19,* 15–33.

Barton, C., Alexander, J. F., Waldron, H., Turner, C. W., & Warburton, J. (1985). Generalizing treatment effects of functional family therapy: Three replications. *American Journal of Family Therapy, 13,* 16–26.

Borduin, C. M., Henggeler, S. W., Blaske, D. M., & Stein, R. J. (1990). Multisystemic treatment of adolescent sexual offenders. *International Journal of Offender Therapy and Comparative Criminology, 34,* 105–113.

Borduin, C. M., Mann, B. J., Cone, L. T., Henggeler, S. W., Fucci, B. R., Blaske, D. M., et al. (1995). Multisystemic treatment of serious juvenile offenders: Long-term prevention of criminality and violence. *Journal of Consulting and Clinical Psychology, 63,* 569–578.

Brown, T. L., Henggeler, S. W., Schoenwald, S. K., Brondino, M. J., & Pickrel, S. G. (1999). Multisystemic treatment of substance abusing and dependent juvenile delinquents: Effects on school attendance at posttreatment and 6-month follow-up. *Children's Services: Social Policy, Research, and Practice, 2,* 81–93.

Bruns, E. J., Suter, J., Burchard, J. D., Force, M., & Dakan, E. (2003). Fidelity to the wraparound process and its association with outcomes. In C. Newman, C. Liberton, K. Kutash, & R. M. Friedman (Eds.), *The 15th Annual Research Conference Proceed-*

ings: *A system of care for children's mental health.* Tampa: University of South Florida, Florida Mental Health Institute Research and Training Center for Children's Mental Health.

Burchard, J. D., Bruns, E. J., & Burchard, S. N. (2002). The wraparound approach. In B. J. Burns & K. Hoagwood (Eds.), *Community treatment for youth: Evidence-based interventions for severe emotional and behavioral disorders* (pp. 69–90). New York: Oxford University Press.

Burns, B. J., & Goldman, S. K. (1999). *Promising practices in wraparound for children with serious emotional disturbance and their families: Vol. IV. Systems of care: Promising practices in children's mental health.* Washington, DC: Center for Effective Collaboration and Practice, American Institutes for Research.

Burns, B. J., Hoagwood, K., & Mrazek, P. J. (1999). Effective treatment for mental disorders in children and adolescents. *Clinical Child and Family Psychology Review, 2,* 199–254.

Center for Substance Abuse Prevention. (2001). *Exemplary substance abuse prevention programs award ceremony.* Washington, DC: Substance Abuse and Mental Health Services Administration, Author.

Chamberlain, P. (1990). Comparative evaluation of specialized foster care for seriously delinquent youths: A first step. *Community Alternatives: International Journal of Family Care, 2,* 21–36.

Chamberlain, P. (2003). *Treating chronic juvenile offenders: Advances made through the Oregon Multidimensional Treatment Foster Care model.* Washington, DC: American Psychological Association.

Chamberlain, P., & Mihalic, S. (1998). *Blueprints for violence prevention: Book Eight. Multidimensional Treatment Foster Care.* Boulder, CO: Center for the Study and Prevention of Violence.

Chamberlain, P., Ray, J., & Moore, K. J. (1996). Characteristics of residential care for adolescent offenders: A comparison of assumptions and practices in two models. *Journal of Child and Family Studies, 5,* 285–297.

Chamberlain, P., & Reid, J. B. (1998). Comparison of two community alternatives to incarceration for chronic juvenile offenders. *Journal of Consulting and Clinical Psychology, 66,* 624–633.

Chambless, D. L., & Hollon, S. D. (1998). Defining empirically supported therapies. *Journal of Consulting and Clinical Psychology, 66,* 7–18.

Elliott, D. S. (Ed.). (1998). *Blueprints for violence prevention.* Boulder, CO: Center for the Study and Prevention of Violence.

Farrington, D. P., & Welsh, B. C. (1999). Delinquency prevention using family-based interventions. *Children and Society, 13,* 287–303.

Gordon, D. A., Arbuthnot, J., Gustafson, K. E., & McGreen, P. (1988). Home-based behavioral-systems family therapy with disadvantaged juvenile delinquents. *American Journal of Family Therapy, 16,* 243–255.

Haley, J. (1987). *Problem-solving therapy* (2nd ed.). San Francisco: Jossey-Bass.

Hann, D. M., & Borek, N. (2001). *Taking stock of risk factors for child/youth externalizing behavior problems* (NIH Publication No. 02-4938). Washington, DC: Department of Health and Human Services, Public Health Service, National Institutes of Health, National Institute of Mental Health.

Hawkins, J. D., Herrenkohl, T., Farrington, D. P., Brewer, D., Catalano, R. F., & Harachi, T. W. (1998). A review of predictors of youth violence. In R. Loeber & D. P. Farrington (Eds.), *Serious and violent juvenile offenders: Risk factors and successful interventions* (pp. 106–146). Thousand Oaks, CA: Sage.

Henggeler, S. W., & Borduin, C. M. (1992). *Multisystemic Therapy Adherence Scales.* Charleston: Medical University of South Carolina, Department of Psychiatry and Behavioral Science.

Henggeler, S. W., Clingempeel, W. G., Brondino, M. J., & Pickrel, S. G. (2002a). Four-year follow-up of multisystemic therapy with substance-abusing and substance-dependent juvenile offenders. *Journal of the American Academy of Child and Adolescent Psychiatry, 41,* 868–874.

Henggeler, S. W., Melton, G. B., Brondino, M. J., Scherer, D. G., & Hanley, J. H. (1997). Multisystemic therapy with violent and chronic juvenile offenders and their families: The role of treatment fidelity in successful dissemination. *Journal of Consulting and Clinical Psychology, 65,* 821–833.

Henggeler, S. W., Melton, G. B., & Smith, L. A. (1992). Family preservation using multi-systemic therapy: An effective alternative to incarcerating serious juvenile offenders. *Journal of Consulting and Clinical Psychology, 60,* 953–961.

Henggeler, S. W., Melton, G. B., Smith, L. A., Schoenwald, S. K., & Hanley, J. H. (1993). Family preservation using multisystemic treatment: Long-term follow-up to a clinical trial with serious juvenile offenders. *Journal of Child and Family Studies, 2,* 283–293.

Henggeler, S. W., Pickrel, S. G., & Brondino, M. J. (1999a). Multisystemic treatment of substance abusing and dependent delinquents: Outcomes, treatment fidelity, and transportability. *Mental Health Services Research, 1,* 171–184.

Henggeler, S. W., Pickrel, S. G., Brondino, M. J., & Crouch, J. L. (1996). Eliminating (almost) treatment dropout of substance abusing or dependent delinquents through home-based multisystemic therapy. *American Journal of Psychiatry, 153,* 427–428.

Henggeler, S. W., Rodick, J. D., Borduin, C. M., Hanson, C. L., Watson, S. M., & Urey, J. R. (1986). Multisystemic treatment of juvenile offenders: Effects on adolescent behavior and family interaction. *Developmental Psychology, 22,* 132–141.

Henggeler, S. W., Rowland, M. D., Randall, J., Ward, D. M., Pickrel, S. G., Cunningham, P. B., et al. (1999b). Home-based multisystemic therapy as an alternative to the hospitalization of youths in psychiatric crisis: Clinical outcomes. *Journal of the American Academy of Child and Adolescent Psychiatry, 38,* 1331–1339.

Henggeler, S. W., & Schoenwald, S. K. (1998). The MST supervisory manual: Promoting quality assurance at the clinical level. Charleston, SC: MST Services.

Henggeler, S. W., & Schoenwald, S. K. (1999). The role of quality assurance in achieving outcomes in MST programs. *Journal of Juvenile Justice and Detention Services, 14,* 1–17.

Henggeler, S. W., Schoenwald, S. K., Borduin, C. M., Rowland, M. D., & Cunningham, P. B. (1998). *Multisystemic treatment of antisocial behavior in children and adolescents.* New York: Guilford Press.

Henggeler, S. W., Schoenwald, S. K., Rowland, M. D., & Cunningham, P. B. (2002b). *Serious emotional disturbance in children and adolescents: Multisystemic therapy.* New York: Guilford Press.

Huey, S. J., Jr., Henggeler, S. W., Brondino, M. J., & Pickrel, S. G. (2000). Mechanisms of change in multisystemic therapy: Reducing delinquent behavior through therapist adherence and improved family and peer functioning. *Journal of Consulting and Clinical Psychology, 68,* 451–467.

Kadish, T. E., Glaser, B. A., Calhoun, G. B., & Risler, E. A. (1999). Counseling juvenile offenders: A program evaluation. *Journal of Addictions and Offender Counseling, 19,* 88–94.

Kazdin, A. E. (1996). Problem solving and parent management in treating aggressive and antisocial behavior. In E. D. Hibbs & P. S. Jensen (Eds.), *Psychosocial treatments for child and adolescent disorders: Empirically based strategies for clinical practice* (pp. 377–408). Rockville, MD: National Institute of Mental Health.

Kazdin, A. E. (1997). Parent management training: Evidence, outcomes, and issues. *Journal of the American Academy of Child and Adolescent Psychiatry, 36,* 1349–1356.

Kazdin, A. E., & Weisz, J. R. (1998). Identifying and developing empirically supported child and adolescent treatments. *Journal of Consulting and Clinical Psychology, 66,* 19–36.

Kendall, P. C., & Braswell, L. (1993). *Cognitive-behavioral therapy for impulsive children* (2nd ed.). New York: Guilford Press.

Lipsey, M. W., & Derzon, J. H. (1998). Predictors of violent or serious delinquency in adolescence and early adulthood: A synthesis of longitudinal research. In R. Loeber & D. P. Farrington (Eds.), *Serious and violent juvenile offenders: Risk factors and successful interventions* (pp. 86–105). Thousand Oaks, CA: Sage.

Lipsey, M. W., & Wilson, D. B. (1998). Effective intervention for serious juvenile offenders: A synthesis of research. In R. Loeber & D. P. Farrington (Eds.), *Serious and violent juvenile offenders: Risk factors and successful interventions* (pp. 313–345). Thousand Oaks, CA: Sage.

Mabe, P. A., Turner, M. K., & Josephson, A. M. (2001). Parent management training. *Child and Adolescent Psychiatric Clinics of North America, 10,* 451–464.

Meyers, J., Kaufman, M., & Goldman, S. K. (1999). *Promising practices: Training strategies for serving children with serious emotional disturbance and their families in a system of care: Vol. V. Systems of care: Promising practices in children's mental health.* Washington, DC: Center for Effective Collaboration and Practice, American Institutes for Research.

Mihalic, S., Irwin, K., Elliott, D., Fagan, A., & Hansen, D. (2001). *Blueprints for violence prevention.* Boulder, CO: Center for the Study and Prevention of Violence.

Minuchin, S. (1974). *Families and family therapy.* Cambridge, MA: Harvard University Press.

Munger, R. L. (1993). *Changing children's behavior quickly.* Lanham, MD: Madison.

National Advisory Mental Health Council Workgroup on Child and Adolescent Mental Health Intervention Development and Deployment. (2001). *Blueprint for change: Research on child and adolescent mental health.* Washington, DC: National Institute of Mental Health.

National Institute on Drug Abuse. (1999). *Principles of drug addiction treatment: A research-based guide* (NIH Publication No. 99-4180). Rockville, MD: U.S. Department of Health and Human Services, National Institutes of Health, Author.

Schoenwald, S. K., Henggeler, S. W., Brondino, M. J., & Rowland, M. D. (2000). Multisystemic therapy: Monitoring treatment fidelity. *Family Process, 39,* 83–103.

Schoenwald, S. K., Sheidow, A. J., & Letourneau, E. J. (2003). Toward effective quality assurance in multisystemic therapy: Links between expert consultation, therapist fidelity, and child outcomes. *Journal of Clinical Child & Adolescent Psychology, 33*(1), 94–104.

Schoenwald, S. K., Sheidow, A. J., Letourneau, E. J., & Liao, J. G. (2003). Transportability of multisystemic therapy: Evidence for multi-level influences. *Mental Health Services Research, 5*(4), 223–239.

Schoenwald, S. K., Ward, D. M., Henggeler, S. W., Pickrel, S. G., & Patel, H. (1996). Multisystemic therapy treatment of substance abusing or dependent adolescent offenders: Costs of reducing incarceration, inpatient, and residential placement. *Journal of Child and Family Studies, 5,* 431–444.

Sexton, T. L., & Alexander, J. F. (2002). Functional family therapy: An empirically supported, family-based intervention model for at-risk adolescents and their families. In T. Patterson (Ed.), *Comprehensive handbook of psychotherapy: Vol. II. Cognitive, behavioral, and functional approaches* (pp. 117–140). New York: Wiley.

Stanton, M. D., & Shadish, W. R. (1997). Outcome, attrition, and family-couples treatment for drug abuse: A meta-analysis and review of the controlled, comparative studies. *Psychological Bulletin, 122,* 170–191.

U.S. Public Health Service. (1999). *Mental health: A report of the Surgeon General.* Rockville, MD: U.S. Department of Health and Human Services, National Institutes of Health, National Institute of Mental Health.

U.S. Public Health Service. (2001). *Youth violence: A report of the Surgeon General.* Washington, DC: Author.

Weisz, J. R., & Jensen, P. S. (1999). Efficacy and effectiveness of child and adolescent psychotherapy and pharmacotherapy. *Mental Health Services Research, 1,* 125–157.

13

RICHARD E. REDDING, FRANCES J. LEXCEN,
AND EILEEN P. RYAN

Mental Health Treatment for Juvenile Offenders in Residential Psychiatric and Juvenile Justice Settings

Recently, there has been an upsurge of interest in what is increasingly acknowledged to be a vast unmet need for mental health services in the juvenile justice population. Many youth in the juvenile justice system have mental health and substance abuse problems, which are risk factors for delinquency. Studies have consistently found very high prevalence rates of mental illness among detained and incarcerated juveniles, and juvenile offenders generally (see Cocozza & Skowyra, 2000; Domolanta, Risser, Roberts, & Risser, 2003; McGarvey & Waite, 2000; Teplin, Abram, McClelland, Dulcan, & Mericle, 2002). While estimates of the percentage of juvenile offenders with mental health problems vary widely (e.g., between about 30 and 90%, depending upon study methodology and definition of mental illness), most estimates are substantially higher than the roughly 20% prevalence rate (see U.S. Department of Health & Human Services, 2001) found in the nondelinquent adolescent population. More juveniles with mental disorders have been entering the juvenile justice system in recent years (see Underwood, Newton, & Jageman, 2001), and they often have mental health needs similar to those of juveniles receiving inpatient or community-based mental health treatment (Evens & Vander Stoep, 1997). However, they are less likely ever to have received mental health treatment (Pumariega et al., 1999). This does not necessarily suggest a causal relationship between lack of access to mental health care and delinquency, but it does suggest that the mental health needs of juvenile offenders often go unrecognized and untreated.

Unfortunately, there has been a trend toward increasing reliance on the justice system to care for juveniles with mental illness (Cocozza & Skowyra, 2000). This trend, combined with the abolition in many states of state hospital care for children and adolescents, has created a population of seriously mentally ill youth for whom adequate services do not exist or cannot be accessed.

In some states, once youth are placed in juvenile detention or correctional facilities, community mental health centers are no longer mandated to provide care. Consequently, there may be little continuity in the provision of mental health services, increasing the risk of recidivism if the juvenile's delinquency is related to a mental illness. Placement in alternative residential facilities may be made in lieu of commitment to a correctional institution, but the juvenile's mental health needs often are not considered, and he or she may be placed alongside other children in state custody for reasons unrelated to delinquency (Gallagher, 1999).

Most juveniles with mental health needs can be cared for adequately within the detention or correctional center environment. For some seriously mentally ill juvenile offenders, however, placement in the correctional population will prove dangerous or iatrogenic in exacerbating behavior problems and psychiatric symptomatology, and hospitalization for acute stabilization or longer-term treatment is necessary. Careful assessment when juveniles enter detention facilities, and a more thorough evaluation at the outset of incarceration, can highlight and determine the specificity of mental health needs, including the need for psychiatric treatment.

Recognizing the specialized treatment needs of particular groups of juvenile offenders is a recent development in residential treatment, particularly in juvenile justice settings. In this chapter, we discuss the mental health treatment options for juvenile offenders placed in residential psychiatric or juvenile justice settings. After discussing the effectiveness and potential risks of residential care, we then discuss the unique treatment, behavioral management, and service delivery issues arising in residential settings and the importance of service integration and aftercare. We conclude with directions for future research and program development in the residential treatment of juvenile offenders.

Effectiveness of Residential Care

While juvenile crime rates were rising, some researchers in juvenile rehabilitation adopted an attitude that "nothing works" in residential (or community) treatment because of the strong evidence of intervention failures and the recognition of serious methodological flaws in studies reporting positive outcomes (Lab & Whitehead, 1988). This view was pervasive, with one study suggesting that day treatment was no worse at reducing recidivism than residential treatment but was significantly less expensive to implement (Velasquez & Lyle, 1985). (See Heilbrun, Lee, & Cottle, ch. 6 in this volume, for a meta-analysis of the effects of residential treatment and correctional interventions on juvenile offenders.)

Yet more recent outcome studies have generally found inpatient psychiatric care for children and adolescents to be effective in treating mental illness (see Gossett, Lewis, & Barhart, 1983; Pfeiffer & Strzelecki, 1990). Compared to community-based programs, residential programs offer greater opportunities for implementing token economies, longer treatment exposure, and more frequent individual or group treatment sessions (Agee, 1979; Denkowski, Denkowski, & Mabli, 1984; Serin & Preston, 2001). Residential programs may also have fewer problems with attendance and homework compliance, issues that are common in community-based treatment (Amini, Zilberg, Burke, & Salasnek, 1982; Meichenbaum & Turk, 1987). However, there is virtually no research on the residential treatment of juvenile offenders with mental disorders, particularly vis-à-vis treatment in correctional or quasi-correctional settings. Unfortunately, "The lack of systematic study of the efficacy of group care coupled with the widespread use of this approach is an excellent example of the rift between clinical practice and research" (Chamberlain & Friman, 1997, p. 422). The few available studies on the residential treatment of juvenile offenders with mental disorders suffer from serious methodological problems, including small sample sizes, unblinded data collectors, use of single measures for dependent variables, lack of validated intervention strategies, lack of control groups, and abbreviated follow-up periods for longitudinal designs (see Basta & Davidson, 1988). Studies also fail to specify the characteristics of the juveniles in terms of relevant offending, risk factor, and psychosocial variables, do not adequately define outcome variables (e.g., antisocial behavior and delinquency, psychiatric symptoms, restrictiveness of living, academic functioning), and fail to adequately assess antisocial behavior (Chamberlain & Friman, 1997).

But as recent meta-analyses have concluded (Lipsey, 1995; Lipsey & Wilson, 1998), treating persistent or serious juvenile offending is not a situation in which "nothing works" (see Martinson, 1974). A recent meta-analysis of 32 studies of juvenile and adult treatment programs, many of them residential, found that recidivism was reduced in 75% of studies (Redondo, Sanchez-Meca, & Garrido, 1999). Behavioral and cognitive-behavioral treatments were the most effective at reducing recidivism. Lipsey and Wilson's (1998) seminal meta-analysis of 83 treatment programs for institutionalized juvenile offenders (74 in juvenile justice facilities; 9 in residential mental health facilities) found that the most effective treatments reduced recidivism by 15 to 20%. The most effective residential treatments were interpersonal skills training and "teaching family homes," followed by behavioral programs, community residential programs, and multiple services programs (see Lipsey & Wilson, 1998, for descriptions of model programs). The most effective treatment programs were of longer duration and demonstrated high fidelity to the treatment model. Programs that were well established and those administered by mental health professionals rather than juvenile justice professionals also had the strongest positive effects. Interestingly, individual characteristics of the juveniles had little effect on outcomes, though most studies included in the meta-analysis were not evaluations of treatment programs designed specifically for mentally disordered offenders. Heilbrun et al.'s more recent meta-analysis, however, did find certain individual characteristics to be important (see Heilbrun, Lee, & Cottle, ch. 6).

Other factors also appear to correlate with better outcomes in residential settings: firmness, warmth, harmony, high expectations, good discipline, and a practical approach to training. (Rutter & Giller, 1984). These factors are not specific to any one treatment philosophy or theoretical orientation. Harris, Cote, & Vipond (1987) described a residential treatment program known to be effective for disturbed delinquent adolescents in Ontario, noting that strong leadership, special education services, work and recreation programs, and good staff and adolescent–staff relations were important factors in program success.

Risks of Residential Care

In addition to the possibility of abuse and neglect and the iatrogenic effects on children of long-term or even short-term psychiatric hospitalization (see Redding, 1992), this section addresses three treatment dilemmas that may cause harm to juveniles in residential treatment: academic, developmental and social delay, lack of family involvement, and the possible iatrogenic effects of exposure to delinquent peers and peer-group treatment.

Academic, Developmental, and Social Delay

Although learning disabilities are common in juvenile offenders, special education services in juvenile correctional facilities frequently are inadequate (Katsiyannis & Murry, 2000; Lynam, Moffitt, & Stouthamer-Loeber, 1993), only exacerbating the academic, social, and developmental delay often present in youthful offenders. Adolescent sex offenders are especially likely to need special education services for serious emotional disturbance (Johnson-Reid & Way, 2001). Juveniles in confinement are guaranteed access to special education services by the Individuals with Disabilities Education Act (IDEA, 1990) and the Americans with Disabilities Act (ADA, 1990). Access to appropriate education is consistent with the traditional rehabilitative goals of the juvenile justice system, but correctional special education is a recently developed field and there is a lack of training for interested teachers (McIntyre, 1993; Rutherford, Griller-Clark, & Anderson, 2001). Special education in residential treatment settings should provide both academic and behavioral education (see Denkowski et al., 1984) and teach functional skills related to basic employment and independent living and appropriate social skills for daily living (Rutherford et al., 2001). Successful methods in correctional special education combine highly structured learning environments and behavior modification to improve functioning in the classroom setting (Forness, Kavale, Blum, & Lloyd, 1997).

Lack of Family Involvement

There always is the danger that residential placement will weaken parent-child bonds (see Mohr, 1998) and produce feelings of "institutionalization" when the juvenile is secluded from family and friends (see Goffman, 1961). Actively maintaining family involvement can reduce these risks, facilitate the juvenile's transition back to the community, and enhance the success of aftercare (Burford & Casson, 1989). Families should be involved in the initial intake and assessment process, family or group therapy, and psychoeducational activities, where appropriate, and regular visits by family members should be encouraged (Burford & Casson, 1989). Parents can be educated about their child's mental health problems and trained in effective parenting skills and behavioral management practices.

Consistent family involvement is important during residential care (see Burford & Casson, 1989; Henggeler, 1999a,b), with family participation in treatment a key predictor of postdischarge outcomes and the generalization of treatment effects (Chamberlain & Friman, 1997; Gossett et al., 1983; Lewis, Lewis, Shanok, Klatskin, & Osborne, 1980; Parmelee, Cohen, Nemil, & Best, 1995). Moreover, Lewis, Yeager, Lovely, Stein, and Cobham-Portorreal's (1994) study of juvenile offenders released to the community found that the best predictor of successful adjustment was return to the family of origin, regardless of how dysfunctional that family may be. They suggested that returning to a social environment provided an opportunity for juveniles to interact with positive attachment figures and more functional role models. Similar results were found in a study of over 500 boys released from a residential program, with those released to their homes less likely to be imprisoned as adults (Kapp, Schwartz, & Epstein, 1994).

Negative Peer Relationships

Association with negative peers is a risk factor for delinquency and substance abuse (Elliott, Huizinga, & Ageton, 1985; Otero-Lopez, Luengo-Martin, Miron-Redondo, Carrillo-De-La-Pena, & Romero-Trinanes, 1994), and residential treatment with other juvenile offenders increases the intensity of exposure to negative peer influences. Treatment results can be diminished by the effects of relationships that develop among peers who are in treatment together or by negative peer relationships that are resumed after discharge (Dishion, McCord, & Poulin, 1999; Eddy & Chamberlain, 2000). In addition, the potential iatrogenic effects of peer-group therapy is a relatively recently documented risk for juvenile offenders (Dishion et al., 1999), which presents a significant new challenge for residential treatment in promoting prosocial behaviors and relationships among youth who may have had limited contact with positive attachment figures. Because longer residential placements may require more community services to remedy the iatrogenic effects of ongoing association with deviant peers while in the residential setting, the duration and intensity of postrelease community services required will not be diminished by longer stays in a treatment or correctional facility.

To address the problem of negative peer influence, Positive Peer Culture (PPC) was developed as a treatment milieu for delinquent youth (Gibbs, 1993; Gibbs, Potter, Barriga, & Liau, 1996; Tannehill, 1987; Vorrath & Brendro, 1974) and has been incorporated into many juvenile residential settings. Positive peer culture is based on the assumption that negative peer influence is one of the major causes of delinquency, but that peer influence can be channeled in positive directions through the use of peer-group modalities that confront and challenge negative behaviors and cognitive distortions (e.g., blaming others, self-serving attributions). While the results of several studies suggest that PPC may be effective in enhancing self-concept and moral development (Davis, Hoffman, & Quigley, 1988), there is little reliable research demonstrating its effectiveness in reducing recidivism or in promoting mental health. A study of the Minnesota Department of Corrections (2000) PPC program showed encouraging results in reducing recidivism but the study has substantial methodological limitations.

Treatment Foster Care

The less restrictive setting of treatment foster care (TFC) is more effective than residential treatment for improving reintegration with families of origin and in reducing recidivism, with family management skills and relations with deviant peers largely mediating these results (Eddy & Chamberlain, 2000). Often used as an alternative to residential psychiatric treatment, TFC is based on the premise that foster parents can serve as major providers of therapy via their daily interactions with the child and that therapy need not be practiced by clinicians alone (Redding, Fried, & Britner, 2000). Therapeutic foster families offer the type of wraparound services found in community-based treatment for chronic offenders, providing youth with consistent supervision in all areas of functioning and improved quality of family life. Effective TFC programs, often based on a social learning approach, include training, supervision, and ongoing support for foster parents and the development of an individualized behavioral program for the child. Treatment foster care provides a good modality to remediate poor parental supervision and discipline practices, which are key risk factors for delinquency.

Recent evaluations of TFC programs for juvenile offenders, which included mental health services and consultation, have shown promising results. Compared to those assigned to alternative diversion programs or group care placements, adolescent boys randomly assigned by the juvenile court to TFC had higher rates of program completion and lower posttreatment arrest and incarceration rates (Chamberlain, 1996; Chamberlain & Moore, 1998). Treatment foster care offers an appealing alternative to more restrictive residential placements, which are more costly and increase a juvenile's exposure to deviant peers (Schoenwald, Scherer, & Brondino, 1995). However, substantial further research is required, as there are few rigorous program evaluations of TFC program effectiveness (see Redding et al., 2000).

Behavioral Management Issues

Efficacious behavior management is a component of treatment that respects each child's dignity and humanity. Detention and correctional environments are always stressful and sometimes dangerous places, with juveniles depending on staff for their protection and well-being. Juveniles may be rendered more vulnerable to emotional, physical, or sexual abuse by virtue of their mental illness and as a result suffer acute exacerbation of their symptomatology. In addition, juveniles with comorbid attention-deficit/hyperactivity disorder, bipolar disorder, or substance abuse disorder are at increased risk for suicidality and aggressive acting-out behaviors, and thus present a considerable risk to others.

In this section, we discuss three key behavioral management concerns in residential settings: fostering prosocial behavior, managing self-injurious or suicidal juveniles, and determining the proper use of seclusion and restraint techniques with such juveniles.

Fostering Prosocial Behavior

It is important to have a consistently implemented behavioral program that is rich in positive reinforcement for adaptive prosocial behavior. Correctional environments, for instance, focus on limit setting and punishment. But mentally ill juvenile offenders are particularly vulnerable to the negative effects of neglectful, punitive environments. Many have been neglected or physically, emotionally, and/or sexually abused in their families of origin (see Loeber, 1990; McManus, Alessi, Grapentine, & Brickman, 1984; Widom, 1994; Yaeger & Lewis, 1996). Others have suffered abuse and neglect in the very systems designed to protect and nurture them. Their previous victimizations render them more vulnerable to revictimization and to the negative emotional consequences of neglectful or abusive practices. Consider the psychotic adolescent who is experiencing paranoid delusions and refusing to leave his room because he is convinced that there is a conspiracy against him. Such a juvenile will not respond well to escalating punishments designed to obtain compliance. He likely will regress further and become more defiant or aggressive. Also consider the quietly psychotic adolescent who regresses in response to a relatively minor incident. Such behavior can easily be misinterpreted by staff as manipulative and result in the use of methods such as isolation that may include sensory deprivation of a level likely to exacerbate the psychotic thinking or depression.

Staff members may be unaware of the negative effects that various interventions may have on seriously mentally ill offenders, and it can be difficult for correctional staff members to determine when disciplinary violations reflect mental health problems and thus whether to punish the juvenile or consult a mental health professional. Punishment for negative behavior may be temporarily effective in decreasing or extinguishing negative behavior, but it is unlikely that negative behaviors will be eliminated solely by punishment, particularly when those behaviors are driven by severe emotional distress. Especially where rehabilitation is a goal, tangible emotional and material reinforcers are necessary components of any successful behavioral program. Reinforcers may include additional telephone time, visitor time, the ability to earn bonus points to purchase items from a facility "bonus store," or extra 1:1 time with a staff member with whom the juvenile has developed a supportive relationship. A well-designed behavioral program individualized to the needs of each juvenile will also be beneficial for the staff. For instance, effectively managed assaultive behavior will result in improved staff morale and retention of staff members having positive and caring instincts, decreased staff and juvenile injuries, decreased liability, and less monetary expenditure for staff injuries and sick time.

In adult prisons, psychopathic individuals tend to flourish and assume leadership roles among the inmate population, often preying upon weaker individuals without reaping negative consequences. For such inmates, who wreak havoc on therapeutic environments and seldom profit from traditional treatment programs, the fruits of dominating and exploiting others are their own rewards. Although budding psychopaths may be present in the juvenile correctional system, caretakers should remember several caveats. First, delinquency and conduct disorder are not synonymous with antisocial personality disorder (APD) or psychopathy. Most adolescents with conduct disorder do *not* develop APD (though most adults with APD will have met criteria for conduct disorder during their adolescence). The *Diagnostic and Statistical Manual of Mental Disorders (DSM-IV)* criteria defining conduct disorder provide no information about the underlying psychiatric and/or neurologic disorders and vulnerabilities, and we have yet to discover the future long-term effects that the stronger emphasis on punishment and harsher sentencing laws will have on those juveniles incarcerated in our correctional facilities today. Second, delinquent or disruptive behavior does not confer immunity against the development of a mental illness. On the contrary, juveniles with conduct disorder have high rates of comorbid psychiatric disorders.

Self-Injurious Behavior and Suicide

In any correctional environment, particularly when mental health and monitoring resources are lacking, some juveniles will engage in self-injurious behavior, often as a manipulative attempt to gain release, increased privileges, or transfer to a noncorrectional setting. Many detained youth have a history of suicidal ideation or behavior (Davis, Bean, Schumacher, & Stringer, 1991; Dembo et al., 1990; Hayes, 2000). Rohde, Mace, and Seeley (1997) found suicide attempts in a delinquent population to be 19.4%, compared to only 6% in the nondelinquent population. In a study of incarcerated adolescents in Virginia correctional facilities, 30.5% of committed females and 7% of committed males had a history of documented suicide attempts resulting in hospitalization (McGarvey & Waite, 2000). Every year at least 11,000 detained juveniles exhibit suicidal behavior in juvenile facilities (Parent et al., 1994). Completed suicide in juvenile detention and correctional facilities is 4 *times* more common than that in the general juvenile population (Memory, 1989).

All self-injurious and destructive behaviors should be taken seriously enough to merit an evaluation. It is important to assess the seriousness and potential lethality of such behaviors and the presence of psychopathology and other risk factors for suicide, which will dictate how and where the juvenile should be managed and treated. But focusing primarily on the question of whether the juvenile is really suicidal encourages two highly problematic outcomes. First, a genuine cry for help may be dismissed as manipulative when recurrent or not potentially lethal (e.g., superficial cutting; tying sheets around the neck in full view of staff or prior to known staff checks). Second, it may send a message to the juvenile that his/her self-injury is unworthy of serious consideration, resulting in a perceived need to "up the ante." This may have disastrous consequences for the truly suicidal adolescent or the adolescent who inadvertently commits suicide. Chronically self-injurious juveniles who are intermittently suicidal present a major dilemma for juvenile justice facilities, presenting liability risks for the staff and systems charged with their care. They are often seriously aggressive to others and are frequently incarcerated for violent offenses. The line between instrumental and dangerous self-injury may become blurred even for the most experienced clinician. These juveniles may engender strong feelings of frustration, anxiety, and fear in their caretakers, feelings that often mirror the emotions of the juvenile and drive their self-destructive behaviors.

The capability to continuously monitor juveniles who exhibit suicidal behavior is necessary for their successful management and treatment. Correctional environments may fall short due to physical plant limitations and staffing deficits, resulting in inadequate responses to dangerous behavior or unnecessary hospitalization. Particularly when a juvenile voices suicidal ideation, especially if he or she has a potentially successful plan in mind, continuous observation is usually recommended until an evaluation can be obtained. However, staff members with whom the juvenile has a good relationship may be able to develop a management strategy in collaboration with the adolescent, without the need for continuous observation.

Correctional staff members must be trained on how to recognize the early signs and symptoms of suicidality, the risk factors for suicide (including characteristics of the residential environment that may foster suicidal behavior), effective suicide prevention and monitoring practices, and legal liability issues. Suicide screening and prevention protocols are necessary, particularly during high-risk periods (e.g., admission, following adjudication or disposition, while in seclusion) (National Commission on Correctional Health Care, 1999; see Hayes, 2000); the National Juvenile Detention Association's detention staff training curriculum includes suicide prevention training (Hayes, 2000). Unfortunately, an Office of Juvenile Justice and Delinquency Prevention study of suicide prevention in juvenile correctional facilities found that only 25% of incarcerated juveniles were in facilities conforming to suicide assessment and prevention criteria (written procedures, intake screening, staff training, and close observation) (Hayes, 2000; Parent et al., 1994). The study found less suicidal behavior in facilities with staff members trained in suicide prevention and intake screening for suicidality and more suicidal behavior among youth in isolation. Ivanoff and Hayes (2001) describe a juvenile center in Ohio that had three suicides in the 1980s. The third suicide became the catalyst for an extensive revamping of their policies, procedures, and practices for assessing and managing potentially suicidal youth. Those changes included yearly suicide assessment and prevention training for staff; several layers of mental health and suicide screening and assessment; increasing the observation of all youth to 15-min intervals (with high-risk youth being observed at 5-min intervals), and the administrative review of every suicide attempt in the facility (Ivanoff & Hayes, 2001).

Seclusion and Restraint

The use of seclusion and restraint has recently received a great deal of critical scrutiny. Limitations on the use of all restrictive treatments have occurred in response to the abuse of such interventions. However, out-of-control aggressive or self-injurious behavior may be impossible to manage without the use of seclusion or restraint, but a one-size-fits-all response is neither helpful nor safe. Seclusion or restraint (whether via mechanical, physical, or psychopharmacological modalities; see 42 CFR § 441, 483) should never be used as a punishment and should be for as brief a period as possible, with concrete release criteria repeatedly clarified for the juvenile. Developmental considerations as well as the specific psychopathology related to the out-of-control behavior must be considered for each juvenile. For example, a mentally retarded, psychotic juvenile may become more regressed and disorganized if secluded, and thus physical restraint may be more advantageous (along with the administration of a pharmacologic agent to decrease agitation and anxiety).

In addition to being familiar with the legal standards of care that must be adhered to in correctional and residential settings (see Coffin, 1999; Haney & Specter, 2001), all staff members should be trained in the use of an institutionally approved behavioral management program. Staff members also should receive regular retraining and recertification to ensure consistency in the implementation of seclusion and restraint procedures, particularly vis-à-vis those behaviors and circumstances for which it is not appropriate. Psychiatrists should consider the relative and absolute medical and psychological contraindications to seclusion and restraint and alert nursing and other staff members. A relative contraindication is a condition conferring additional risk of an adverse reaction. The necessity and potential benefits of the intervention may outweigh the potential risks or vice versa. An absolute contraindication is a condition precluding the use of an intervention. (For instance, a history of asthma or seizure disorder may be a relative medical contraindication for seclusion, whereas wheezing or respiratory distress is an absolute contraindication for seclusion or restraint). Careful vigilance through continuous observation is recommended even in routine cases, since the individual's status may deteriorate rapidly. Unforeseeable deaths occur (for example, secondary to a lethal cardiac arrhythmia in an adolescent with a never-diagnosed congenital cardiac abnormality), but often are preventable. Facilities utilizing restraints and seclusion should have:

1. Staff well trained in effective verbal maneuvers for de-escalating agitated juveniles and, in the event those techniques are unsuccessful, the safe and effective implementation of seclusion and/or restraint utilizing the least amount of force
2. Continuous observation of restrained or secluded juveniles, including monitoring of vital signs (especially for those on medication)
3. Rapid termination of the seclusion or restraint after the emergency has passed

4. Clinical/administrative review of all seclusion and restraint incidents to ensure proper and appropriate utilization

New federal regulations (effective in 2001) govern the use of seclusion and restraint with youth under 21 in psychiatric residential treatment facilities participating in the Medicaid program (42 CFR § 441, 483 [2003]). They require that seclusion or restraint may only be used in emergency situations to ensure safety and must terminate when the emergency ends, that the least restrictive alternative be used, and that seclusion or restraint be used for a maximum of 1–4 hours (depending on the age of the child). Clinical staff must continually monitor the child's physical and psychological status, and the regulations prohibit the use of "as needed" orders. The regulations also require that there be notification of parents when seclusion or restraint is used, debriefing sessions with the juvenile and involved staff, and staff training on the use of seclusion and restraints.

Mental Health Service Delivery Issues in Residential Settings

Juvenile justice officials regard the care of youth with serious mental illness as among their greatest challenges (Cocozza & Skowyra, 2000). Although even seriously mentally ill youth need limit setting and consequences for their illegal behavior, correctional facilities are often unable to provide adequate treatment for their mental health problems. The more closely interrelated the psychiatric disorder and behavioral disturbance that led to the legal involvement, the less useful incarceration will be as a deterrent to future delinquency. If resources for adequate mental health assessment and intervention are unavailable in the correctional facility, the child is unlikely to profit from any "lesson" to be learned and the potential for dire consequences can be significant. The National Commission on Correctional Health Care (1999) standards, requiring that mental health services be provided in juvenile correctional settings, mandate the development and implementation of policy and procedure manuals, communication between custodial and mental health care staff about juveniles' mental health needs, designated line staff members who are trained in mental health issues, intake screening (followed by a more comprehensive assessment within 2 weeks of admission, if indicated), the development of individualized treatment plans for juveniles with mental health problems, and a quality improvement program.

Staff Training

To ensure a safe, rehabilitative environment where youth are not victimized by staff members or other juveniles, facilities must provide the staff ratios necessary to adequately treat and supervise youth. Facilities must also provide ongoing training to all staff members on mental health, safety, and behavioral control issues and the proper use of medication (Coalition for Juvenile Justice, 2000).

Unfortunately, the clinical staff may have little interaction with the mainline correctional staff, promoting a sense of suspicion and mistrust. Frontline correctional staff members who maintain order in a correctional facility and are chronically at risk for injuries may be skeptical of a mental health professional perceived as making recommendations from the safe confines of an office. Mental health professionals, therefore, should be integrated into the facility so as to be perceived by frontline staff member as a valuable resource assisting them in their work. Staff education about the signs and symptoms of mental illness and the interventions likely to ameliorate or exacerbate a mental health crisis is an important role for mental health professionals, as are standardized training manuals in residential settings treating mentally ill juvenile offenders. Mental health clinicians can also provide guidance and support to staff, particularly around the management of juveniles whose aggressive or defiant behaviors present challenges to the staff members' ability to remain calm and evenhanded in their interactions.

It also is important to recognize the therapeutic potential of correctional officers and other line staff members who can potentially have a substantial psychological impact on juveniles (Hafemeister, Hall, & Dvoskin, 2001). Since line staff members spend the greatest amount of time with the youth, they have many opportunities to notice early signs of psychological problems and to interact with them in ways that are therapeutically beneficial. But they also have opportunities to abuse the juveniles under their care. Line staff members should be selected who have a nonpunitive orientation. (Research suggests that older applicants and female applicants for juvenile correctional positions are less likely to be punitive [Bazemore, Dicker, & Al-Gadheeb, 1994].) Staff members can assist mental health professionals and promote juveniles' mental health by observing behavior, talking with youth, implementing behavioral treatment programs, watching for signs and symptoms of psychiatric distress, suicidality, and reactions to medications, and helping youth cope with the stresses of incarceration (Hafemeister et al., 2001).

Cultural Sensitivity

Treatment placement and planning should be culturally sensitive (see Wierson & Forehand, 1995). The Coalition for Juvenile Justice (2000) recommends that residential staff members receive "specific mental heath training in cultural, racial, gender, sexual orientation and developmental issues" (p. 81).

Research suggests that juvenile courts are more likely to refer female and White juvenile offenders for psychiatric hospitalization, while males and non-Whites are more likely to be incarcerated (Lewis, Balla, & Shanok, 1979; Snyder & Sickmund, 1995), and that mental health problems are less likely to be diagnosed in African American youth (Lewis et al., 1979). This highlights the need to consider gender and ethnicity issues in placement selection and treatment planning. Perhaps mental health professionals and courts are less likely to recognize the mental health basis for delinquent behavior in males and minorities (see

Lewis et al., 1979; Thomas & Stubbe, 1996), which would indicate a need to train mental health and juvenile justice professionals on these issues.

Mental Health Screening

The National Commission on Correctional Health Care (1999) standards require intake screening within the first 24 hours of confinement, followed by a psychological evaluation within 2 weeks if indicated by the initial screening. The use of mental health screening instruments can reduce the risk of harm to the youth and others, reduce potential legal liability, prevent and alleviate suffering, and provide useful additional information about the youth. For many facilities, particularly detention facilities lacking sufficient mental health personnel on staff, mental health screening instruments can help ensure that youth needing services are identified. In the context of juvenile detention, substance abusing, aggressive, and suicidal youth are of particular concern (Reppucci & Redding, 2000).

To be useful, however, an instrument must be brief in administration and staff untrained in mental health must be able to administer, score, and utilize the results as a guide for referral to mental health professionals. In addition, the instrument must screen for risk of suicide. Two such instruments, the Massachusetts Youth Screening Instrument (MAYSI; Grisso & Barnum, 2000; Grisso, Barnum, Fletcher, Cauffman, & Peuschold, 2001) and the Brief Symptom Inventory (BSI; Derogatis, 1979), show promise (Reppucci & Redding, 2000). Screening instruments such as the BSI and the MAYSI are relatively easy to use and can provide valuable information. Juveniles identified as potentially being in psychological distress may warrant more intensive monitoring, added safety or security measures, the gathering of additional information on their mental health and medical history and status, or a referral for mental health evaluation or treatment.

It is critically important, however, that staff members not rely solely on any screening instrument, particularly because some juveniles may deny their symptoms when answering questions on a quick screening instrument. Additional and collateral information must be obtained, such as medical and mental health history, prior treatment records, information from parents or guardians, school records, and records of other involved agencies. Whatever screening instrument is used, it is essential that the staff receives adequate training and practice in its use.

Psychiatric and Medical Services

Incarcerated juveniles need psychiatric services acutely as well as on an ongoing basis. Unfortunately, there is great variability in the level of services provided in juvenile correctional facilities and the extent to which mental health problems are identified and treated. Internalizing disorders (e.g., anxiety, depression) are less likely to be identified, particularly when there is a shortage of mental health professionals on staff. Services must go beyond pharmacologic treatments, which are rarely recommended as the sole treatment. The identification and monitoring (e.g., blood work, EKGs) of specific target symptoms for pharmacological intervention (e.g., aggression, social withdrawal, sleep and appetite disturbance) is often difficult to accomplish in a correctional facility, although crucial for ensuring that juveniles are not unnecessarily continued on medications having potential side effects. But, while facilities must be careful not to overmedicate juveniles for behavioral control purposes, it is equally important not to undermedicate juveniles who require medications as part of the efficacious treatment of their mental disorder.

Unfortunately, even long-term juvenile correctional centers may not have access to child and adolescent psychiatrists for consultation and treatment. Psychiatrists who consult to juvenile justice facilities are typically available part-time, often for only a few hours weekly or monthly, thereby limiting the quantity and quality of treatment that can be provided on site to acutely ill juvenile offenders. If a facility cannot provide the services necessary for the management of a juvenile's psychopharmacological treatment, then the juvenile should be transferred to another correctional or treatment facility.

Psychiatric Hospitalization

Studies suggest that hospitalized and incarcerated juveniles are very similar populations in terms of psychopathology (Friman, Evans, Larzelere, Williams, & Daly, 1993). Hospitalized adolescents frequently carry disruptive behavior disorder diagnoses (e.g., ADHD and/or conduct disorder) that create management problems because of their aggressive and destructive behaviors. Hospital staff members frequently experience feelings of helplessness when faced with an assaultive mentally ill adolescent transferred from a correctional environment. In states that have maintained state hospital services for children and adolescents, seriously ill youth with regressed or repeatedly serious suicidal behavior in correctional environments may be transferred to a hospital. A "ping-pong" effect often ensues in which the juvenile is transferred back and forth between facilities.

Yet few pediatric psychiatric facilities, including state hospitals, have security commensurate with the correctional environment from which the juvenile was transferred. For example, a juvenile may be transferred from a correctional facility, where confinement to a room without any stimulation for 23 of 24 hours as a consequence for misbehavior is commonplace, to a hospital where a restriction program for assaultive behavior is not allowed. Hospitals are limited by a myriad of regulatory codes concerning the use of restrictive interventions. Frequently hospitals are unable to manage seriously disruptive or aggressive conduct-disordered youth who, while seriously mentally ill, also require firm limits and consequences for dangerously assaultive behavior. The development of psychiatric units for seriously mentally ill offenders in juvenile correctional facilities with appropriate staffing and security could circumvent some of these problems. Such residential treatment units have proven successful with adult inmates in reducing symptomatology, hospital transfers, disciplinary violations, and staff assaults (Condelli, Bradigan, & Holanchock, 1997; Condelli, Dvoskin, & Holanchock, 1994; Lovell, Allen, Johnson, & Jemelka, 2001).

Treatment for serious psychiatric disorders should be provided in the least restrictive setting that is safe and effective. Factors to be considered in determining whether hospitalization is necessary include the availability of a safe environment (i.e., whether a detention facility can provide 1:1 observation for a juvenile threatening suicide), the severity of the illness (psychosis and/or severe neurovegetative symptoms typically indicate the need for hospitalization), the availability of adequate crisis intervention and psychiatric and psychological consultation, and the severity of comorbid psychiatric or medical conditions.

Service Integration and Collaboration

Juvenile offenders often have a myriad of psychiatric disorders and other problems, necessitating the development of a multimodal treatment plan allowing flexibility and creativity in implementation. This often requires effective collaboration between the multiple agencies and facilities serving juvenile offenders with mental illness. Services need to be coordinated and tailored to the needs of the juveniles as well as to the agency or system charged with their guardianship. Because the risk factors for delinquency exist across multiple systems and contexts, including the child, home, school, peers, and neighborhood environments (see Henggeler, Schoenwald, Borduin, Rowland, & Cunningham, 1998), residential treatment and rehabilitation programs will be most effective when coordinated with community-based services with close cooperation among juvenile justice, mental health, and social service agencies (see Henggeler et al., 1998; Stroul & Friedman, 1986).

A recent study (Redding, 2001) of barriers in the juvenile justice system to serving juvenile offenders' mental health needs identified a variety of problems in service integration and interagency collaboration. Although the study was conducted in Virginia, the barriers identified are common in many states. Three of the barriers are particularly relevant for residential juvenile justice settings. First, correctional center staff members often feel conflicted about their role in working with juvenile offenders. Are they rehabilitating juvenile offenders, punishing them, securing their confinement, or some combination thereof? Such role confusion is commonly experienced by juvenile justice professionals (Holt, 2001). Since parole officers as well as state and local juvenile justice and social services agencies may share the responsibility for facility-to-community transitions and aftercare, there often are interagency conflicts over the issue of rehabilitation versus public safety (Altschuler, 1998) and whether an offender is mentally ill or "bad." At the heart of the issue is uncertainty about the extent to which the system's goal is to punish or rehabilitate juveniles. Here again, staff training is important. Mental health professionals working in the juvenile justice system can play an important role in training and mentoring juvenile justice professionals on how effectively to integrate their custodial and public safety roles with appropriate treatment and rehabilitative goals.

A second barrier to effective collaboration is that the juvenile justice system may be a "dumping ground" for mentally ill juveniles. Many offenders with a history of involvement with the mental health system migrate to the juvenile justice system because the mental health system has failed to serve their needs. Many times the mental health system cannot access needed residential treatment, whereas the juvenile justice system cannot access needed community-based treatments, producing a revolving door of mentally ill juveniles migrating back and forth for services between the juvenile justice and mental health systems. Perhaps the most significant obstacle to providing mental health services to juvenile offenders is that adequate funding often is not provided to the local community mental health centers serving these youth. Instead, "court intervention is seen as the only means to access mental health service for clients" (Virginia Commission on Youth, 1996, p. 2). However, in many locations, the juvenile justice system also lacks sufficient resources to serve the needs of mentally ill juveniles. The juvenile court may be insufficiently attentive to mental health issues, with judges and court-intake officers lacking knowledge in this area. (At detention hearings and reviews, for example, a juvenile's mental health status may be a reason to continue detention, though typically few mental health services are provided in detention.)

Juvenile detention and correctional centers are not well staffed to serve mentally ill juveniles and often have difficulty finding an inpatient facility willing and able to accept seriously mentally ill juveniles from these facilities. Frequently, no bed is available or the waiting time is substantial. Ultimately, many of these juveniles are referred to the juvenile justice system in the hope that the justice system will be able to monitor the juvenile and provided needed services. More juveniles with mental health problems are being detained, in part, due to a lack of insurance for treatment services, producing a net-widening effect of juveniles who come to detention. This may be producing a "criminalization of the mental ill" (Teplin, 1984) among the juvenile population.

A third significant barrier is the lack of diagnostic and treatment services typically available in predispositional detention facilities. Mental health treatment services should be provided in detention centers and made more programmatically specific so that detention centers can provide specialized treatment while the juvenile is in crisis or in the "active" phase of problems. Detention often is a time when both the juvenile and his parents are the most highly motivated to participate in treatment. Even in cases where the juvenile's stay in detention is short, it still may provide a good platform from which to develop a supportive and therapeutic network for juveniles and their families. Detention centers, however, should not be used as community dumping grounds through which to obtain mental health treatment or emergency services for court-involved juveniles.

Aftercare

Behavioral treatments for delinquent youth are often in the residential facility but the behavioral changes frequently do not generalize to the community after discharge (Quinsey, Harris, Rice, & Cormier, 1998). Collaboration between residential care facilities and community-based services must include planning for aftercare services, which are necessary to ensure continuity of care, ongoing treatment services in the community, and reduced recidivism vis-à-vis the need for future residential care. Community programs offer the opportunity to practice newly acquired skills in vivo, promoting accommodations in significant relationships that are consistent with positive changes in the adolescent's behavior. Given the multidetermined nature of delinquency and adolescent mental illness, the most effective aftercare will reflect a system-of-care concept that provides "a comprehensive spectrum of mental health and other necessary services which are organized into a coordinated network to meet the changing needs of children and adolescents with severe emotional disturbances and their families" (Stroul & Friedman, 1986, p. iv). Promising approaches to aftercare consistent with this model include the intensive aftercare program (IAP), wraparound services, and multisystemic therapy (MST).

Designed for chronic and incarcerated serious juvenile offenders, IAP is based on a graduated sanctions approach (see Wilson & Howell, 1995) consisting of three components: (a) prerelease planning; (b) a structured transition involving institutional and aftercare staff prior to, and following, release; and (c) long-term reintegrative activities to facilitate service delivery and social control (Altschuler & Armstrong, 1997). But recent studies (see Altschuler, 1998) of intensive aftercare have produced mixed results, showing no positive effects or reductions in the number of rearrests, but not in the propensity to reoffend. Many of the IAP programs evaluated to date have poorly implemented IAP principles and goals, particularly with respect to providing appropriate and adequate treatment services, with many programs functioning "much more as a surveillance enhancement than treatment enhancement" (Altschuler, 1998, p. 374), leaving few data about the effects of a properly implemented IAP program.

"Wraparound services" promote flexible and highly individualized services and interagency collaboration (see Tate & Redding, ch. 7 in this volume). Funding follows the child's treatment needs rather than being targeted according to particular services or programs (Brown, Borduin, & Henggeler, 2001). The individuals and systems impacting the child and family are brought together to determine what is needed (Burchard & Burns, 1998). "Instead of having professionals try to fit the child into existing service categorical services, the people who are most influential to the child and family tailor the services to fit the child and family" (Burchard & Burns, 1998, p. 364), resulting in an individualized service plan. An excellent example of wraparound services designed to serve emotionally disturbed youth in the juvenile justice system is Wraparound Milwaukee, designed to facilitate the return to the community of juveniles in residential treatment centers. Families are court-ordered into the program, which utilizes "care coordinators" to help the family obtain services and facilitate the development of a team of resource people and natural supports. Evaluations of Wraparound Milwaukee have shown it to be effective in improving psychosocial functioning, in reducing recidivism and the number of psychiatric hospitalizations, and in improving service integration between child welfare, juvenile justice, and mental health systems (Goldman & Faw, 1999; Kamradt, 1998). This also has produced significantly reduced costs (Goldman & Faw, 1999).

Multisystemic therapy (MST; see Henggeler et al., 1998) has become a model for communities that wish to provide cost-effective, nonresidential treatment for persistent offenders. MST includes intervention in home, school, and community settings and has generated impressive reductions in recidivism in previously incarcerated chronic offenders released to the community (Brown et al., 2001; Henggeler, 1996; Henggeler, Melton, & Smith, 1992). MST also is effective at reducing the number of drug-related arrests and substance abuse in chronic juvenile offenders (Henggeler et al., 1991, 1992). After discharge from residential care, youth might benefit from sustained outpatient treatment such as MST. Follow-up care that assertively seeks out the youth and his family members (Henggeler, Pickrel, Brondino, & Crouch, 1996) can cost-effectively work to overcome the circumstances of daily life that can undermine successful treatment maintenance in the community.

Future Directions for Research

The dual purposes of the juvenile system, community safety and rehabilitation, make evaluating the effectiveness of residential treatment complicated. Researchers' attempts to satisfy the dual goals of juvenile justice have produced study designs that begin with a rehabilitation goal of treatment gains but conclude by assessing for the correctional goal of recidivism. For example, a youth arrested for a property offense associated with symptoms of substance abuse might make treatment gains that contribute to a successful reintegration into the community as an adolescent after release. If the same person is arrested as an adult for a sex offense, for which he had no treatment, then the new offense might disguise the otherwise effective treatment for substance abuse. In this case, the treatment gains for substance abuse, a rehabilitation goal, are being measured against the outcome of rearrest, a correctional failure. An equally deceptive outcome could occur if a youth who was treated and released never offended again due to natural desistance rather than to treatment effects. A follow-up study might consider this youth a treatment success even if he continued to suffer mental health symptoms related to the original arrest.

In addition to conflicting goals, methodological issues challenge the interpretation and generalization of results. There is a lack of consistency in the types of outcomes assessed in studies of residential treatment. Outcomes measured often include one or more of the following: gains in physical health and mental health functioning, including decreased substance abuse, an expanded repertoire of interpersonal skills for more positive family and peer relations, progress in educational attainment and occupational preparation, and decreased delinquency. Few studies include all of these outcomes. Additionally, there are few mental health assessment instruments that have been validated for assessing treatment outcomes with juvenile offenders (Novaco, 1994). The instruments usually lack validity scales and rely on items with transparent content (Hughes, 1993). Many are self-report, without corroboration from secondary sources, a questionable strategy for obtaining reliable responses from youthful offenders.

Self-report instruments that do not include validity or response set scales are vulnerable to distortion. Collaboration from secondary sources, such as parents, caregivers, or teachers, can provide confirming or disconfirming data about a youth's mental health symptoms. Youth tend to report symptoms of internalizing disorders, while other observers report a greater number of externalizing symptoms (Youngstrom, Loeber, & Stouthamer-Loeber, 2000). In addition, self-report instruments in forensic settings are especially likely to misrepresent the types of symptoms and behaviors that others observe in an individual (Hare, 2003).

The lack of accurate descriptions of the similarities and differences between offenders raises additional concerns about interpreting the results of treatment outcomes. In general, there is a lack of consistency in the diagnostic categories and descriptive dimensions used in research related to child psychopathology (McClellan & Werry, 2000), including the disorders that are often seen in juvenile offenders, and there is almost no information on how specific cognitive, psychological and behavioral disorders contribute to particular offense characteristics.

The following questions summarize key issues that should be considered when evaluating the effectiveness of residential treatment for juvenile offenders:

- Which youth seem to benefit from residential treatment?
- Are those benefits rehabilitation goals or correctional goals?
- What characteristics (e.g., offense types, cognitive deficits, mental health symptoms) consistently and accurately describe those youth who seem to benefit?
- What standardized measures can be readily used to identify youth with those characteristics?
- What standardized treatments produce specific rehabilitation or correctional outcomes?
- What is the connection between offender characteristics, treatments implemented, treatment gains, and correctional gains?
- How long do the gains persist?
- Would these youth have desisted from offending regardless of treatment?

Until available models are evaluated vis-à-vis both rehabilitation and corrections outcomes, it is difficult to say which models of residential treatment are superior. Describing treatment gains as a result of a specific treatment and explaining how treatment goals may impact correctional goals may help to lessen the confusion about effective interventions for juvenile offenders. Treatment and corrections goals need to be defined by researchers prior to designing a study. Program development should begin with mental health and psychosocial assessments using instruments reliable and valid for use with juvenile offenders, followed by program planning that includes both treatment and corrections goals. Treatments should be part of a design that tests their effects on offense-related behaviors and should be delivered in a manner consistent with any cognitive impairments, learning disabilities, or physical disabilities that the juveniles may have. Treatment effectiveness also must be evaluated in the context of aftercare (Saxe, Cross, & Silverman, 1988); a meta-analysis of 34 studies of residential psychiatric treatment for children and adolescents found the availability of after-care to be a key determinant of treatment outcomes (Pfeiffer & Strzelecki, 1990).

The improvement of methodologies might begin with establishing types of offenders who are committed to residential treatment. A substantial body of past research on the characteristics of juvenile offenders, such as mental health or behavioral disorders associated with offense types, has attempted to create meaningful typologies of offender groups. In an example of positive outcomes using generally sound methods, Swenson and Kennedy (1995) documented a decrease in negative incidents in a large sample of adolescent males after only 3–4 months of residential treatment. The extended sampling of negative behaviors improved the chance that the measurement would be representative of the outcome, especially when compared to a single measurement at a given point in time. The Child Behavior Checklist (Achenbach, 1991), a valid and reliable child mental health instrument, was used to create a typology of youth (externalizers vs. internalizers) to assess treatment response. They used a before-and-after treatment design that compared negative behaviors recorded by program teachers for 2-week periods. Another typology based on observed psychological characteristics was successful at predicting preincarceration experiences and behaviors, as well as responses to specific treatment program components (Gold, Mattlin, & Osgood, 1989). The typology was based on symptoms of depression and anxiety as reported by the investigators, a less than ideal method since it is difficult for other researchers to replicate. But the attempt to relate treatment responses of offender types to specific parts of the treatment program is forward thinking and should be considered for future designs. These two examples begin to address the initial methodological problem of identifying types of offenders who can then be followed for their responses to treatment programs or program components.

In addition, severe delinquent behavior (and the comorbid mental disorders frequently associated with delinquency) is similar to a chronic, relapsing condition requiring long-term supervision and support rather than an acute syndrome that responds to single or multiple episodes of short-term intervention (see Wolfe, Braukmann, & Ramp, 1987). Residential treatment could play an important role in a reconceptualized approach to treating juvenile offenders that is premised on the need for continuing support to prevent relapse into mental illness or recidivism. Follow-up outcome measures of recidivism should be adapted to be consistent with the model of a chronic, relapsing disease. Setbacks can be differentiated from failures, and acute exacerbations addressed by prompt and aggressive treatment. Treatment success should not be reported in results that do not account for natural resistance from offending behavior. Adopting a more realistic approach to behavioral problems that have proven unresponsive to episodic intervention may subtly alter the types of measurements that are used to assess treatment outcomes for juvenile offenders in ways that provide for improved empirical results, ultimately leading to improved treatment programs. Describing treatment gains as a result of a specific treatment and explaining how treatment goals may impact correctional goals may help to lessen the confusion about effective interventions for juvenile offenders.

At present, however, there is insufficient empirical evidence that residential treatment can divert a persistent juvenile offender into a less negative life course trajectory, and little is known about which treatments are effective for diverting specific types of offenders, particularly those with mental disorders. Conversely, there is little way of knowing whether juvenile offenders who report successful adjustment after community release have prospered because of treatment or because of a natural propensity to desist. Studies generally fail to acknowledge the limitations of their results in light of natural desistance. For example, measuring changes and outcomes in time periods that can be meaningfully compared may provide better indications of the benefits of residential treatment. More successful outcomes may be identified if researchers evaluate time periods during which youth report being relatively unimpaired by mental health and behavior disorders and periods of time when offending behavior diminishes or disappears altogether. A staggered strategy that measures improvement during placement compared to the period immediately prior to placement, or comparing early placement outcomes with later placement outcomes, might improve the understanding of how and when changes occur in response to treatment. It would also provide valuable feedback for developing a youth's treatment plan. This strategy could be applied to any characteristic of interest, including mental health symptoms, behavioral performance, academic progress, or peer relationships.

Most significantly, there is a need for research that identifies how specific mental health symptoms contribute to offense characteristics and whether appropriate treatment of those symptoms reduces aspects of offending. Paradoxically, when residential placement is selected by offense characteristics rather than treatment needs, the effectiveness of treatment modalities for reducing recidivism may be obscured. A residential treatment program's ability to meet the correctional goal of reduced recidivism cannot be appraised at follow-up if the individual's treatment needs were not matched to the treatment program initially, even if treatment gains were made in education, mental health, or other areas of psychosocial functioning (Serin & Preston, 2001).

Conclusion

We have attempted to delineate what the research and clinical literatures tell us about what constitutes "best practices" in the delivery of mental health treatment in residential treatment and juvenile justice settings. Unfortunately, the conclusions that may be drawn are limited by the state of the research on residential treatment of mental illness in juvenile offenders. Research on the residential treatment of juvenile offenders with mental disorders is virtually nonexistent. There also is little research testing the efficacy of pychopharmacological and psychotherapeutic treatments for various mental illnesses in the juvenile offender population. Moreover, existing research often fails to distinguish between delinquency risk factors and mental illness and between correctional versus treatment settings, and it suffers from a variety of methodological limitations; particularly problematic has been the definition and measurement of outcomes.

We hope that methodologically sound research will identify and test best practices for the delivery of mental health services for juvenile offenders in residential treatment and juvenile justice settings. Programmatic research in this area is essential for a successful juvenile justice system, particularly given the unmet but substantial mental health needs of juvenile offenders and the increasing number of offenders entering the juvenile justice system with comorbid mental disorders.

References

Achenbach, T. M. (1991). *Manual for the Youth Self Report and 1991 Profile*. Burlington: University of Vermont Department of Psychiatry.

Agee, V. L. (1979). *Treatment of the violent incorrigible adolescent*. Lexington, MA: Lexington Books.

Altschuler, D. M. (1998). Intermediate sanctions and community treatment for serious and violent juvenile offenders. In R. Loeber & D. P. Farrington (Eds.), *Serious and violent juvenile offenders: Risk factors and successful interventions* (pp. 367–388). Thousand Oaks, CA: Sage.

Altschuler, D. M., & Armstrong, T. L. (1997). Aftercare not afterthought: Testing the IAP model. *Juvenile Justice, 3*(1),115–122.

Americans with Disabilities Act of 1990, Public Law No. 101-336. 42 U.S.C. § 12101 *et seq.*

Amini, F., Zilberg, N. J., Burke, E. L., & Salasnek, S. (1982). A controlled study of inpatient vs. outpatient treatment of delinquent drug abusing adolescents: One year results. *Comprehensive Psychiatry, 23,* 436–444.

Basta, J. M., & Davidson, W. S. (1988). Treatment of juvenile offenders: Study outcomes since 1980. *Behavioral Sciences and the Law, 6,* 355–384.

Bazemore, G., Dicker, T. J., & Al-Gadheeb, H. (1994). The treatment ideal and detention reality: Demographic, professional/occupational and organizational influences on detention worker punitiveness. *American Journal of Criminal Justice, 19,* 21–41.

Brown, T. L., Borduin, C. M., & Henggeler, S. W. (2001). Treating juvenile offenders in community settings. In J. Ashford, B. Sales, & W. Reid (Eds.) *Treating adult and juvenile offenders with special needs* (pp. 445–464). Washington, DC: American Psychological Association.

Burchard, J. D., & Burns, E. J. (1998). The role of the case study in the evaluation of individualized services. In N. H. Epstein, J. Kutash, & A. Duchnowski (Eds.), *Outcomes for children and youth with emotional and behavioral disorders and their families: Programs and evaluation best practices* (pp. 363–383). Austin, TX: PRO-ED.

Burford, G., & Casson, S. F. (1989). Including families in residential work: Educational and agency tasks. *British Journal of Social Work, 19,* 17–37.

Chamberlain, P. (1996). Community-based residential treatments for adolescents with conduct disorder. In T. H. Ollendick & R. J. Prinz (Eds.), *Advances in clinical child psychology* (Vol. 18, pp. 63–89.) New York: Plenum.

Chamberlain, P., & Friman, P. C. (1997). Residential programs for antisocial children and adolescents. In D. Stoff, J. Breiling, & J. Maser (Eds.), *Handbook of antisocial behavior* (pp. 416–424). New York: Wiley.

Chamberlain, P., & Moore, K. (1998). A clinical model for parenting juvenile offenders: A comparison of group care versus family care. *Clinical Child Psychology and Psychiatry, 3,* 1359–1045.

Coalition for Juvenile Justice. (2000). *Handle with care: Serving the mental health needs of young offenders*. Washington, DC: Author.

Cocozza, J. J., & Skowyra, K. R. (2000). Youth with mental health disorders: Issues and emerging responses. *Juvenile Justice*, 7, 3–13.

Coffin, C. L. (1999). Case law & clinical considerations involving physical restraint and seclusion for institutionalized persons with mental disabilities. *Mental and Physical Disability Law Reporter*, 23, 597–602.

Condelli, W. S., Bradigan, B., & Holanchock, H. (1997). Intermediate care programs to reduce risk and better manage inmates with psychiatric disorders. *Behavioral Sciences and the Law*, 15, 460–467.

Condelli, W. S., Dvoskin, J. A., & Holanchock, H. (1994). Intermediate care programs for inmates with psychiatric disorders. *Bulletin of the American Academy of Psychiatry and Law*, 22, 63–70.

Davis, D. L., Bean, G. L., Schumacher, J. E., & Stringer, T. L. (1991). Prevalence of emotional disorders in a juvenile justice institutional population. *American Journal of Forensic Psychology*, 9, 1–13.

Davis, G., Hoffman, R.G., & Quigley, R. (1988). Self-concept change and positive peer culture in adjudicated delinquents. *Child and Youth Care Quarterly*, 17(3), 137–145.

Dembo, R., Williams, L., Wish, E. D., Berry, E., Getreu, A. M., Washburn, M., et al. (1990). Examination of the relationships among drug use, emotional/psychological problems, and crime among youth entering a juvenile detention center. *International Journal of the Addictions*, 25, 1301–1340.

Denkowski, G. C., Denkowski, K. M., & Mabli, J. (1984). A residential treatment model for MR adolescent offenders. *Hospital and Community Psychiatry*, 35, 279–281.

Derogatis, L. R. (1979). *Brief Symptom Inventory*. Minneapolis, MN: National Computer Systems.

Dishion, T. J., McCord, J., & Poulin, F. (1999). When interventions harm: Peer groups and problem behavior. *American Psychologist*, 54, 755–764.

Domolanta, D. D., Risser, W. L., Roberts, R. E., & Risser, J. M. (2003). Prevalence of depression and other psychiatric disorders among incarcerated youth. *Journal of the American Academy of Child and Adolescent Psychiatry*, 42, 477–484.

Eddy, J. M., & Chamberlain, P. (2000). Family management and deviant peer association as mediators of the impact of treatment condition on youth antisocial behavior. *Journal of Consulting and Clinical Psychology*, 68, 857–863.

Elliott, D. S., Huizinga, D., and Ageton, S. S. (1985). *Explaining delinquency and drug use*. Newbury Park, CA: Sage.

Evens, C. C., & Vander Stoep, A. (1997). Risk factors for juvenile justice system referral among children in a public mental health system. *Journal of Mental Health Administration*, 24, 443–455.

Forness, S. R., Kavale, K. A., Blum, I. M., & Lloyd, J. W. (1997). Mega-analysis of meta-analysis: What works in special education and related services. *Teaching Exceptional Children*, 29, 4–10.

Friman, P. C., Evans, J., Larzelere, R., Williams, G., & Daly, D. L. (1993). Correspondence between child dysfunction and program intensiveness: Evidence of a continuum of care across five mental health programs. *Journal of Community Psychology*, 21, 227–233.

Gallagher, C. A. (1999). Juvenile offenders in residential placement, 1997. In S. Bilchik (Ed.), *OJJDDP fact sheet*. Washington, DC: U.S. Department of Justice.

Gibbs, J. C. (1993). Moral-cognitive interventions. In A. P. Goldstein & C. R. Huff (Eds.), *The gang intervention handbook* (pp. 159–185). Champaign-Urbana, IL: Research Press.

Gibbs, J. C., Potter, G. B., Barriga, A. Q., & Liau, A. K. (1996). Developing the helping skills and prosocial motivation of aggressive adolescents in peer group programs. *Aggression and Violent Behavior, 1,* 283–305.

Goffman, E. (1961). *Asylums.* Garden City, NY: Doubleday.

Gold, M., Mattlin, J., & Osgood, D. W. (1989). Background characteristics and responses to treatment of two types of institutionalized delinquent boys. *Criminal Justice and Behavior, 6,* 5–33.

Goldman, S. K., & Faw, L. (1999). Three wraparound models as promising approaches. In B. J. Burns & S. K. Goldman (Eds.), *Promising practices in wraparound for children with serious emotional disturbance and their families: Vol. IV. Systems of care: Promising practices in childrens' mental health, 1998 Series.* Washington, DC: American Institutes for Research, Center for Effective Collaboration and Practice.

Gossett, J. F., Lewis, J. M., & Barhart, F. D. (1983). *To find a way: The outcome of hospital treatment of disturbed adolescents.* New York: Brunner/Mazel.

Grisso, T., Barnum, R., Fletcher, K. E., Cauffman, E., & Peuschold, D. (2001). Massachusetts Youth Screening Instrument for mental health needs of juvenile justice youth. *Journal of the American Academy of Child and Adolescent Psychiatry, 40*(5), 541–548.

Grisso, T. J., & Barnum, R. (2000). *Massachusetts Youth Screening Instrument-2: User's manual and technical report.* Worcester: University of Massachusetts Medical Center.

Hafemeister, T. L., Hall, S. R., & Dvoskin, J. A. (2001). Administrative concerns associated with the treatment of offenders with mental illness. In J. Ashford, B. Sales, & W. Reid (Eds.), *Treating adult and juvenile offenders with special needs* (pp. 419–444). Washington, DC: American Psychological Association.

Haney, C., & Specter, D. (2001). Treatment rights in uncertain legal times. In J. B. Ashford, B. D. Sales, & W. H. Reid (Eds.), *Treating adult and juvenile offenders with special needs* (pp. 51–79). Washington, DC: American Psychological Association.

Hare, R. D. (2003). *The Hare Psychopathy Checklist—Revised* (2nd ed.). North Tonawanda, NY: Multi-Health Systems.

Harris, D. P., Cote, J. E., & Vipond, E. M. (1987). Residential treatment of disturbed delinquents: Description of a centre and identification of therapeutic factors. *American Journal of Psychiatry, 32,* 579–583.

Hayes, L. M. (2000). Suicide prevention in juvenile facilities. *Juvenile Justice, 8,* 24–32.

Henggeler, S. W. (1996). Treatment of violent juvenile offenders—We have the knowledge: Comment on Gorman-Smith et al. *Journal of Family Psychology, 10,* 137–141.

Henggeler, S. W. (1999a). Multisystemic therapy: An overview of clinical procedures. *Child Psychology and Psychiatry Review, 4,* 2–10.

Henggeler, S. W. (1999b). Multisystemic treatment of serious clinical problems in children and adolescents. *Clinician's Research Digest* (Supplemental Bulletin 21).

Henggeler, S. W., Borduin, C. M., Melton, G. B., Mann, B. J., Smith, L. A., Hall, J. A., et al. (1991). Effects of multisystemic therapy on drug use and abuse in serious juvenile offenders: A progress report from two outcome studies. *Family Dynamics of Addiction Quarterly, 1,* 40–51.

Henggeler, S. W., Melton, G. B., & Smith, L. A. (1992). Family preservation using multisystemic therapy: An effective alternative to incarcerating serious juvenile offenders. *Journal of Consulting and Clinical Psychology, 60,* 953–961.

Henggeler, S. W., Pickrel, S. G., Brondino, M. J., & Crouch, J. L. (1996). Eliminating (almost) treatment dropout of substance abusing or dependent delinquents through home-based multisystem therapy. *American Journal of Psychiatry, 153,* 427–428.

Henggeler, S. W., Schoenwald, S. K., Borduin, C. M., Rowland, M. D., & Cunningham,

P. B. (1998). *Multisystemic treatment of antisocial behavior in children and adolescents.* New York: Guilford Press.

Holt, C. (2001). The correctional officer's role in mental health treatment of youthful offenders. *Issues in Mental Health Nursing, 22,* 173–180.

Hughes, G. V. (1993). Anger management program outcomes. *Forum on Corrections Research, 5,* 3–5.

Individuals with Disabilities Education Act. (1990). Public Law No.101-476, 20 U.S.C. § 1400.

Ivanoff, A. & Hayes, L. M. (2001). Preventing, managing, and treating suicidal actions in high-risk offenders. In J. B. Ashford, B. D. Sales, & W. H. Reid (Eds.), *Treating adult and juvenile offenders with special needs* (pp. 313–331). Washington, DC: American Psychological Association.

Johnson-Reid, M., & Way, I. (2001). Adolescent sexual offenders: Incidence of childhood maltreatment, serious emotional disturbance, and prior offenses. *American Journal of Orthopsychiatry, 71,* 120–130.

Kamradt, B. J. (1998). The 25 kid project: How Milwaukee utilized a pilot project to change their system of care. *A TA brief from the National Resource Network.* Washington, DC: U.S. Department of Justice, Office of Juvenile Justice and Delinquency Prevention.

Kapp, S. A., Schwartz, I., & Epstein, I. (1994). Adult imprisonment of males released from residential childcare: A longitudinal study. *Residential Treatment for Children and Youth, 12,* 19–36.

Katsiyannis, A. Y., & Murry, F. (2000). Young offenders with disabilities: Legal requirements and reform considerations. *Journal of Child and Family Studies, 9,* 75–86.

Lab, S. P., & Whitehead, J. T. (1988). An analysis of juvenile correctional treatment. *Crime & Delinquency, 34,* 60–83.

Lewis, D. O., Balla, D. A., & Shanok, S. S. (1979). Some evidence of race bias in the diagnosis and treatment of the juvenile offender. *American Journal of Orthopsychiatry, 33,* 518–528.

Lewis, D. O., Yeager, C. A., Lovely, R., Stein, A., & Cobham-Portorreal, C. S. (1994). A clinical follow-up of delinquent males: Ignored vulnerabilities, unmet needs and the perpetuation of violence. *Journal of the American Academy of Child and Adolescent Psychiatry, 33,* 518–528.

Lewis, M., Lewis, D. O., Shanok, S. S., Klatskin, E., & Osborne, J. R. (1980). The undoing of residential treatment. *Journal of the American Academy of Child Psychiatry, 19,* 160–171.

Lipsey, M. W. (1995). What do we learn from 400 research studies on the effectiveness of treatment with juvenile delinquents? In J. McGuire (Ed.), *What works? Reducing reoffending* (pp. 63–78). New York: Wiley.

Lipsey, M. W., & Wilson, D. B. (1998). Effective intervention for serious juvenile offenders: A synthesis of research. In R. Loeber & D. Farrington (Eds.), *Serious and violent juvenile offenders; Risk factors and successful interventions* (pp.313–345). Thousand Oaks, CA: Sage.

Loeber, R. (1990). Development and risk factors of juvenile antisocial behavior and delinquency. *Clinical Psychology Review, 10,* 1–41.

Lovell, D., Allen, D., Johnson, C., & Jemelka, R. (2001). Evaluating the effectiveness of residential treatment for prisoners with mental illness. *Criminal Justice Behavior, 28,* 83–104.

Lynam, D., Moffitt, T., & Stouthamer-Loeber, M. (1993). Explaining the relation between IQ and delinquency: Class, race, test motivation, school failure, or self control? *Journal of Abnormal Psychology, 102,* 187–196.

Martinson, R. (1974). What works? Questions and answers about prison reform. *The Public Interest, 35,* 22–54.

McClellan, J. M., & Werry, J. S. (2000). Introduction—research psychiatric diagnostic interviews for children and adolescents. *Journal of the American Academy of Child & Adolescent Psychiatry, 39,* 1, 19–27.

McGarvey, E. L., & Waite, D. (2000). Mental health needs among juveniles committed to the Virginia Department of Juvenile Justice. *Developments in Mental Health Law, 20,* 1–24.

McIntyre, T. (1993). Behaviorally disordered youth in correctional settings: Prevalence, programming, and teacher training. *Behavioral Disorders, 18,* 167–176.

McManus, M., Alessi, N. E., Grapentine, W. L., & Brickman, A. (1984). Psychiatric disturbances in serious delinquents. *Journal of the American Academy of Child and Adolescent Psychiatry, 23,* 602–615.

Meichenbaum, D., & Turk, D. C. (1987). *Facilitating treatment adherence: A practitioner's guidebook.* New York: Plenum.

Memory, J. (1989). Juvenile suicides in secure detention facilities: Correction of published rates. *Death Studies, 13,* 455–463.

Minnesota Department of Corrections. (2000). *1999 performance report: Juvenile recidivism in Minnesota.* St. Paul, MN: Research and Evaluation Unit.

Mohr, W. (1998). Experiences of patients hospitalized during the Texas mental health scandal. *Perspectives on Psychiatric Care, 34,* 5–17.

National Commission on Correctional Health Care. (1999). *Standards for health services in juvenile detention and confinement facilities.* Chicago: Author.

Novaco, R. W. (1994). Anger as a risk factor for violence among the mentally disordered. In J. Monahan & H. J. Steadman (Eds.), *Violence and mental disorder: Developments in risk assessment* (pp. 21–59). Chicago: University of Chicago Press.

Otero-Lopez, J. M., Luengo-Martin, A., Miron-Redondo, L., Carrillo-De-La-Pena, M. T., & Romero-Trinanes, E. (1994). An empirical study of the relations between drug abuse and delinquency among adolescents. *British Journal of Criminology, 34,* 459–478.

Parent, D. G., Leiter, V., Kennedy, S., Livens, L., Wentworth, D., & Wilcox, S. (1994). *Conditions of confinement: Juvenile detention and corrections facilities.* Washington, DC: U.S. Department of Justice, Office of Justice Programs, Office of Juvenile Justice and Delinquency Prevention.

Parmelee, D. X., Cohen, R., Nemil, M., & Best, A. M. (1995). Children and adolescents discharged from public psychiatric hospitals: Evaluation of outcome in a continuum of care. *Journal of Child and Family Studies, 4,* 43–55.

Pfeiffer, S. I., & Strzelecki, C. C. (1990). Inpatient psychiatric treatment of children and adolescents: A review of outcome studies. *Journal of the American Academy of Child and Adolescent Psychiatry, 29,* 847–853.

Pumariega, A. J., Atkins, D. L., Rogers, K., Montgomery, L., Nybro, C., Caesar, R., et al. (1999). Mental health and incarcerated youth. II: Service utilization. *Journal of Child and Family Studies, 8,* 205–215.

Quinsey, V. L., Harris, G. T., Rice, M. E., & Cormier, C. A. (1998). *Violent offenders: Appraising and managing risk.* Washington, DC: American Psychological Association.

Redding, R. E. (1992). Children's competence to provide informed consent to mental health treatment. *Washington and Lee Law Review, 50,* 695–753.

Redding, R. E. (2001). Barriers to meeting the mental health needs of offenders in the juvenile justice system. *Juvenile Correctional Mental Health Report, 1,* 17–18, 26–30.

Redding, R. E., Fried, C., & Britner, P. A. (2000). Predictors of placement outcomes in treatment foster care: Implications for foster parent selection and service delivery. *Journal of Child and Family Studies, 9,* 425–447.

Redondo, S., Sanchez-Meca, J., & Garrido, V. (1999). The influence of treatment programs on the recidivism of juvenile and adult offenders: A European meta-analytic review. *Psychology, Crime and Law, 5,* 251–278.

Reppucci, N. D., & Redding, R. E. (2000, November/December). Screening instruments for mental health problems in juvenile offenders. *Correctional Mental Health Report,* 52–53.

Rohde, P., Mace, D. E., & Seeley, J. R. (1997). The association of psychiatric disorders with suicide attempts in a juvenile delinquent sample. *Criminal Behavior and Mental Health, 7,* 187–200.

Rutherford, R. B., Griller-Clark, H. M., & Anderson, C. W. (2001). Treating offenders with educational disabilities. In J. B. Ashford & B. D. Sales (Eds.), *Treating adult and juvenile offenders with special needs* (pp. 221–245). Washington, DC: American Psychological Association.

Rutter, M., & Giller, H. (1984). *Juvenile delinquency: Trends and perspectives.* New York: Guilford Press.

Saxe, L., Cross, T., & Silverman, N. (1988). Children's mental health: The gap between what we know and what we do. *American Psychologist, 43,* 800–807.

Serin, R. C., & Preston, D. L. (2001). Managing and treating violent offenders. In J. B. Ashford & B. D. Sales (Eds.), *Treating adult and juvenile offenders with special needs* (pp. 249–271). Washington, DC: American Psychological Association.

Schoenwald, S. K., Scherer, D. G., & Brondino, M. J. (1995). Effective community-based treatments for serious juvenile offenders. In S. W. Henggeler & A. B. Santos (Eds.), *Innovative approaches for difficult-to-treat populations* (pp. 65–82). Washington, DC: American Psychiatric Press.

Snyder, H. N., & Sickmund, M. (1995). *Juvenile offenders and victims: A focus on violence.* Pittsburgh, PA: National Center for Juvenile Justice.

Stroul, B., & Friedman, R. (1986). *A system of care for children and youth with severe emotional disturbances.* Washington, DC: Georgetown University, Child Development Center.

Swenson, C. C., & Kennedy, W. A. (1995). Perceived control and treatment outcome of chronic adolescent offenders. *Adolescence, 30,* 565–578.

Tannehill, R. L. (1987). Employing a modified positive peer culture treatment approach in a state youth center. *Journal of Offender Counseling, Services and Rehabilitation, 12,* 113–129.

Teplin, L. A. (1984). Criminalizing mental disorder: The comparative arrest rate of the mentally ill. *American Psychologist, 39,* 794–803.

Teplin, L. A., Abram, K. M., McClelland, G. M., Dulcan, M. K., & Mericle, A. A. (2002). Psychiatric disorders in youth in juvenile detention. *Archives of General Psychiatry, 59,* 1133–1143.

Thomas, W. J., & Stubbe, D. E. (1996, Fall). A comparison of correctional and mental health referrals in the juvenile court. *Journal of Psychiatry & Law, 24,* 379–400.

Underwood, L. A., Newton, J. A., & Jageman, M. A. (2001). Integrating juvenile correctional and community mental health approaches: A promising program for juvenile offenders with mental health disorders. *Juvenile Correctional Mental Health Report, 1,* 33–34, 42, 46–47.

U.S. Department of Health and Human Services. (2001). *Mental health: A report of the Surgeon General*. Rockville, MD: USDHHS, National Institute of Mental Health, Center for Mental Health Services.

Velasquez, J. S., & Lyle, C. G. (1985). Day versus residential treatment for juvenile offenders. The impact of program evaluation. *Child Welfare, 64*, 145–157.

Virginia Commission on Youth. (1996). *The study of juvenile justice system reform* (House Document No. 37). Richmond: Commonwealth of Virginia, Virginia General Assembly.

Vorrath, H. H., & Brendro, L. K. (1974). *Positive peer culture*. New York: Aldine.

Widom, C. S. (1994). Childhood victimization and adolescent problem behavior. In R. D. Ketterlinus & M. E. Lamb (Eds.), *Adolescent problem behaviors: Issues and research* (pp. 127–164). Hillsdale, NJ: Erlbaum.

Wierson, M., & Forehand, R. (1995). Predicting recidivism in juvenile delinquents: The role of mental health diagnosis and the qualification of conclusion by race. *Behaviour Research & Therapy, 33*, 63–67.

Wilson, J. J., & Howell, J. C. (1995). Comprehensive strategy for serious, violent and chronic juvenile offenders. In J. C. Howell, B. Krisberg, J. D. Hawkins, & J. J. Wilson (Eds.), *Sourcebook on serious, violent, and chronic juvenile offenders* (pp. 35–46). Thousand Oaks, CA: Sage.

Wolfe, M. M., Braukmann, C. J., & Ramp, K. A. (1987). Serious delinquent behavior as part of a significantly handicapping condition: Cures and supportive environments. *Journal of Applied Behavior Analysis, 20*, 347–359.

Yaeger, C. A., & Lewis, D. O. (1996). The intergenerational transmission of violence and dissociation. *Child and Adolescent Psychiatric Clinics of North America, 5*, 393–430.

Youngstrom, E., Loeber, R., & Stouthamer-Loeber, M. (2000). Patterns and correlates of agreement between parent, teacher, and male adolescent ratings of externalizing and internalizing problems. *Journal of Consulting & Clinical Psychology, 68*(6), 1038–1050.

14

LOURDES M. ROSADO

Training Mental Health and Juvenile Justice Professionals in Juvenile Forensic Assessment

Juvenile and criminal court professionals—judges, prosecutors, defense attorneys, and probation officers—use forensic assessments to aid them in critical decision making with regard to youth who become involved in the justice system. On one level, these professionals often call on the expertise of psychologists and psychiatrists to help them answer key legal questions regarding individual youth who come before the court, including issues of competence, culpability, amenability to rehabilitation and treatment, and appropriate treatment planning. On a second level, forensic psychologists and psychiatrists help to guide court professionals in the latter's distinct roles as policy-makers and resource allocators for the justice system. For example, their findings concerning the mental, emotional, and behavioral disorders prevalent among court-involved youth, as well as their knowledge of evidence-based interventions, inform decision making about what types of programming the court should seek and/or develop to appropriately treat youth.

Often, however, these collaborations do not work as effectively as they could because court professionals and forensic evaluators lack a sufficient shared knowledge base from which to operate. For example, judges and lawyers rarely receive formal education or training in adolescent development and psychology. Consequently, they do not know how to interpret an evaluation and apply it to the key legal question at hand or how to judge the quality of an evaluation.

At an even more basic level, they may lack awareness of the factors that suggest a youth should be referred for evaluation in the first place. Many mental health professionals receive no formal training on the law pertaining to the specific legal questions on which they are asked to opine. While forensic training is more widely available for psychiatrists and psychologists today than it was a decade ago, such training is not universal, and the availability of *juvenile* forensic training is even more limited (Otto & Heilbrun, 2002).[1]

---

1. Among the entities currently offering comprehensive juvenile forensic training are the Institute of Law, Psychiatry, and Public Policy at the University of Virginia, www.ilppp.virginia.edu, and

The challenge is to expand the shared base of substantive knowledge for use by both sets of professionals in and out of court. This chapter explores professional education and training of judges, lawyers, and probation officers as an important strategy for expanding that base. Clinicians with expertise in assessing juvenile offenders can play a critical role in training legal professionals to more effectively use that expertise to address the overarching goals of ensuring better outcomes for court-involved youth while promoting public safety. In the first part of the chapter, we explore the relationship between forensic assessment and legal decision making in the juvenile court process. The second part of the chapter describes the development of a unique curriculum designed specifically to train juvenile court professionals on forensic assessment, adolescent development, and psychology generally. The remainder of the chapter outlines the current use of the curriculum in the United States, as well as future plans for its revision and expansion.

Legal Decision Making and Forensic Evaluation: Why Do Judges, Lawyers, and Probation Officers Need to Understand Adolescent Development and Psychology?

As an individual youth's case proceeds through the different stages of the court process, court professionals must make a number of critical decisions. An understanding of adolescent development generally, as well as specific information about the individual youth in question—such as his/her level of development in different domains and whether the youth has any learning disabilities, special education needs, or mental health diagnoses—can and should inform such decisions. Thus, for example, when a youth is first arrested, probation or other court officers assess the youth's potential for diversion from the justice system. Depending on the youth's alleged offense, history, needs, and circumstances, the intake officer may decide that it is in both the public's and the youth's best interests not to proceed with the court case and, instead, to refer the youth to community service or other special programming (Woolard, Gross, Mulvey, & Reppucci, 1992).

If a youth is not diverted out of the court system, the agency responsible for filing a charging document with the court (in some jurisdictions it will be the probation department, and in others it will be the prosecutor's office) must decide what offenses to charge. A related decision made at this stage is whether the youth will proceed in juvenile versus adult criminal court; mechanisms in different states differ in where they vest this decision-making authority. For example, under some state schemes, the juvenile court judge must make the decision whether to "waive" juvenile court jurisdiction and transfer a case to adult court,

the Department of Mental Health Law and Policy of the Louis de la Parte Florida Mental Health Institute at the University of South Florida, www.fmhi.usf.edu/mhlp/training/statement.htm.

although the degree of judicial autonomy also varies among so-called "waiver" states. In other jurisdictions, the prosecutor is empowered to decide whether to initiate or "direct file" a case in juvenile or adult criminal court. A number of state schemes also allow juveniles who are being prosecuted as adults to petition the criminal court to transfer their case to juvenile court; this has been called "reverse waiver" or "decertification" in different jurisdictions. In making these decisions, prosecutors and/or judges must consider a number of factors; typically included are the youth's age and previous delinquency record, the alleged offense, and the youth's amenability to treatment and rehabilitation within the juvenile justice system (Griffen, Torbet, & Szymanski, 1998).

Whether the case proceeds in juvenile or adult court, questions may arise about the youth's competence to stand trial, to enter a guilty plea, or to have made a knowing, voluntary, and informed waiver of his rights under *Miranda v. Arizona* (1966) prior to making a statement to police. At the adjudicatory phase, the court must determine the youth's culpability in the alleged offense. At the final disposition or sentencing stage, the court must assess the youth's amenability to treatment and rehabilitation, special needs, and capacity to develop competencies (as in the mastery of skills) in fashioning an appropriate disposition plan or sentence (Woolard et al., 1992).

It is not surprising, then, that many juvenile court professionals routinely order or request forensic evaluations to aid them in making these critical decisions. However, such professionals are usually doing so without any formal education or training in

- The role of the juvenile court professional in the evaluation process (e.g., informing the evaluator about what legal questions the evaluation will be used to answer, supplying records and information for the evaluator's consideration, and the like) and how the court professional can play a role that does not undermine the autonomy and credibility of the evaluator
- The information collected and the testing performed in these evaluations
- The meaning/relevance of tests performed with regard to the legal question that has to be answered
- How to distinguish a good from a poor quality evaluation (i.e., juvenile court professionals as discriminating consumers of evaluations)
- What conclusions can validly be drawn—and not drawn—from what is described in the evaluation

This lack of formal training in forensic assessment puts the juvenile court professional at risk of both underutilization of and overreliance on these evaluations in legal decision making. It also hinders the development of institutional capacity (i.e., the creation of appropriate forensic resources on which judges, lawyers, and probation officers may rely).

The Development of *Understanding Adolescents: A Juvenile Court Training Curriculum*

It was this deficit in training on forensic assessment, as well as adolescent development and psychology generally, which spurred the creation of an interdisciplinary curriculum for juvenile court professionals. *Understanding Adolescents: A Juvenile Court Training Curriculum* (Rosado, 2000) is a joint project of three organizations—the American Bar Association Juvenile Justice Center in Washington, DC; the Juvenile Law Center, which is based in Philadelphia, Pennsylvania; and the Youth Law Center, which has offices in San Francisco and Washington, DC. The curriculum project built on the work of these same three organizations in conducting the first national study in the United States of access to defense counsel and quality of representation in juvenile court. This study (Puritz, Burrell, Schwartz, Soler, & Warboys, 1995) identified several critical areas in which defender training was inadequate or nonexistent. While juvenile defenders received training in adult criminal procedure, they received little or no education in subject areas specific to juvenile court practice, including child and adolescent development (Puritz et al., 1995).

With funding from the John D. and Catherine T. MacArthur Foundation, in 1996 the project team embarked on a multiyear project to fill the void in professional legal education. The project team was assisted by a multidisciplinary advisory group that included psychologists, psychiatrists, social workers, special education experts, adult education consultants, professional trainers, and social scientists representing a wide range of disciplines, as well as juvenile court judges, prosecutors, defense attorneys, and probation officers. In the project's first phase, the team gathered training curricula and materials from national and state professional organizations that represent and serve defense attorneys, as well as judges, prosecutors, and probation officers. The team and its advisors assessed the materials to identify additional subject areas that would augment the training that juvenile court professionals already received from these other traditional sources. The project team found that juvenile court professionals typically lacked training opportunities to learn about the process of forensic assessment and its application to legal decision making.

The review of current training curricula also demonstrated a gap in formal education about certain groups that are increasing in numbers within the juvenile justice population. These special populations include:

- *Youth with mental health disorders.* The precise prevalence of mental health disorders in the juvenile justice system is currently unknown, as few large-scale empirical studies had been conducted until recently. Several small studies showed that the rate of mental health disorders was higher among court-involved youth. Depending on the methodology used, these studies showed that the percentage of youth in the justice system meeting diagnostic criteria for mood disorders had a range of 10 to 88%, compared to 5 to 9% for the youth population generally; for attention-deficit/hyperactivity disorder, 2 to 76% as

contrasted to 3 to 7% in the youth population as a whole; for psychotic disorders, 1 to 16% versus 1 to 5%; for conduct disorder, 32 to
100% versus 1 to 10%; and substance abuse/dependence, 46 to 88% as
contrasted to 5 to 9% in the general youth population. In addition, a
high percentage of these youth suffered from more than one mental
health disorder and/or had a co-occurring substance abuse problem
(Boesky, 2002; Cocozza & Skowyra, 2000; Grisso, 1999; Otto, Greenstein, Johnson, & Friedman, 1992). Recently, some larger empirical
studies have confirmed the higher prevalence rates of these disorders
among the juvenile justice population. For example, in a random
study of 1,829 youth arrested and detained in Cook County, Illinois,
researchers found that nearly two thirds of males and three quarters
of females met the diagnostic criteria for one or more psychiatric disorders, and about one half of both males and females had a substance abuse disorder (Teplin, Abram, McClellan, Dulcan, & Mericle, 2002).

- *Youth with learning disabilities.* Estimates of the rate of learning disorders among the juvenile court population are in the range of 36 to
  53% compared to 4 to 9% for the general population, and for mental
  retardation the rate is about 13% versus 1% generally (Boesky, 2002;
  Smykla & Willis, 1981).
- *Females.* The juvenile justice system has witnessed an increase in
  the number of girls who become involved, including the number of
  females entering residential facilities. Empirical studies, as well as
  anecdotal evidence, suggest that females in the system have a higher
  prevalence of mental health disorders than their male counterparts,
  particularly with respect to depression and anxiety disorders. Moreover, some studies show that the great majority of females in the
  juvenile justice system have been victims of physical or sexual abuse
  and/or witnessed traumatic events (Acoca, 1999; Boesky, 2002;
  Cauffman, Feldman, Waterman, & Steiner, 1998; National Mental
  Health Association, 2000; Teplin et al., 2002; Timmons-Mitchell et
  al., 1997).

In addition to needing relevant information on these groups to address the issues above, these special populations require the juvenile court to interact with
other systems, such as mental health and education, about which juvenile court
professionals may have limited knowledge. For example, many disabled youth
qualify for special education under the Federal Individuals with Disabilities
Education Act, 20 U.S.C. § 1400 *et seq.* (IDEA; National Council on Disability,
2003). However, juvenile justice professionals have not been routinely trained on
the IDEA, including the entitlement and rights it accords to eligible children.

At an even more basic level, the team also found that court professionals
lacked a foundation in what is *normative* adolescent development. How do
teenagers develop their cognitive skills, moral framework, social relations, and
sense of identity? What aspects of youthful offending can be viewed as sympto-

matic of normal adolescent development, as opposed to pathological/abnormal? If some offending behavior can indeed be characterized as within the range of normal adolescent development, what are the implications for juvenile court practice, in both individual cases and overall policy making? The answers to these questions are relevant to the legal decisions that must be made at different stages of the court process, as described in the previous section. For example, in assessing a youth's culpability in an offense, the court should consider the youth's level of cognitive processing. In fashioning a rehabilitation plan for an adjudicated youth, it would be helpful for the court to be informed about that youth's moral development and the role that family and peers play in his/her life.

These subjects typically are not covered comprehensively in continuing education for juvenile court judges, prosecutors, defense attorneys, and probation officers. Thus, the project team set out to create an interdisciplinary curriculum that would not only educate juvenile court professionals on all of these issues, but also inform clinicians about what juvenile court professionals need to know from them in these areas. The team wanted to put the clinician in the role of educator, so that the clinician would be able to more effectively interact with juvenile court professionals in the clinician's role as evaluator. The main purpose of such a curriculum would be to teach juvenile court practitioners how they could apply research on adolescent development and related areas to improve decision making at every stage of the court process. The curriculum also would be designed to give juvenile court professionals the background information to conduct global planning in their jurisdictions (e.g., develop prevention and diversion programming, develop/contract with appropriate programming for adjudicated youth), and legislative and regulatory advocacy (e.g., enacting/amending statutes that set forth the criteria for juvenile vs. adult criminal court jurisdiction or that govern residential programs for adjudicated youth).

In the project's second phase, the team negotiated with the juvenile courts in West Palm Beach, Florida, and Oakland, California, to become pilot sites for the curriculum's development. The pilot sites were the laboratories in which the team and its national advisory board tested subject matter to include in the final curriculum and the format in which it would be delivered. Team members met with stakeholders at both sites to develop a list of prospective training topics and solicit specific questions that the trainees wanted the experts to answer in each of these topic areas. In developing the topic list, the project team also was aware that, to some extent, the prospective trainees were not aware of their training needs. To address this issue, the team supplemented the list with input from clinicians and social scientists who work in and have familiarity with the juvenile justice system.

With the subject areas determined, the project team then recruited experts from around the United States to develop and present initial trainings to the juvenile court professionals at the pilot sites. The trainings were delivered in installments from 1997 through 1999. At both training sites, the presiding juvenile court judge set aside specific dates for the trainings in advance and either closed the courts or lengthened the lunch recess so all court professionals could attend. Most of the trainings were 3 hours long, and all of the trainings were cross-disciplinary—judges, prosecutors, defense attorneys, and probation staff were trained at the same time.

The team applied the feedback from these pilot sites to the next stage of the project: writing a curriculum for national publication and distribution. The team faced a number of challenges in drafting the final version of the curriculum. First, the team sought to design a curriculum with maximum flexibility and broad applicability. The team wanted the clinicians who would teach from the curriculum to be able to personalize the modules to reflect their own expertise and research interests and to tailor, to some degree, the modules to the particular audience, including commentary on relevant state law and local practice. Adaptability also was critical because of the mixed knowledge base among potential trainees, as well as different audience preferences for training methodology (e.g., some lawyers think that role-playing is an invaluable learning tool, while others think it's silly). At the same time, the team sought to minimize bias and idiosyncrasies in the material content without making it too generic.

The team also had to take the material one step further than some of the pilot presenters were able to do. The curriculum needed to elucidate the connection between the information presented and actual juvenile court practice, so juvenile court professionals would see the relevance and potential applications of the materials. Consistent feedback from both pilot sites indicated that the trainees wanted information and materials to use in court the next day. To achieve this, the team built a number of features into the curriculum. For example, included in the curriculum are "tool kits" from which trainers can draw to engage the juvenile court professionals more effectively in the training sessions. The tool kits feature checklists and questionnaires that participants could immediately use in their daily practice in juvenile court, as well as realistic interactive exercises. Finally, the team structured the modules so that they could be delivered by teams of attorneys and clinicians. Some pilot site trainees commented that they found initial sessions "informative but not useful." Attorneys as cotrainers could describe the relevance of the training material to daily practice in a way that clinicians alone could not.

Published in 2000, the curriculum consists of six separate modules:

1. Kids are different: How knowledge of adolescent development theory can aid decision making in court
2. Talking to teens in the justice system: Strategies for interviewing adolescent defendants, witnesses, and victims
3. Mental health assessments in the justice system: How to get high-quality evaluations and what to do with them in court
4. The pathways to juvenile violence: How child maltreatment and other risk factors lead children to chronically aggressive behavior
5. Special ed kids in the justice system: How to recognize and treat young people with disabilities that compromise their ability to comprehend, learn, and behave
6. Evaluating youth competence in the justice system

The modules can be downloaded at no cost from the American Bar Association Juvenile Justice Center's Web site (http://www.abanet.org/crimjust/juvjus/macarthur.html). Individuals with expertise in the covered subject areas may use the curriculum modules, again at no cost, to teach juvenile court professionals and forensic evaluators by registering with the American Bar Association Juvenile Justice Center at the above Web site. Since the modules are written as teaching guides, they must be taught by individuals with expertise in that particular topic. The modules each stand alone, so jurisdictions can organize a session on a single module or put together a training program featuring a combination of modules.

Modules 3 and 6 of the curriculum most directly address the use of forensic evaluations in the court process, and the training team for each of these modules must include an experienced forensic evaluator who has specifically worked in juvenile court (or assessed adolescents in the context of adult criminal court proceedings). The goal of module 3 is to train juvenile court professionals on what mental health professionals should be doing when they serve as consultants to the court and how they should be doing their consulting to produce mental health evaluations that aid court personnel in key decision making. Upon completion of the training, participants should be better informed consumers of mental health evaluations. To accomplish this, the module first instructs the clinician-trainer regarding the substantive information about the mental health field to convey to juvenile court professionals. Thus, the trainer reviews the

- Legal contexts in which a mental health evaluation may be indicated
- Distinctions between mental health professionals (how does a psychiatrist differ from a psychologist, and what are their respective areas of expertise? When would it be appropriate for a youth to be evaluated by a psychologist, a psychiatrist, or both?)
- Role of the fourth edition of the *Diagnostic and Statistical Manual of Mental Disorders* (*DSM-IV*) as a classification system in forensic evaluations, including the meaning of the different domains or "axes" used in the system and descriptions of the disorders most prevalent among children in the juvenile justice system
- Various psychological tests and instruments administered to youth that are most relevant to the legal questions that juvenile court professionals must answer regarding youth

The module then has the clinician-trainer discuss how, as a court practitioner, one should think about, request, and review a forensic evaluation. The clinician-trainer should describe how a juvenile court practitioners could assess the qualifications and expertise of a mental health professional they are considering hiring. In fact, the module provides an outline that juvenile court professionals can use to assess an expert witness. With respect to preparation, the legal participants are taught how to identify and discuss with the evaluator the law and psychological factors, legal issue(s), and the youth's relevant mental states, capacities, behaviors, knowledge, and skills. Participants are taught how to review a completed evaluation and assess its quality and usefulness in helping to answer the pertinent legal questions. Participants also receive another handout—a checklist of the minimum criteria of a good forensic evaluation—that they can use in their daily practice.

Finally, the clinician-trainer leads the participants through a number of exercises that simulate how to use forensic evaluations and work with evaluators in court cases. For example, the court practitioners are asked to draft a court order that will provide the best possible guidance to the mental health professional about the issues to address in the report to the court. The trainer then examines the drafted orders and explains how the evaluation—both the methods and tests used to gather and analyze information and the final product delivered to the court—would differ depending on the stated purpose of the evaluation. The objective of another exercise is to help participants develop a system for analyzing a forensic evaluation under time pressure. Specifically, participants read an actual evaluation and then complete a work sheet identifying their goal for the examination of the mental health professional on the stand and the areas of the evaluation that either support or do not support their goal. The exercise also directs them to formulate questions that illustrate the link between the diagnosis in the evaluation and its supporting components and reveal whether the evaluator's diagnosis was based on adequate information and skilled interpretation. The clinician-trainer can role-play the evaluator on the witness stand and at the same time offer feedback to the juvenile court professionals on their questions.

Module 6 focuses on the use of forensic evaluation in assessing the competencies necessary for youth to perform different tasks in the juvenile and adult criminal court process, particularly competence to have waived *Miranda* rights at the time of a statement and competence to stand trial. Trainers first review the relevant legal standards for these competencies. The module then directs the clinician-trainer to review with participants the principles of forensic assessment relevant to evaluating these competencies, including the instruments and tests that can be used, the records that should be reviewed, and the interviews that should be conducted by the evaluator. As with the module on forensic evaluation generally, the module on evaluating youth competence takes the juvenile court practitioners through a series of exercises that mimic real-life court tasks, including how to analyze a competence evaluation and prepare for an examination of the evaluator in a hearing.

The remaining four modules in the series, while not directly addressing the art of forensic assessment, convey to juvenile court practitioners valuable information that should facilitate the use of forensic evaluations in their work. For example, module 1 provides an overview of adolescent development, focusing on how teenagers develop their cognitive skills, moral framework, social relations, and identity. Juvenile court professionals learn about how adolescent thinking differs from that of children and adults and how adolescent thinking increases the likelihood of taking risks and engaging in undesirable behaviors. Participants also are taught about adolescent identity development, including the role that family, peers, and the larger community play in this development. With respect to moral development, the module reviews how adolescents develop and express concepts of right and wrong and the influence of peers and family on the development of moral reasoning.

Other modules focus on special needs groups within the juvenile justice population. Juvenile court practitioners often call on forensic evaluators to help identify youth with special needs and weigh in on a number of legal decisions that the court will eventually have to make with respect to such issues as competence, amenability to rehabilitation, and appropriate treatment planning. In module 4, legal professionals learn how they can better recognize and treat youth in the justice system who have disabilities that compromise their abilities to comprehend, learn, and/or behave in socially acceptable ways. The module reviews the types of disabilities commonly found among court-involved youth, as well as different theories about the possible relationship between disabling conditions and delinquency (e.g., are there different attributes of these disabling conditions that may predispose youth to offending behaviors?). Importantly, the module also covers the federal legal entitlements to special education (for children both within and outside of the juvenile justice system), including their rights to continue their education when they get into trouble at school.

Similarly, module 4 examines the relationship between childhood trauma and maltreatment and the chronic violent behavior exhibited by some youth in the justice system. Participants learn about the developmental dynamics of violent offending—the risk factors related to the onset of aggressive behavior in children and its further development into chronic violent behavior as these youth become young adults. Participants are also taught about the protective factors that may help keep children exposed to these risk factors from becoming chronically violent. Developmentally appropriate interventions are also reviewed for teaching young people who have already engaged in violence to learn to deal with potentially threatening situations with nonviolent action.

How the *Understanding Adolescents* Curriculum Is Currently Being Used

Since its publication in September 2000, more than 1,000 juvenile court judges, prosecutors, defense attorneys, probation officers, and forensic mental health professionals in approximately 20 states have been trained in the *Understanding Adolescents* curriculum. Portions of the curriculum have been taught at national training venues for legal and mental health professionals, including the National Council of Juvenile and Family Court Judges, the National Juvenile Defender, and the National Mental Health Association. However, much of the training has taken place at the state and local levels, as juvenile courts and probation offices have sought to expand the training opportunities available to their professionals.

Indeed, the project team continues to work to facilitate the curriculum's use around the country. The project team will help training organizations and individual juvenile courts to identify and cultivate experts to deliver the trainings. Rather than recruiting a nationally known clinician-trainer to a locale for a particular training, the project team will help juvenile court professionals identify individuals in their jurisdictions with the requisite expertise to teach the courses. The advantage of this approach is that the juvenile court develops local resources who can be tapped after the training is complete. The project team will help prepare these identified professionals to teach the curriculum by lending them videotapes of curriculum training sessions conducted by others, providing feedback on which material and exercises have and have not been successful with particular audiences, and pointing out connections between material in the curriculum and the expert's known research and teaching interests so that the expert can make the curriculum his or her own. The project team also will work with the clinician-trainer and training organizers to tailor the material to the local audience. For example, the team can advise trainers how to incorporate information about local law and practice into the training and which interactive exercises would be most relevant to that particular audience.

The project team can also advise organizations and jurisdictions on certain decisions that must be made when organizing trainings based on the curriculum. For example, from the beginning, the project team considered the advantages and disadvantages of conducting trainings with "mixed" audiences that included judges, prosecutors, defense attorneys, and probation officers versus training more homogeneous professional groups separately. On the one hand, cross-disciplinary trainings ensure that all juvenile court practitioners are exposed to the same information and tools. Issues raised and insights gained from the trainings may lead to changes in practice, which should be more successful if there is a shared understanding and consensus among juvenile court professionals. Training the professions together also presents the opportunity for lively discussions among practitioners who have different roles in and perspectives of the juvenile court process.

On the other hand, the juvenile justice system is based on an adversarial model, and professionals may be inhibited from candid discussion when adversaries are in the room. As one criminologist who served on the national advisory board commented, "Training with adversaries is not a difficult problem, it's an impossible problem." There is also some advantage to tailoring the presentation of information to specific professional groups because members of each group are likely to use the information differently. Because there is no one best answer to this question, the project team advises individuals who are organizing trainings to consult with the professionals in their jurisdictions and select the means of delivering the trainings accordingly.

Another major task on the project team's post-publication agenda is finding better ways to assess the impact of the curriculum on actual decision making. How do we know whether professionals actually apply what they learn to daily practice? The project team has collected some anecdotal evidence of changes in practice that followed curriculum trainings. For example, in one jurisdiction, members of the probation department met with the juvenile court master immediately following a training on the special education module and established a new policy such that any time a school-referred juvenile case is before the master, the court will require the school to demonstrate that it has fulfilled its legal obligations when the student may be eligible for special education. The juvenile court professionals learned about schools' legal obligations at the training; they are planning to use this knowledge as a tool to reduce inappropriate school-based referrals to the court. With respect to the mental health assessment module, the project team will know that the curriculum has had a favorable impact if there is an improvement in the quality and usefulness of court-ordered evaluations. The challenge is to find a means to make this assessment.

Conclusion: Next Steps in Expanding the Shared Knowledge Base

At about the same time that it funded the curriculum project, the MacArthur Foundation launched its Research Network on Adolescent Development and Juvenile Justice, a group of some of the country's leading scientific and legal researches in the area of children and the law. The Network's mission is to develop new knowledge regarding the assumptions on which the juvenile justice system functions and, like the curriculum, improve legal practice and policy making with accurate information about adolescent development derived from a solid foundation of science and scholarship. As the Network reports new findings regarding adolescent development, the curriculum will need to be updated. For example, in 2003 the Network released the findings of a major study on juvenile adjudicative competence (Grisso et al., 2003; http://www.mac-adoldev-juvjustice.org). The results of the study indicate that, compared to adults, a significant proportion of juveniles in the community who are aged 15 and younger have meaningful impairments in functional abilities underlying competence to proceed to adjudication in criminal proceedings. The findings suggest that states that transfer large numbers of youth 15 and younger to adult court may be subjecting a significant portion of such youth to trials for which they lack the basic capacities that are essential for competent participation as defendants. The study may also have implications for the ways in which forensic psychologists conduct competence examinations of court-involved youth. The curriculum will be updated to reflect this and other relevant studies that advance our knowledge of adolescent development and its implications for the functioning of the court system.

The curriculum is an excellent vehicle through which to convey to both juvenile court professionals and forensic evaluators updated research on adolescent development and the practice of forensic assessment. It also creates an opportunity for mental health and legal professionals to build a shared knowledge base about the juvenile justice population. The project team will continue to work with both national and local groups to organize trainings around the country.

References

Acoca, L. (1999). Investing in girls: A 21st century strategy. *Juvenile Justice, 6*, 3–13.
Boesky, L. M. (2002). *Juvenile offenders with mental health disorders: Who are they and what do we do with them?* Lanham, MD: American Correctional Association.

Cauffman, E., Feldman, S., Waterman, J., & Steiner, H. (1998). Posttraumatic stress disorder among female juvenile offenders. *Journal of the American Academy of Child and Adolescent Psychiatry*, 37, 1209–1216.

Cocozza, J. J., & Skowyra, K. R. (2000). Youth with mental health disorders: Issues and emerging responses. *Juvenile Justice*, 7, 3–13.

Griffin, P., Torbet, P., & Szymanski, L. (1998). *Trying juveniles as adults in criminal court: An analysis of state transfer provisions*. Washington, DC: Office of Juvenile Justice and Delinquency Prevention.

Grisso, T. (1999). Juvenile offenders and mental illness. *Psychiatry, Psychology and Law*, 6, 143–151.

Grisso, T., Steinberg, L., Woolard, J., Cauffman, E., Scott, E., Graham, S., et al. (2003). Juveniles' competence to stand trial: A comparison of adolescents' and adults' capacities as trial defendants. *Law and Human Behavior*, 27, 333–363.

Miranda v. Arizona, 384 U.S. 436 (1966).

National Council on Disability. (2003). *Addressing the needs of youth with disabilities in the juvenile justice system: The current status of evidence-based research*. Washington, DC: Author.

National Mental Health Association. (2000). *Fact sheet: Mental health and adolescent girls in the justice system*. Washington, DC: Author..

Otto, R. K., Greenstein, J. J., Johnson, M. K., & Friedman, R. M. (1992). Prevalence of mental disorders among youth in the juvenile justice system. In J. Cocozza (Ed.), *Responding to the mental health needs of youth in the juvenile justice system* (pp. 7–48). Seattle, WA: The National Coalition for the Mentally Ill in the Criminal Justice System.

Otto, R. K., & Heilbrun, K. (2002). The practice of forensic psychology: A look toward the future in light of the past. *American Psychologist*, 57, 5–18.

Puritz, P., Burrell, S., Schwartz, R., Soler, M., & Warboys, L. (1995). *A call for justice: An assessment of access to counsel and quality of representation in delinquency proceedings*. Washington, DC: American Bar Association Juvenile Justice Center.

Rosado, L. (2000). *Understanding adolescents: A juvenile court training curriculum*. Washington, DC: American Bar Association Juvenile Justice Center.

Smykla, J. O., & Willis, T. W. (1981). The incidence of learning disabilities and mental retardation in youth under the jurisdiction of the juvenile court. *Journal of Criminal Justice*, 9, 219–225.

Teplin, L. A., Abram, K. M., McClelland, G. M., Dulcan, M. K., & Mericle, A. A. (2002). Psychiatric disorders in youth in juvenile detention. *Archives of General Psychiatry*, 59, 1133–1143.

Timmons-Mitchell, J., Brown, C., Schulz, S. C., Webster, S. E., Underwood, L. A., & Semple, W. E. (1997). Comparing the mental health needs of female and male incarcerated delinquents. *Behavioral Sciences and the Law*, 15, 195–202.

Woolard, J. L., Gross, S. L., Mulvey, E. P., & Reppucci, N. D. (1992). Legal issues affecting mentally disordered youth in the juvenile justice system. In J. Cocozza (Ed.), *Responding to the mental health needs of youth in the juvenile justice system* (pp. 90–106). Seattle, WA: The National Coalition for the Mentally Ill in the Criminal Justice System.

15

KIRK HEILBRUN, NAOMI E. SEVIN GOLDSTEIN,
AND RICHARD E. REDDING

Emerging Directions

Implications for Research, Policy, and Practice

In this final chapter, we highlight and discuss some of the important implications from the previous chapters. Our discussion addresses the broad domains of prevention, assessment, and intervention relevant to juvenile offending and adolescent antisocial behavior. Within each of these domains, we address some particularly important implications for the areas of research, policy, and practice and describe how these implications may affect the larger goal of using research to better inform policy and practice.

Prevention: Implications for Research

The first research implication in the area of prevention involves what might be investigated to promote the earlier identification of young children who eventually become serious, violent, or chronic offenders. Younger age at first contact with and first commitment to the juvenile system are significant predictors of later offending, according to the research described in the chapter 6 meta-analysis (Heilbrun, Lee, & Cottle, in this volume). Some ongoing research attempts to use a single disorder or construct that has been associated with offending in adults (e.g., psychopathy; see Barry et al., 2000; Frick & Silverthorn, 2001; see also substance abuse; Department of Health and Human Services [DHHS], 2001). However, the research strategies discussed by Mulvey (ch. 10 in this volume) may be more likely to accurately identify a higher percentage of children at risk for later offending (a) using cumulative risk rather than single risk factors; (b) empirically distinguishing between risk markers and risk factors, to better identify the latter in order to help shape risk reducing interventions; and (c) distinguishing risk state variables, particularly once higher risk status has been more firmly established in a much younger group.

Another crucial area for the prevention of juvenile offending, thus far understudied, involves the role of protective factors. Longitudinal research on a large group of high-risk young children would identify some who eventually become offenders and misidentify others who do not. What would distinguish these subgroups? The impact of naturally occurring protective factors might guide the development of risk-reducing interventions delivered to those in higher risk status groups. This might be particularly useful if such protective interventions also reduced the risk of other problematic outcomes (e.g., poor school adjustment, childhood and adolescent victimization through physical abuse, sexual abuse, and school bullying) without stigmatizing young children in the course of delivery. It would also be valuable to consider the role of gender in such research, as the prevalence of juvenile offending attributable to girls has increased in recent years. Furthermore, given the prevalence of mental health disorders among delinquent youth, identifying links between mental health problems and offending could be useful in the development of prevention programs (see Sevin Goldstein, Olubadewo, Redding, & Lexcen, ch. 5 in this volume). Finally, it would be useful to learn more about resilience and pathways to desistence. Why do some adolescents persist in offending over the life span, while the majority desist in early adulthood?

Prevention: Implications for Policy

Accurate data can make a crucial contribution to informed policy making. Significant family problems are both a risk factor for juvenile offending (see De-Matteo & Marczyk, ch. 2 in this volume) and a target for risk-reducing interventions (see Sheidow & Henggeler, ch. 12 in this volume), so further research will refine what we know about the relationship between family functioning and juvenile offending. However, it seems clear that social policy that promotes strengthening of families and effectiveness of parenting is likely to pay dividends of delinquency risk reduction.

One of the most exciting areas of research in recent years has focused on the variety of ways in which adolescents differ from adults related to judgment and decision making. Overseen by the MacArthur Research Network on Juvenile Justice and Adolescent Development, such research has been described at length elsewhere (see, e.g., Fagan & Zimring, 2000; Grisso & Schwartz, 2000; Grisso et al., 2003), but clearly has implications for mental health interventions for adolescents in the juvenile justice system (see Sevin Goldstein et al., ch. 5), the assessment of competence to stand trial in criminal court (see Otto & Goldstein, ch. 9 in this volume), adolescent violence risk assessment (see Mulvey, ch. 10), and legal decision making more generally involving adolescents in the juvenile justice system (see Redding & Mrozoski, ch. 11 in this volume). These research findings have important implications for policy that recognizes distinctions between adolescents and adults in these areas, particularly when adolescents are faced with a demand (such as standing trial in criminal court) that is usually applied only to adults.

Some kinds of adolescent violence are very rare. However frightening, school shootings are extremely unusual (see Cornell, ch. 3 in this volume) and call for policy that balances the gravity of serious threats against the empirical reality of their extreme infrequency. Such policy might involve promoting (a) open communication between students and school administrators, addressing less serious but far more frequent forms of school-based aggression (such as bullying, a genuine school-based problem in this area) that can motivate some victimized youth to retaliate; (b) structured threat assessment; and (c) a range of risk-reducing interventions appropriate to the level of the threat (Fein et al., 2002; Mulvey & Cauffman, 2001). However, policy that does not incorporate flexibility, communication, information gathering, and intervention based on such information—policy that instead substitutes "zero tolerance" for the threat of violence—is in many respects harmful to adolescents who violate such policy but would not present a risk of serious violence in school.

Prevention: Implications for Practice

A number of known risk factors for juvenile offending and adolescent violence have been identified in various chapters in this volume (see, in particular, Krisberg & Wolf, ch. 4). Focusing on such risk factors in the delivery of prevention-oriented services is likely to reduce these kinds of target behaviors (DeMatteo & Marczyk, ch. 2) and may also improve functioning in other areas as well. Concurrently, however, the empirical evaluation of prevention programs is very important. Some existing programs appear to work well, while others are demonstrably ineffective and a few may even be harmful (DHHS, 2001). A focus on both individual risk factors and social/environmental factors (e.g., family, school, and peers) have generally marked such effective programs, although strong risk factors such as antisocial peers and gang involvement remain to be addressed effectively (DHHS, 2001).

Assessment: Implications for Research

A number of noteworthy advances in assessment with juveniles have been described in this volume. These generally fall into three areas: (a) risk/needs tools (Mulvey, ch. 10), (b) mental health screening (Sevin Goldstein et al., ch. 5), and (c) specialized forensic mental health assessment tools (Otto & Goldstein, ch. 9). The research needs for tools of this kind require their adaptation for use with adolescents, as both content and norms differ between adolescents and adults. Tools in each of these areas are also relatively new, however, and their success needs to be replicated in different jurisdictions to strengthen their empirical base and add to their generalizability.

There are two additional research needs identified by contributors. First, influences that are specific to adolescence, such as psychosocial maturity, appear relevant to clinical-legal issues such as competence to stand trial (Grisso et al., 2003). However, additional research (particularly using empirically supported structured tools) would be helpful to gauge the strength and extensiveness of such influences. Second, threats and violence that occur in schools are substantially different in prevalence and etiology from most other types of juvenile offending. Validating research on school-based threat assessment, and its linkage with risk-reducing interventions, is a second need (Cornell, ch. 3).

Assessment: Implications for Policy

Policy-makers and juvenile administrators should take a hard look at the accuracy and cost-effectiveness of the assessment tools currently used in the juvenile justice system. The use of tools that are relevant to the specific legal question(s), supported by well-designed and replicated empirical research, and reasonable in their cost is a luxury that may soon become fully available. However, those who make decisions about which tests to use must be informed and attentive to these issues.

The disposition of juvenile cases has often been guided primarily by the nature of the offense and the availability of services for adjudicated juveniles. To some extent, this is a function of community values and will undoubtedly continue. However, as variables such as juveniles' risk for reoffending and risk-relevant needs are measured more accurately, it will become possible to weigh values such as community safety, rehabilitation, retribution, and cost-effectiveness with more "knowns" and fewer questions.

Assessment: Implications for Practice

One of the more important developments during the last decade has been the construction and beginning stages of validation of risk–needs tools for adolescents. Such tools allow those conducting assessment of juvenile offenders to gauge the adolescent's functioning in a variety of dynamic, risk-relevant areas — and to place this information in the context of the adolescent's reoffense risk status. Tools such as the Youth Level of Service/Case Management Inventory (Hoge & Andrews, 2002), the Structured Assessment of Violence Risk in Youth (Borum, Bartel, & Forth, 2002), and the Washington State Juvenile Assessment (Barnoski, 2002) show considerable promise, once fully validated, for informing decision-makers about both risk status and the more stable aspects of risk state (see Mulvey, ch. 10).

Information about the clinical functioning of adolescents involved in the juvenile justice system has become more valuable with the recent introduction of efficient screening tools such as the Massachusetts Youth Screening Instrument-2 (Grisso & Barnum, 2000), accompanied by evidence of relatively high rates of disorders such as depression, learning disorders, attention deficit disorder, and substance abuse. It will be important to consider the link between treating such disorders and reducing reoffense risk through further research, particularly longitudinal research that allows us to distinguish those who desist from offending in young adulthood from those who persist for many more years. Particularly for youth who are likely to desist, the promotion of improved functioning through skills-based and multisystemic interventions across multiple domains, including clinical, family, social, and educational, represent the strategy that is most likely to succeed in promoting and hastening such desistance. Hence, standardized screening for mental health disorders most prominent among adolescent offenders should become an integral part of the assessment of juveniles.

Such advances may take some time to become integrated into juvenile courts. Judges and attorneys who work with juveniles can be greatly assisted in learning about and integrating information that has been provided through research focused on adolescents in the juvenile system. For this reason, a curriculum such as that developed by specialized juvenile groups and supported by the MacArthur Foundation (see Rosado, ch. 14 in this volume) has the potential to change the practice of juvenile law considerably. Developed in modular format to promote efficiency, available online and free of charge, informed by significant relevant research in human development as well as juvenile offending, and updated regularly, the MacArthur juvenile curriculum provides a model of how interdisciplinary collaboration and modern technology can be combined to yield a powerful educational tool. Moreover, attorneys and judges who are trained using this curriculum may subsequently demand a high level of relevance and sophistication in the evaluations of juveniles conducted by mental health professionals.

Intervention: Implications for Research

There are several particularly salient research implications to be drawn from the chapters in this volume. The first continues the developing emphasis on "best practice" or "empirically validated treatment" that has become prominent in medicine and psychology during the last decade. The importance of good research on the validation of interventions can hardly be overstated. Among other things, this continuing emphasis would involve (a) increased use of meta-analysis (which reveals, as may be seen in Heilbrun et al., ch. 6, that we really have insufficient evidence at present to gauge the effectiveness of specialized interventions for adolescent sexual offenders); (b) the development and testing of more interventions, such as multisystemic therapy (MST), that are manualized and allow careful attention to treatment fidelity, in turn permitting good validation research; (c) the use of broad-based outcomes across multiple domains, including reoffending but also encompassing family, social, educational, and vocational functioning; and (d) more frequent use of longitudinal designs and appropriate control groups, to allow consideration of naturally occurring influences such as desistance, but also allowing conclusions about whether a given set of interventions hastens desistance from offending.

Such research is difficult, expensive, and labor-intensive. However, even if appropriate resources are invested in this enterprise, there remains the important question of what precisely is to be investigated. Single interventions, even when promising, are not likely to influence adolescents as strongly as necessary when trying to move them away from involvement (particularly chronic or serious) in juvenile offending. The strategy of evaluating systems of care, involving multiple interventions across different domains, is probably more effective. This approach has yielded encouraging results with MST, but it is time to expand it by incorporating additional individual variables, including gender, age, and degree of chronicity, as well as system-level variables such as diversion, transfer to criminal court, and blended sentencing.

Indeed, some of the most pressing research needs can be seen in relation to such system-level variables. Blended sentencing (see Redding & Mrozoski, ch. 11) permits combining juvenile commitment with a subsequent adult sentence when the individual reaches a certain age. A number of important questions regarding blended sentencing must be addressed through research in coming years. Does the use of blended sentencing widen or narrow the net of adult sanctions? Does it affect the fairness and developmental appropriateness of juvenile case dispositions? Does it reduce subsequent reoffending following the end of the sentence? What kinds of cases are most appropriate for blended sentencing?

In a related vein, there is a clear need for further research on the process of transferring juvenile offenders to criminal court. Do transfer laws have a significant deterrent function? Can the impact of incarceration in adult facilities versus commitment to juvenile facilities be documented across multiple domains (e.g., rearrest, vocational functioning, social functioning) in large, multisite, extended longitudinal studies? Researchers focusing on variables that are more limited in scope have more control over their designs, but those investigating system-level decisions, such as blended sentencing and transfer, are working with powerful interventions that have the potential to substantially affect the lives of many juveniles.

Finally, research is needed on mental health services and their impact on adolescent functioning and recidivism risk (see Tate & Redding, ch. 7 in this volume). While it may be that many current services can be delivered as safely and effectively in the community, there will always be a need for residential placement for some juveniles (see Redding, Lexcen, & Ryan, ch. 13 in this volume). Research is needed on when such placement is needed, both for maximum rehabilitative impact and public safety, and on when an adolescent may be placed in a less secure and remote setting without loss of rehabilitative impact or public safety.

Intervention: Implications for Policy

A range of sanctions described in this volume can be applied to adolescents at various stages of the juvenile process. The use of graduated sanctions, depending not only on the nature of the offense but on community needs and the adolescent's needs and level of development, has been a model consistent with the goals of balanced and restorative justice. However, such a model can also more easily incorporate new findings regarding adolescent development and intervention effectiveness as they emerge. The broad range of sanctions for adolescents should include diversion under some circumstances (see Chapin & Griffin, ch. 8 in this volume), empirically validated community-based interventions, residential treatment, discretionary transfer to criminal court that includes consideration of whether the defendant is competent to stand trial as an adult, and blended sentencing options. Enhanced judicial discretion (as contrasted with automatic transfer procedures) can facilitate the incorporation of relevant information and hence individualize the decision regarding a particular juvenile. This is feasible particularly when there are explicit statutory guidance and decision-making criteria for judges, developed to improve accuracy and uniformity of transfer decisions and relying in part on actuarial models of recidivism based on various characteristics of the offender, the offense history, and the offense itself.

Particular jurisdictions must decide about the resources that will be invested in their juvenile system. One of the important considerations in determining whether a given resource will be cost-effective relates to Mulvey's (ch. 10) point regarding risk markers versus risk factors—cost-effective interventions are more likely to target risk factors and promote protective factors. A second consideration is the demonstrated effectiveness of an intervention. It may be that interventions such as MST, which have demonstrated effectiveness with less serious offenders, can also be delivered efficaciously (with no elevated risk to the community) with some serious juvenile offenders.

The kind of interdisciplinary training for lawyers and judges described by Rosado (ch. 14) can easily incorporate important information on interventions as well. The nature of the placement (e.g., community-based vs. residential) and the types of interventions delivered in different placements can provide important information for judges and attorneys regarding existing resources. Being informed about the "state of the art" may also provide juvenile legal professionals with greater incentive to encourage policy-makers to provide practitioners with more resources.

Intervention: Implications for Practice

Finally, these chapters have implications for the practice of certain interventions with juveniles. The use of best-practice/empirically supported treatments has been mentioned a number of times in this chapter and needs no elaboration beyond noting that implementing such interventions is often less time-consuming and labor-intensive than might be imagined.

It is becoming increasingly clear that girls are offending more frequently, and more seriously, than they have in the past. Many of the interventions in the present juvenile system may be inappropriate for girls. As discussed by Sevin Goldstein et al. (ch. 5), however, the remedy for this difficulty may involve the design, implementation, and outcome measurement of interventions that are gender specific.

It can be helpful to train legal professionals by updating them on cutting-edge research. It may also be quite helpful to ensure that mental health professionals involved in the juvenile system remain updated on advances through such training. However, perhaps the most useful approach to training would involve juvenile justice professionals from a variety of disciplines in the same community working their way through a structured curriculum and discussing its implications for practice and quality improvement in their own jurisdiction.

References

Barnoski, R. (2002). Monitoring vital signs: Integrating a standardized assessment into Washington state's juvenile justice system. In R. Corrado, R. Roesch, S. Hart, & J. Gierowski (Eds.), *Multi-problem violent youth: A foundation for comparative research on needs, interventions, and outcomes*. Washington, DC: IOS Press.

Barry, C. T., Frick, P. J., Grooms, T., McCoy, M. G., Ellis, M. L., & Loney, B. R. (2000). The importance of callous-unemotional traits for extending the concept of psychopathy to children. *Journal of Abnormal Psychology, 109*, 335–340.

Borum, R., Bartel, P., & Forth, A. (2002). *Manual for the Structured Assessment of Violence Risk in Youth (SAVRY)*. Tampa: University of South Florida.

Department of Health and Human Services. (2001). *Youth violence: A report of the Surgeon General*. Washington, DC: Author.

Fagan, J., & Zimring, F. (Eds.). (2000). *The changing borders of juvenile justice: Transfer of adolescents to the criminal court*. Chicago: University of Chicago Press.

Fein, R. A., Vossekuil, F., Pollack, W. S., Borum, R., Modzeleski, W., & Reddy, M. (2002). *Threat assessment in schools: A guide to managing threatening situations and to creating safe school climates*. Washington, DC: U.S. Secret Service and U.S. Department of Education.

Frick, P. J., & Silverthorn, P. (2001). Behavior disorders in children. In H. E. Adams & P. B. Sutker (Eds.), *Comprehensive handbook of psychopathology* (3rd ed., pp. 879–919). New York: Plenum.

Grisso, T., & Barnum, R. (2000). *Massachusetts Youth Screening Instrument–second version: User's manual and technical report*. Worcester: University of Massachusetts Medical School.

Grisso, T., & Schwartz, R. (Eds.) (2000). *Youth on trial: A developmental perspective on juvenile justice*. Chicago: University of Chicago Press.

Grisso, S., Steinberg, L., Woolard, J., Cauffman, E., Scott, E., Graham, S., et al. (2003). Juveniles' competence to stand trial: A comparison of adolescents' and adults' capacities as trial defendants. *Law and Human Behavior, 27*, 333–363.

Hoge, R., & Andrews, D. (2002). *The Youth Level of Service/Case Management Inventory (YLS/CMI) user's manual*. North Tonawanda, NY: Multi-Health Systems.

Mulvey, E. P., & Cauffman, E. (2001). The inherent limits of predicting school violence. *American Psychologist, 56*, 797–802.

Index

Please note that page numbers for the authors/scholars indexed below reflect pages on which they are discussed in detail in text. Please see the reference sections in individual chapters for additional citations.

331